T0296494

# CANNABIS DEPENDENCE

Its Nature, Consequences, and Treatment

Cannabis dependence is controversial. Does it occur or is it a myth put forth by those who oppose legalization? What are the signs of cannabis dependence? How many people are affected? What are the health and behavioral risks of becoming cannabis dependent? What counseling approaches have been tested with adults and adolescents, and how effective are they? What are the arguments for legalization, regulation, or prohibition? Looking back and toward the future, what do we know and what do we need to learn?

This state of the science review sets out to answer all those questions, beginning with an historical examination and moving into diagnosis, classification, epidemiology, public health, policy, issues relating to regulation and prohibition, and evidence-based interventions.

ROGER A. ROFFMAN is a Professor of Social Work at the University of Washington. Along with Robert Stephens he has conducted a series of controlled trials to investigate the efficacy of behavioral interventions with adult and adolescent cannabis users. His research also focuses on HIV prevention with several populations and early intervention with perpetrators of domestic violence.

ROBERT S. STEPHENS is an Associate Professor of Psychology at Virginia Tech. His work includes collaborations with Roger A. Roffman on the treatment of cannabis dependence, research on social cognitive determinants of drinking and drug use, and behavioral interventions to improve substance abuse treatment aftercare attendance.

INTERNATIONAL RESEARCH MONOGRAPHS IN THE ADDICTIONS
(IRMA)

*Series Editor*
Professor Griffith Edwards
*National Addiction Centre*
*Institute of Psychiatry, London*

Volumes in this series present important research from major centers around the world on the basic sciences, both biological and behavioral, that have a bearing on the addictions. They also address the clinical and public health applications of such research. The series will cover alcohol, illicit drugs, psychotropics, and tobacco. It is an important resource for clinicians, researchers, and policy-makers.

Also in this series

Cannabis and Cognitive Functioning
*Nadia Solowij*
ISBN 0 521 159114 7

A Community Reinforcement Approach to Addiction Treatment
*Robert J. Meyers and William R. Miller*
ISBN 0 521 77107 2

Circles of Recovery: Self-help Organizations for Addictions
*Keith N. Humphreys*
ISBN 0 521 79299 0

Alcohol and the Community: A Systems Approach to Prevention
*Harold D. Holder*
ISBN 0 521 59187 2

Treatment Matching in Alcoholism
*Thomas F. Babor and Frances K. Del Boca*
ISBN 0 521 65112 3

Gambling as an Addictive Behaviour: Impaired Control, Harm Minimization, Treatment, and Prevention
*Mark Dickerson and John O'Connor*
ISBN 0 521 84701 X

# CANNABIS DEPENDENCE

Its Nature, Consequences, and Treatment

Edited by

## ROGER A. ROFFMAN

*Innovative Programs Research Group*
*University of Washington School of Social Work*

## ROBERT S. STEPHENS

*Department of Psychology*
*Virginia Polytechnic Institute and State University*

Foreword by

## G. ALAN MARLATT

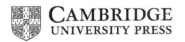
CAMBRIDGE
UNIVERSITY PRESS

CAMBRIDGE UNIVERSITY PRESS
Cambridge, New York, Melbourne, Madrid, Cape Town, Singapore,
São Paulo, Delhi, Dubai, Tokyo

Cambridge University Press
The Edinburgh Building, Cambridge CB2 8RU, UK

Published in the United States of America by Cambridge University Press, New York

www.cambridge.org
Information on this title: www.cambridge.org/9780521891363

First published 2006
This digitally printed version 2009

*A catalogue record for this publication is available from the British Library*

ISBN 978-0-521-81447-8 Hardback
ISBN 978-0-521-89136-3 Paperback

## Dedication

To my wife, Cheryl Richey, for her love, friendship, and support.

R.A.R.

To my wife, Amy Forsyth-Stephens, for endless amounts of patience and support, and for always believing in me.

R.S.S.

The old orchid hunter lay back on his pillow, his body limp with the effort of talking so long. He coughed and a ripple of pain ran through the wasted length of him beneath the covers. Still his eyes burned unwaveringly bright with the memory of the places he had seen and the things he had done, bright with an unquenchable passion for the life he would never suffer or enjoy again.

"You'll curse the insects," he said at last, "and you'll curse the natives. Your lips will crack and you'll lick them and taste the salt of your own sweat. The sun will burn you by day and the cold will shrivel you by night. You'll be racked by fever and tormented by a hundred discomforts, but you'll go on. For when a man falls in love with orchids, he'll do anything to possess the one he wants. It's like chasing a green-eyed woman or taking cocaine. A sort of madness...."

Prologue to:

Norman MacDonald
The Orchid Hunters: A Jungle Adventure
New York: Farrar & Rinehart
1939

Printed in the USA by Quinn & Boden Company, Inc., Rahway, N.J.

# Contents

## Part II: Interventions with Cannabis-Dependent Adults

### 6 *Cognitive-Behavioral and Motivational Enhancement Treatments for Cannabis Dependence*

ROBERT S. STEPHENS, ROGER A. ROFFMAN,
JAN COPELAND AND WENDY SWIFT

### 7 *Contingency-Management Interventions for Cannabis Dependence*

ALAN J. BUDNEY, BRENT A. MOORE, STACEY C. SIGMON
AND STEPHEN T. HIGGINS

## 8   *The Marijuana Check-Up*

ROBERT S. STEPHENS AND ROGER A. ROFFMAN

## 9   *Guided Self-Change: A Brief Motivational Intervention for Cannabis Abuse*

LINDA C. SOBELL, MARK B. SOBELL, ERIC F. WAGNER,
SANGEETA AGRAWAL AND TIMOTHY P. ELLINGSTAD

**Part IV: Policy**

**Part V: Conclusion**

# Contributors

**Sangeeta Agrawal**, M.Sc.
Research Analyst/Instructor
College of Nursing
University of Nebraska
Omaha, Nebraska, USA

**James C. Anthony**, Ph.D
Chairperson
Department of Epidemiology
College of Human Medicine
Michigan State University
East Lansing, Michigan, USA

**Thomas F. Babor**, Ph.D, M.P.H
Department of Community Medicine and
 Health Care
School of Medicine
University of Connecticut Health Center
Farmington, Connecticut, USA

**James Berghuis**, Ph.D
Community Health Centers of King
 County
Kent, Washington, USA

**Alan J. Budney**, Ph.D
Department of Psychiatry
University of Arkansas for Medical
 Sciences
Little Rock, Arkansas, USA

**Kathleen Carroll**, Ph.D
Department of Psychiatry
Director of Psychosocial Research
Division of Substance Abuse
School of Medicine
Yale University
New Haven, Connecticut, USA

**Jan Copeland**, Ph.D
National Drug and Alcohol Research
 Centre
School of Community Medicine and
 Public Health
University of New South Wales
Sydney, NSW, Australia

**Michael L. Dennis**, Ph.D
Chestnut Health Systems
Bloomington, Illinois, USA

**Guy Diamond**, Ph.D
Children's Hospital of Philadelphia and
 the University of Pennsylvania
Philadelphia, Pennsylvania, USA

**Caroline Easton**, Ph.D
Department of Psychiatry
School of Medicine
Yale University
New Haven, Connecticut, USA

**Timothy P. Ellingstad**, Ph.D
Clinical Psychologist
Aurora Behavioral Health
Burlington, Wisconsin, USA

**Susan H. Godley**, Rh.D
Chestnut Health Systems
Bloomington, Illinois, USA

**Brin Grenyer**, Ph.D
Illawarra Institute for Mental Health and
  Department of Psychology
University of Wollongong
NSW, Australia

**Wayne Hall**, Ph.D
Institute for Molecular Bioscience
University of Queensland
St Lucia, Queensland, Australia

**Stephen T. Higgins**
Human Behavioral Pharmacology
  Laboratory
University of Vermont
Burlington, Vermont, USA

**Jodi Leckrone**, M.Ed
Children's Hospital of Philadelphia
Philadelphia, Pennsylvania, USA

**Aron H. Lichtman**, Ph.D
Department of Pharmacology and
  Toxicology
Virginia Commonwealth University
Richmond, Virginia, USA

**Billy R. Martin**, Ph.D
Department of Pharmacology and
  Toxicology
Virginia Commonwealth University
Richmond, Virginia, USA

**Brent A. Moore**, Ph.D
Department of Psychiatry
Yale School of Medicine
New Haven, Connecticut, USA

**Roger A. Roffman**, D.S.W
School of Social Work
University of Washington
Seattle, Washington, USA

**Sam Schwartz**, M.S.W
School of Social Work
University of Washington
Seattle, Washington, USA

**Stacey C. Sigmon**
Department of Psychiatry
University of Vermont
Burlington, Vermont, USA

**Rajita Sinha**, Ph.D
Department of Psychiatry
School of Medicine
Yale University
New Haven, Connecticut, USA

**Linda C. Sobell**, Ph.D
Center for Psychological Studies
Nova Southeastern University
Ft. Lauderdale, Florida, USA

**Mark B. Sobell**, Ph.D
Center for Psychological Studies
Nova Southeastern University
Ft. Lauderdale, Florida, USA

**Nadia Solowij**, Ph.D
Illawarra Institute for Mental Health and
  Department of Psychology
University of Wollongong
NSW, Australia

**Robert Stephens**, Ph.D
Department of Psychology,
Virginia Polytechnic Institute and State
  University
Blacksburg, Virginia, USA

**Wendy Swift**, Ph.D
National Drug and Alcohol Research
  Centre
School of Community Medicine and
  Public Health
University of New South Wales
Sydney, NSW, Australia

**Eric F. Wagner**, Ph.D
College of Health and Urban Affairs
Florida International University
North Miami, Florida, USA

# Acknowledgments

We have many to thank for the contributions they have made to our research on cannabis dependence and to the preparation of this volume. Professors Tom Babor and Wayne Hall offered invaluable advice as we began to plan the book's purposes and consider its potential audience. Professor Griffith Edwards, editor of the IRMA series, warmly welcomed our inquiry about the prospect of a book with this theme and then helped us to refine our early ideas concerning its contents. We benefited greatly by Professor Edwards' tutelage and encouragement.

Richard Barling, Pauline Graham, and Jayne Aldhouse at Cambridge University Press offered enthusiastic support along the way and helped us to understand and appreciate the requirements of book production. We are privileged in having our work put into print by this highly esteemed publishing house.

We very much appreciate having had the opportunity to work with the Project Management staff at Charon Tec where the copy editing, typesetting, and correspondence with authors concerning editing queries were completed.

The contributors to this volume, leaders in cannabis studies in their respective disciplines, willingly trekked with us by preparing brief concept pieces concerning their chapters, moving from concept to outline, attending to our feedback, completing initial drafts, and again being responsive to our requests and suggestions in preparing the final manuscripts. We appreciate the quality of their scholarship and their patience with us as co-editors.

Over a number of years, many faculty, staff, and student colleagues at the University of Washington and Virginia Polytechnic Institute and State University played key roles in implementing the intervention trials discussed in Parts II and III. We are particularly grateful to Julia McGraw and Mckenzie Winters who edited each chapter to meet the publisher's citation and formatting requirements.

Our colleague and friend, Professor Alan Marlatt, was gracious in agreeing to read the book and offer his reflections in the Foreword. As is true for many who study addictive disorders, we have been inspired by Alan's creativity and enormously influential work.

We wish to express our gratitude to the National Institute on Drug Abuse and to the Center for Substance Abuse Treatment for the funding that has supported our cannabis intervention trials. Finally, as is the case with all who study human behavior, we are indebted to the participants in these trials for permitting us to learn through their experiences.

# Executive Summary

At the time of this volume's completion in 2005, important advances had been made in understanding the etiology and epidemiology of cannabis dependence, describing its neuropharmacology and the physiology of the endocannabinoid system, identifying associated consequences that impact health and behavior, and developing and evaluating the relative effectiveness of a variety of counseling interventions for adults and adolescents with cannabis abuse disorders. Many of these advances built on recent progress in the neuroscience of the endogenous cannabinoid system, in more precise classification and diagnostic paradigms for drug use disorders, and in the development and testing of theories of human behavior change.

This volume is organized into four sections. Part I focuses on the nature of cannabis dependence, with chapters devoted to the history of the concept, diagnosis and classification, pharmacology and physiology, epidemiology, and adverse health and behavioral consequences. Part II discusses intervention trials based on several theoretical frameworks with cannabis-dependent adults. Therapeutic interventions with adolescents and young probation-referred adults, again drawing from similar theories of behavior change, are the focus of Part III. Policy considerations vis-à-vis cannabis dependence are the focus of Part IV, and the volume concludes in Part V with commentary that offers a summary and synthesis of what is currently known about dependence on cannabis. Below we have listed some of the primary conclusions that can be drawn from each of the chapters in these areas.

## Part I: The Nature of Cannabis Dependence

Our understanding of the existence and nature of cannabis dependence has long been shaped by social and political forces that have polarized opinions and policies. The explosion of scientific research on the phenomena in recent years is starting to build a consensus that a small but significant subset of cannabis users develops a dependence syndrome, many of whom need treatment.

Standard nomenclatures and classification systems, such as ICD and DSM, provide reliable and valid operational criteria for cannabis dependence. With these tools it has become possible to characterize participants in clinical research and to obtain population estimates of cannabis use disorders.

The elucidation of the structure of delta-9-tetrahydrocannabinol, the discovery of anandamide and cannabinoid receptors, and the synthesis of cannabinoid agonists and antagonists support the existence of an endocannabinoid system in the central nervous system that is believed to modulate cannabis dependence.

There is considerable evidence from animal and human models that physical dependence on cannabis, as identified by tolerance and withdrawal phenomena, can be induced via prolonged exposure.

Current research is focused on which regions of the brain mediate physical dependence and the nature of the underlying cellular mechanisms of action. Research focusing on the $CB_1$ receptor and the action of antagonists such as SR141716A in precipitating withdrawal has potential relevance to the eventual development of pharmacotherapies for the treatment of cannabis dependence.

In the USA, within the first 24 months of cannabis use initiation, 2–4% of users (or 50–80 people each day) progress to cannabis dependence. Annually, that amounts to 20,000–30,000 individuals. Cannabis dependence occurs in 1 in 9 to 11 individuals who have ever used the drug, and 11–16% (1.6–2.3 million individuals) of the 14 million current users.

Converging evidence from the USA, Australia, and New Zealand, although limited due to sample differences, supports an estimate that 1 in 6 or 7 adolescents and young adult cannabis users become cannabis dependent by their early to mid-twenties: *USA*: 1 in 6–7 (16%); *New Zealand*: 1 in 7 or 7.5 (13–14%); *Australia*: 1 in 6 (16.7%). It is uncertain why a lower risk is reflected in data from Germany: 1 in 20–25 (4–5%).

More than 90% of cannabis dependence cases in the USA occur between the ages of 15 and 35 years, typically within the first 10 years of use. Male cannabis users have more commonly become dependent on the drug, although the gender gap has lessened. With reference to race and ethnicity, Native Americans disproportionately report persistent cannabis use, and there is some evidence that young African Americans and young Hispanic males had disproportionately greater increases in the prevalence of cannabis use disorders in the 1990s.

Risk factors for cannabis dependence may include mood disorders, residing in neighborhoods with greater magnitudes of daily users, and having a history of alcohol use disorder. Common vulnerability traits that contribute to cannabis dependence, as well as other disorders, may result from either genetic or environmental factors or their interaction. In the future, it is likely that studies of community and family contextual effects, when examined along with individual-level risk factors, will further our understanding of the etiology of cannabis dependence.

### The Adverse Health and Psychological Consequences of Cannabis Dependence

Understanding of the health consequences of cannabis dependence is based on studies with heavy users rather than with the more specific population of those who are cannabis dependent.

Increased risk of chronic bronchitis and histopathological changes in the respiratory system that may precede malignancy are related to the method of administration (smoking). There is some evidence that heavy cannabis smokers are at greater risk for infectious diseases such as pneumonia. Clarification of the relationship between cannabis smoking and cancer risk will necessitate larger cohort studies and larger case control studies.

Some research supports the existence of subtle types of cognitive impairment (attention; memory; and impaired verbal learning, retention, and retrieval) in long-term heavy cannabis users. Competing explanations for these findings include residual effects from recent use, residues of the drug that are stored in the body after abstinence is attained, and the nervous system's re-adaptation to abstinence following chronic exposure. Research on the recovery of cognitive functioning following cessation is needed. Functional brain imaging studies will be important in future investigations of cannabis-related cognitive deficits.

The risk of cannabis dependence appears to be increased in those who initiate use at earlier ages. Early use also has been shown to be associated with earlier withdrawal from school, earlier sexual activity, pregnancy during adolescence, unemployment, and leaving the family home early. Adolescents who smoke cannabis heavily appear to be at increased risk of using "harder drugs." The causal relationship of cannabis use to these outcomes is not well established because young users often have multiple risk factors.

Subgroups of cannabis-dependent persons at increased health risk include:

• adults with cardiovascular disease who may precipitate myocardial infarctions by smoking cannabis;
• adolescents whose school performance and psychosocial development may be adversely affected and who may be at increased risk of using other illicit drugs;

- persons with schizophrenia and other psychoses whose illnesses may be exacerbated by continued use of cannabis;
- persons with a family history of psychoses in whom regular cannabis use may precipitate the onset of a psychosis.

## Part II: Interventions with Cannabis-Dependent Adults

A variety of treatments for cannabis-dependent adults have been tested in randomized controlled trials. All are adaptations of therapeutic models that have shown efficacy in the treatment of alcohol, tobacco, or other drug problems. Chapters in this and the following section present the theoretical background, treatment techniques, and issues in the adaptation and implementation of these approaches with cannabis-dependent adults, as well as the results of treatment-outcome studies completed to date.

Motivational enhancement therapy (MET) and cognitive-behavioral therapy (CBT) have received the most research attention and have often been combined with MET strategies used in early sessions and CBT strategies in later sessions. Results have been uniformly positive in showing reduced marijuana use and associated problems following treatment, but long-term abstinence rates are typically less than 20% and relapse is common.

There is little evidence that either MET or CBT is superior to the other and both are effective in either group or individual formats.

In several trials, very brief (2–4 sessions) MET interventions produced significant reductions in cannabis use but there is some evidence that longer (9–14 sessions) MET/CBT interventions yield better outcomes.

Contingency management (CM), involving the delivery of monetary incentives for urine-verified abstinence, showed promise in increasing rates of continuous abstinence during treatment, but longer-term outcomes after the incentives are discontinued are not yet known. Other novel adaptations of the CM approach are being studied.

A Marijuana Check-Up (MCU) designed to appeal to adult cannabis users who were ambivalent about change or treatment attracted a sample of daily users. They differed little from treatment seekers with the exception of less readiness to change and somewhat fewer self-reported negative consequences. The two-session MET intervention resulted in a greater reduction in the frequency of cannabis use during the follow-up period compared to control conditions. Reductions in use were small in absolute terms, but the approach showed promise in reaching another segment of cannabis-dependent adults who may benefit from treatment.

Supportive–Expressive (SE) psychotherapy, emphasizing the importance of effective interpersonal relationships in overcoming addiction, led to greater rates of abstinence than a single session of advice. Process data indicated that SE led to changes in interpersonal effectiveness that at least partially accounted for the greater abstinence.

## Part III: Interventions with Cannabis-Dependent Adolescents and Young Adults

There is a dearth of controlled treatment-outcome studies with adolescent or young adult cannabis abusers. These groups are at different stages of development and pose different treatment issues compared to adults. Most are coerced into treatment rather than seeking it voluntarily.

The Cannabis Youth Treatment study, a large multi-site investigation, compared five interventions of different durations and intensities. Therapeutic models included various combinations of MET, CBT, and family therapy. Although there were few differences in outcomes between treatments, overall results indicated substantial reductions in cannabis use and problems during the 12 months of follow-up. Analyses addressed issues of comorbidity, retention in treatment, differential response to treatment, and cost-effectiveness.

Two adaptations of the "check-up" model as a method for reaching teenage cannabis users on a voluntary basis were tested in the USA and Australia. The respective projects used somewhat different methods of recruiting participants, but both delivered a two-session MET intervention. Results from these uncontrolled studies showed substantial reductions in cannabis use and positive perceptions of the interventions supporting further development and testing.

An intervention combining MET with monetary incentives for attending treatment sessions increased treatment attendance in young adults referred by probation departments relative to MET alone. Greater reductions in marijuana use were not observed as a consequence, however.

## Part IV: Policy

### *The Policy Implications of Cannabis Dependence*

Public education of the risks of cannabis dependence must present credible consequences of heavy use in order to avoid being rejected.

Prevention efforts should include opportunistic (e.g., primary care) and targeted screening and brief interventions in vulnerable populations. Delivery of more extensive treatment services to meet the needs of cannabis-dependent individuals with comorbid substance abuse or mental health disorders in specialized treatment agencies would provide a more complete continuum of care.

Studies of decriminalization in several countries yield conflicting conclusions regarding effects on rates of cannabis use and do not address effects on heavy use or dependence.

The prevalence of cannabis dependence may increase if legal sanctions for use were decreased or eliminated because lower price and greater availability would result in more people using cannabis regularly and for longer periods in their lives. Greater numbers of individuals, therefore, may experience health and psychological problems, including cannabis dependence.

However legalization would allow for a regulated cannabis market that would permit more widespread harm minimization educational activities and the development of social norms favoring moderation and stigmatizing excess. Adequate data do not exist to predict the net result of such changes in policy.

## Part V: Conclusion

Cannabis dependence exists and is associated with negative consequences that affect millions of users. Many of these individuals need and want help in overcoming dependence.

Despite the apparent validity of a dependence syndrome, the negative consequences of cannabis dependence may not be as severe as for many other drug dependencies. This relative lack of negative consequences may fuel low motivation for change and undermine the effectiveness of treatment interventions.

More research on the nature and consequences of cannabis dependence is needed to inform policy decisions that can prevent its occurrence. More research is also needed on treatment approaches that build and sustain motivation for change.

# Foreword

Marijuana continues to be a hot topic in the news. At the time of this writing (July, 2005), The Seattle Times has published numerous stories about the "green plant" and controversies surrounding its use and potential for abuse. Many featured articles described the debate about medical marijuana and the US Supreme Court's recent decision that federal drug charges can be applied to users and distributors of marijuana even in those states that passed local laws approving cannabis use as a treatment for several disorders (e.g., reduction of nausea associated with chemotherapy, appetite enhancement in the treatment of AIDS, lowering intra-ocular pressure in the treatment of glaucoma, and so on). As Washington is one of the states that voted to approve the medical use of marijuana, press coverage has been sympathetic to the plight of patients who may now be denied access to the healing herb. Based on this press coverage, most readers (as judged by letters to the Editor of the Seattle Times) were outraged by the Supreme Court decision, given the evidence that so many patients reported beneficial effects from smoking pot.

Other stories about marijuana that have been covered in the local press express criticism and concern over its use. Here in the Pacific Northwest, public officials have expressed outrage about the distribution of potent marijuana that has been smuggled into Washington and adjoining states from our Canadian neighbors to the north. Known as "B.C. bud," this strong variety of marijuana is highly sought after by local smokers. Recently, several B.C. residents were arrested after they were discovered smuggling large quantities of B.C. bud through a sophisticated 360-foot tunnel buried under the Canada–USA border near Langley, B.C. The three men arrested were monitored in the underground pathway carrying hockey bags and garbage sacks containing 93 pounds of B.C. bud. Political tension between the two countries has also been exacerbated by the recent announcement by the mayor of Vancouver, B.C. that efforts would soon be made to decriminalize marijuana sales in the province and to provide additional tax revenues as a result. Marijuana sales would be regulated in the same manner as tobacco and alcohol, according to the mayor. Public opinion sways back and forth on both sides of the border. Is marijuana use helpful (as a medicine) or harmful (as an addictive drug)? Confusion and debate continue about the potential for abuse and dependence among marijuana smokers. Some see it as a relatively benign substance compared to other drugs of abuse, while others see it as a "stepping stone" that leads to further illegal drug use.

Despite the continuing controversy and public ambivalence, one fact stands out clearly: marijuana is the most commonly used illicit drug in the world. In "A Closing Note" at the conclusion of Chapter 1 of the current volume, the authors cite a United Nations report issued in 2004 indicating that cannabis is the most widely used illicit drug worldwide "with an estimated 146.2 million people having consumed cannabis at least once in the previous 12-month period. Although this report suggested that the spread of drug abuse is losing momentum globally, the one notable exception was cannabis which was described as spreading at an accelerated pace." According to a recent Research Report on Marijuana Abuse published by the National Institute on Drug Abuse (July, 2005), marijuana is also the most commonly used illicit drug in the US. The report concludes that more than 94 million Americans (40% of the population) aged 12 years and older have tried marijuana at least once. Data from the 2004 Monitoring the Future Survey, summarized in the NIDA report, indicated that 46% of high-school seniors had tried marijuana at some time and that 20% were current users. A study conducted by the National Institute of Justice's Arrestee Drug Abuse Monitoring Program (also cited in the NIDA report) found that 57% of juvenile male and 32% of juvenile female arrestees tested positive for marijuana. The NIDA report also summarized findings from the 2003 National Survey on Drug Use and Health, indicating that an estimated 21.6 million Americans aged 12 or older were classified with substance dependence or abuse (9.1% of the total population); of the estimated 6.9 million Americans classified with abuse or dependence on illicit drugs, 4.2 million were dependent on or abused marijuana. In 2002, 15% of people entering drug abuse treatment programs reported that marijuana was their primary drug of abuse, according to the NIDA report. Epidemiological data described in the current book also indicates that many users are at risk for developing a diagnosis of cannabis dependence. Among current users (i.e., used at least once in the prior month), roughly 11–16% (1.6–2.3 million individuals) qualify for the diagnosis of cannabis dependence, as reported in Chapter 1.

Although marijuana may be less harmful in terms of health consequences and addiction potential compared to other illicit drugs (such as heroin or crystal meth) or licit substances (alcohol and tobacco), the information reported on the high rates of use and associated risks for marijuana dependency represents a major public health challenge for health professionals. Surprisingly little information currently exists regarding treatment approaches for cannabis dependence. In response to this growing need, the present volume is both timely and relevant. As a colleague and friend of both Roger Roffman and Robert Stephens for many years, I congratulate them for their excellent work in co-editing this new book on cannabis dependence. They are both pioneers in the field of marijuana research and associated treatment and intervention programs. Together, they have invited an impressive list of authors to contribute their expertise and clinical experience to further our understanding of this important topic. As a result, they have brought together a wealth of information and insight that readers will find invaluable.

The fifteen chapters in this book are divided into five parts. Part I contains five chapters devoted to describing the nature of cannabis dependence. Chapter 1 (Roffman, Schwartz, and Stephens) provides a history of cannabis dependence themes that have appeared in the past and that continue to have influence on how this concept will be defined in the future. In Chapter 2, Babor provides an incisive overview of the diagnostic criteria for cannabis dependence, including its etiology, course, and natural history. The pharmacology and physiology of this dependency is presented in Chapter 3 (Lichtman and Martin), based on results from both animal and human studies that indicate a reciprocal relationship between cannabinoid and opioid systems in drug dependence. The epidemiology and etiology of cannabis dependence are reviewed in Chapter 4 by James Anthony, with a focus on recent evidence from field studies. In Chapter 5, the final chapter in this section, Hall and Solowij provide a review of evidence related to the adverse health and psychological consequences, with an emphasis on studies of long-term daily cannabis users.

Part II consists of five chapters devoted to treatment interventions for cannabis-dependent adults. Given the need for more information on evidence-based treatment approaches, the authors are to be commended for their cutting-edge empirical work and the presentation of treatment-outcome data in many of the chapters. Chapter 6 (Stephens, Roffman, Copeland and Swift) provides an overview of both cognitive-behavioral (e.g., relapse prevention) and motivational enhancement (e.g., motivational interviewing) treatment approaches, both of which have been relatively effective and well received by adult clients. Another promising intervention, contingency management, is described in Chapter 7 (Budney, Moore, Signon and Higgins) and has been found effective in enhancing initial abstinence rates in treatment-outcome studies. For adult marijuana users who have questions or concerns about their use, the "Marijuana Check-up" described in Chapter 8 by Stephens and Roffman is highly recommended, consisting of a brief two-session assessment and feedback intervention patterned after the "Drinkers' Check-up" designed to promote change in alcohol users who are unlikely to seek formal treatment. Another treatment approach first developed for use with problem drinkers and now modified as a brief motivational intervention for cannabis abuse is guided self-change, described in Chapter 9 (Sobell, Sobell, Wagner, Agrawal and Ellingstad). This intervention may be particularly helpful for cannabis users with less severe problems or who are ambivalent about treatment goals (reduced use versus abstinence). In Chapter 10, Grenyer and Solowij describe supportive–expressive psychotherapy, a dynamic approach that emphasizes the importance of effective interpersonal relationships as an important mediating factor in treatment outcome.

Three chapters are presented in Part III, each describing promising interventions for adolescents and young adults. Chapter 11 (Diamond, Leckrone, Dennis and Godley) provides preliminary findings from the Cannabis Youth Treatment Study that evaluated the impact of five brief intervention programs, including various combinations of cognitive-behavioral, motivational enhancement, family support networks, a community reinforcement approach, and multidimensional family therapy in the outpatient treatment of adolescents with marijuana problems. Preliminary results indicate that these brief interventions can be helpful for many adolescent clients; treatment was found to be effective overall (although few differences were reported across the different treatment conditions), showing good retention rates and lower costs. The "Teen Cannabis Check-Up" program for adolescent clients, similar in content and format to the check-up program for adult users, is described in Chapter 12 (Berghuis, Swift, Roffman, Stephens and Copeland), with encouraging results in terms of reduced cannabis use among teens studied in both Australia and the USA. The final chapter (Chapter 13) in this section presents promising findings in the treatment of young probation-referred marijuana-abusing individuals (Carroll, Sinha, and Easton), in which motivational enhancement therapy and contingency management were evaluated.

Part IV consists of a single chapter (Chapter 14) outlining the public policy implications of cannabis dependence, and discussing implications for both the public health sector and the specialized treatment arena. Hall and Swift also discuss additional hot policy topics, including cannabis decriminalization. Part V concludes the book with a final wrap-up chapter by the editors (Chapter 15 by Stephens and Roffman), integrating the treatment findings presented in the preceding chapters and discussing implications for future research. Although they conclude that reductions in cannabis use resulting from treatment were often substantial (consistent with a harm-reduction approach), long-term abstinence rates remain relatively low (80% relapse rate). Clearly there is still a room for improvement in our treatment approaches for cannabis dependence, but the material presented throughout this valuable text should pave the way for future advances in the field. Hats-off and thumbs-up to Roger Roffman and Robert Stephens for opening up the highway!

G. ALAN MARLATT
*University of Washington*

# Part I

The Nature of Cannabis Dependence

# 1

# Themes in the History of Cannabis Dependence

ROGER A. ROFFMAN, SAM SCHWARTZ AND ROBERT S. STEPHENS

In the foreword to the 1972 trade book edition of *Marihuana: A Signal of Misunderstanding*, the official report to the US President and Congress of the National Commission on Marihuana and Drug Abuse, the Commission's chairman wrote:

If public need is an appropriate purpose for publishing a book, and surely it must be, I cannot readily imagine a more legitimate book than the one at hand. For seldom in the nation's history has there been a phenomenon more divisive, more misunderstood, more fraught with impact on family, personal, and community relationships than the marihuana phenomenon.

As the Commission noted more than 30 years ago, the concept of cannabis dependence also had been highly subject to misunderstanding. That challenge is ongoing. Over time, its very existence has been both vigorously asserted and robustly denied in legislative hearings, books and articles in the popular literature, scientific writings, and in the pronouncements of medical and legal experts. In this chapter, we examine the history of this concept, particularly emphasizing key themes that have contributed to how cannabis dependence has been perceived by the general public, by the scientific community, and by policy-makers.

At the outset we ought to acknowledge that many kinds of influence have shaped these perceptions at different points in time. Legend, cannabis users' autobiographical accounts, findings of commissions of inquiry, expert opinion, colorful newspaper stories and Hollywood films, the shifting meanings of such terms as "narcotic" and "addict," nomenclatures for classifying drug and alcohol problems, various iterations of diagnostic guidelines, epidemiological studies of cannabis users, research on brain physiology, and treatment outcome studies have all contributed to how cannabis dependence has been and currently is perceived. This list is not exhaustive, however, since one factor it does not yet include is the impact of advocacy by diverse stakeholders

3

(e.g., governmental entities such as the Drug Enforcement Administration and the National Institute on Drug Abuse, and drug reform groups such as the Marijuana Policy Project and the National Organization for the Reform of Marijuana Laws) in their efforts to achieve hegemony in influencing public attitudes about cannabis use and whether and how it ought to be dealt with in the law, in education, and in treatment.

The contributors to this volume offer current findings of various scientific disciplines in seeking meaning of the cannabis dependence concept. One might anticipate, however, that political and cultural factors that have played a role in defining this concept in the past will likely evolve and continue to have influence on how this phenomenon is understood in the future.

Studying the salience of factors that shape the meaning of cannabis dependence is not simply an intellectual exercise. Rather, examining these sources of influence helps to illuminate how consensus for varying conceptualizations of cannabis dependence grows or recedes in the attitudes of the general public, among legislators, in fields of science, and in the human services (Edwards, 1968). Ultimately, these perceptions shape the nature of research inquiry, social policy reflected in the law, decisions concerning the expenditure of public funds, and the design of educational and therapeutic approaches. To illustrate the point, we might consider the implications of three quite different profiles of cannabis dependence:

1. an addiction to a narcotic by societal outcasts who will likely become violent and insane,
2. a disease of the brain brought about by altered neurotransmission, or
3. a social construction based on cultural conflict.

A good place to start in this effort to understand the evolution of the meaning of cannabis dependence is to acknowledge the diversity of the product itself.

## Diversity of Cannabis Preparations

Variations in cannabis plant species, preparations, and methods of administration result in a wide range of behavioral effects associated with the regular use of this drug. As a consequence, understanding the nature of cannabis dependence requires specification of a context. Which cannabis product is being considered, how has it been prepared, and how is it being consumed?

Linnaeus named the hemp plant Cannabis sativa and classified it as a member of a plant family known as *Cannabinaceae* (Earleywine, 2002). Later, Lamarck distinguished between hemp grown in Europe from the plant variety grown in India, with the name *Cannabis indica* given to the latter. Yet another variety of hemp was given the name *Cannabis ruderalis*. While each plant variety is distinguished from the others in terms of the quantity of resin produced, it remains uncertain whether these types are separate species or variations of one plant (Schultes *et al.*, 1975).

Varying preparations of cannabis and alternative methods with which they are consumed further add to the diverse profiles associated with regular cannabis use. As an example, three cannabis products used in India include ganja (the flowering tops of the cannabis plant), charas (the plant's resin), and bhang (either a combination of the flowering tops and small stems or a beverage made from the leaves). Ganja and charas are smoked, thus resulting in a faster delivery of tetrahydrocannabinol (THC) to the brain. Bhang is eaten or consumed as a beverage, both of which result in a slower delivery of THC.

Illustrating how the process of plant cultivation can add to variation in the product's effects, Abel (1980) notes that in India plants used to produce bhang are given relatively little attention during the growing season whereas plants grown to produce ganja or charas are carefully cultivated to maximize their THC content. Thus, the plant cultivation procedures, the products that result, and alternative modes of administration all contribute to the wide variations in effects. Just one example of the many different cannabis concoctions is dawamesc, a confection in Arab countries made from hashish, butter, cantharides, pistachio, musk, sugar, cinnamon, ginger, and cloves (Abel, 1980).

Given the influence of these factors, it is not surprising that the addiction potential of cannabis was characterized quite differently in America, Asia, and Europe (Bromberg, 1939). In the early 1900s as cannabis use in the US increased, American writers tended to see the drug as habit-forming while writers in parts of the world where more potent forms were consumed perceived it as producing a physical addiction.

## The Influence of Tales, Legend, Myth, and Lore

Vivid and evocative imagery, often conveyed in popular literature and the media, has been among the key contributors to the public's perceptions of cannabis, its dependence liability, and the consequences of becoming dependent. Prominent themes have included portraying the cannabis-dependent individual as menacing the public through theft, murder, rape, or the seduction of children; the user's will being entirely taken over; and his/her moral standards being subjugated. Not uncommonly, racist associations were embedded in accounts of the drug's effects. In these portrayals, neither moderate patterns of use nor use with only positive consequences were generally acknowledged.

Just a few examples will illustrate this contributing factor to the cannabis dependence phenomenon.

First, from the Arab world come stories of cannabis both as an instrument of political murder and as an aid to attaining spiritual vision. Marco Polo wrote in the late 13th century of a ruthless Persian ruler (the Old Man of the Mountains) whose disciples committed religiously motivated murders. Subsequent chroniclers reported that these followers, encouraged to develop insatiable appetites for hashish in order to fortify their courage, consequently came to be known as Hashshashin, allegedly the derivation of the term assassin. Contemporary historians describe a reign of terror in which leaders of a sect of the Shiite branch of Islam did indeed recruit and train a unit of men to commit secret assassinations of their political opponents. What is questioned, however, is there being any basis for their fanaticism and brutality having been induced by hashish (Mandel, 1966). In his recent book *Cannabis: A History*, Booth (2003) comments on the likely historical misattribution:

So it was that, gradually, by association with the Assassins … hashish came to be considered a drug capable of generating bedlam, undermining society, creating chaos and turning otherwise merciful men into merciless murderers. And this grossly erroneous myth has been perpetuated ever since, right up to the modern day… (p. 55).

While cannabis was first used for religious purposes in India, in the 12th century AD the Sufis, a mystical movement of ascetics in the Arab world whose religious principles were contrary to Islamic orthodoxy similarly encouraged the seeking of spiritual insights through the use of hashish. Their critics, decrying the heretical ideas espoused by this offshoot religious group, claimed that use of hashish was driven by a physical addiction to the drug, leading the addict to be preoccupied with searching for new sources (Rosenthal, 1971). Additionally, the Sufi use of hashish was seen as not only a challenge to traditional forms of Islam at the time, but also as a challenge to society as a whole, because users were more interested in searching for mystical experiences than working within the traditional roles of society.

Finally, stories from Africa tell of induced dependence on cannabis as a means of holding people captive or for the purpose of greatly enhancing their capabilities. In the late 18th century, African white landowners were described as having intentionally addicted Bushmen at an early age to dagga, another name for cannabis. The goal was to create an irresistible inducement for Bushmen to remain in the landowner's service (Thompson, 1967). In the mid-1800s, young Zulu warriors were described as being capable of accomplishing hazardous feats due to stimulation from dagga. A. T. Bryant, a white explorer who wrote *The Zulu People*, portrayed the Zulus as addicted to dagga (Bryant, 1970).

As will be noted later in this chapter, the telling of colorful and often frightening tales about the addiction liability of cannabis and its consequences continued into the 20th century. These examples from as early as a thousand years ago make it evident that cannabis hyperbole is not an invention of our time.

## Memoirs and Writings of Key Literary Figures and Artists

Another major influence on the public's perceptions of cannabis dependence has come from descriptions by writers and artists of their personal experiences. There is an extensive literature of this genre, and two specific examples will be illustrative.

In the mid-1800s, a group of French writers and artists, referring to themselves as Le Club des Hachichins (The Hashish Eaters' Club), met monthly in Paris, experimented with an eaten cannabis concoction, and mused about its effects on their creative imaginations. Among the club's members were Fernand Boissard de Boisdenier, Théophile Gautier, Gérard de Nerval, Charles Baudelaire, Victor Hugo, Honoré de Balzac, and Honoré-Victorin Daumier, and their writings about hashish led to greater public awareness of cannabis in Europe. The corpus of their published work conveyed vivid portrayals of altered states of consciousness as well as warnings that the user needed to be in a positive psychological disposition before consuming the drug. Based on his personal experience, Baudelaire eventually came to be highly critical of hashish when its use was motivated to attain heightened states of consciousness, stating that it ultimately risked the destruction of man's will.

Also in the mid-1800s, an American writer by the name of Fitz Hugh Ludlow published an autobiography titled, *The Hasheesh Eater: Being Passages from the Life of a Pythagorean*. Ludlow described his youth as having been spent in a constant state of cannabis intoxication, and noted that he eventually became psychologically dependent on the drug. He wrote of the lessons learned from hashish use, including terrifying hallucinogenic experiences that led to short-lived vows to abstain. He concluded, however, that society ought not to judge those who seek self-awareness through its use. When he eventually tried to quit, efforts to combat his dependence by taking laudanum and later alcohol proved unsuccessful. He found himself unable to stop either abruptly or through tapering, and ultimately needed the help of a physician to successfully overcome cannabis dependence (Ludlow, 1857).

## Commissions of Inquiry Concerning Cannabis Dependence

Formal boards of inquiry have been established periodically in order to summarize existing knowledge concerning cannabis, recommend policy, and – in some cases – to conduct new research. As will be noted in this section, the findings of these various boards and commissions *vis-à-vis* the addiction potential of cannabis have varied considerably.

### The 1893–1894 Indian Hemp Drugs Commission

Established in 1893 by the British Secretary of State for India, this commission was charged with identifying the consequences of cannabis use, particularly focusing on its possible impact on the moral and social life of the people of India, and the pros and cons of cannabis prohibition. While commerce in cannabis was legal at the time, concern arose among both British and native Indian administrators that cannabis use was eroding the efficiency of native troops employed by the British and members of the lower working class who performed most of the manual labor in the country. A Member of Parliament who had called for an official inquiry had asserted that ganja was far more harmful than opium.

More than a thousand individuals offered testimony to the commission which issued its findings in a seven-volume report. Among the conclusions were an acknowledgement that understanding cannabis' effects necessitated taking into account both the frequency of usage and the potency of the specific preparation being considered. Moreover, because cannabis concoctions frequently contained other substances (e.g., opium, datura, and hyoscyamis), determining whether any adverse effects were due to cannabis was extremely difficult.

The commission found that cannabis use for recreational, medical, and religious purposes was more widespread than had been estimated; that it was not a cause of criminal behavior; that moderate use was not a cause of mental illness or immoral behavior; and that banning its use would adversely affect religious observance and cause civil unrest. The commission's witnesses tended to believe that moderate cannabis usage eventually developed into excessive usage with a consequent heightened likelihood of moral degradation and mental instability, but they perceived this vulnerability toward progression to be held in common by all intoxicants. The commissioners recommended against prohibiting cannabis, suggesting that if discouragement of use were desirable, taxation would be a preferable approach. At the time of its issuance, the report of the Indian Hemp Drugs Commission (1969) was the most comprehensive inquiry to ever have been conducted about cannabis.

In the years that followed, the beginning of the twentieth century witnessed a greater emphasis on drug prevention, with calls for international restrictions on cultivation and commerce in cannabis due to its presumed addictive nature. Representatives from Egypt and Turkey, at a 1924 meeting of the International

Opium Conference, claimed that chronic hashishism was occurring in their countries (Booth, 2003). In his autobiography, the British journalist Malcolm Muggeridge noted that many of the students he taught at the University of Cairo were addicted to hashish (Muggeridge, 1972).

## The 1925 Panama Canal Zone Report

Concerns about the potential deleterious effects of cannabis use on American soldiers stationed in the Canal Zone led to the convening of a formal committee of inquiry in April of 1925. Data considered by the committee included a review of the literature, consultation with experts, testimony from army officers, an examination of personnel records to look for a link between cannabis use and unruly behavior, and observations of several soldiers, four physicians, and two policemen while they smoked marijuana under controlled circumstances. The committee concluded that marijuana was neither habit forming nor risky in terms of the user's health and behavior. Two subsequent formal inquiries in the Panama Canal Zone produced essentially the same findings.

## The 1929 Preliminary Report on Indian Hemp and Peyote issued by US Surgeon General Hugh S. Cummings

In the late 1920s, several members of Congress had expressed concern about marijuana, primarily in response to reports from constituents that marijuana was being sold to school children. Congressional attention to cannabis also was heightened following the inclusion of Indian hemp in a 1929 bill authorizing the establishment of two narcotic farms for the treatment of persons addicted to habit-forming drugs. This was the first time that marijuana had been identified as a narcotic in federal legislation.

Surgeon General Cummings' report was ostensibly the first official scientific inquiry of the US government on the effects of marihuana. By current standards, however, its investigative methodology was merely cursory. Neither the empirical literature nor the findings of the earlier government-sponsored boards of inquiry appear to have been considered when the report was drafted. The report's inadequacy may have been related to the fact that cannabis use at the time was largely limited to ethnic minority groups in the southwestern states, the lack of a constituency for a rigorous scientific inquiry, and the subordinate role that government health officials played *vis-à-vis* law enforcement officials in shaping government policy (Bonnie & Whitebread, 1974).

In contrast with the Indian Hemp Drugs Commission's findings, the Surgeon General's report failed to distinguish between moderate and excessive use of cannabis. As to the drug's dependence liability, the report found that cannabis was a narcotic and was habit forming but not addicting (i.e., caused psychological but not physical dependence).

Surgeon General Cummings' report contributed to what has become a potent linguistic ambiguity concerning the meaning of the term "narcotic." From a biological perspective, a narcotic induces narcosis (numbness, sleep) and analgesia (the alleviation of pain). The most notable narcotics are the opiates which have a high addiction potential when used regularly. Over time, however, the term narcotic came to be commonly used in the literature as well as in legislation to refer to: (1) any addicting drug, or (2) any illegal drug. Despite noting that cannabis was habit forming and not addictive, by referring to cannabis as a narcotic the Cummings Report lent official credence to the drug's addiction liability while also misrepresenting its pharmacological effects. The ultimate impact of this definitional confusion was marijuana coming to be indistinguishable from the opiates and cocaine in relation to its legal status. Additionally, the view of the marijuana "addict" changed from the "accidental addict" to the newly defined "dope fiend" and "immoral street user." Thus, this report greatly contributed to negative perceptions of the marijuana user's lifestyle (Bonnie & Whitebread, 1974).

## The 1944 LaGuardia Committee Report ("The Marihuana Problem in the City of New York")

Sensationalistic accounts of young people engaging in criminal activities while under the influence of marijuana led Mayor Fiorello LaGuardia in 1938 to request that the New York Academy of Medicine conduct an investigation of the drug. The in-depth inquiry was conducted by a distinguished panel of medical practitioners and social scientists. The Committee concluded that most of the claims of marijuana's dangers were untrue or exaggerated. It found that marijuana smoking did not lead to addiction in the medical sense of the word (i.e., physical dependence), its use was not a precursor to opiate or cocaine addiction, and most of those who used it for a period of years did not demonstrate mental or physical deterioration (Mayor's Committee on Marihuana, 1944).

These conclusions stood in rather stark contrast with what the public and legislative bodies had been hearing about cannabis in the early to middle decades of the 20th century. In that period, the popularity of cannabis increased, gradually evolving from a southwest regional phenomenon to a national one. Increasingly, stories in the popular literature and legislative testimony conveyed racist conclusions that cannabis use caused crime and insanity in black and Mexican populations. Also, the emergence of jazz and its association with the Prohibition-era speakeasy further fueled public fears, with marijuana ("muggles") smoking quickly becoming iconic of a cultural identity among jazz musicians, most of whom were black.

Harry Anslinger, Director of the Federal Bureau of Narcotics from 1930 to 1962, worked diligently to warn the public that marijuana use presented a serious threat, although most of the harms he claimed existed had no empirical support. Salacious stories and Hollywood portrayals of young people's lives being destroyed by marijuana (Reefer Madness) added to a building sense of urgency. Legislatures in the southwest and south lobbied Washington for federal prohibition, and by 1936 thirty-eight states had added marijuana to their lists of dangerous drugs in the Uniform State Narcotics Acts. Then, enactment of the 1937 Marijuana Tax Act brought federal sanctions to bear on the problem. The subsequent 1951 Boggs Act and the 1956 Narcotic Control Act greatly increased criminal penalties for cannabis possession and sale. One argument put forth to support greater penalties was the claim that marijuana use was a precursor to heroin addiction, perhaps the first time that the "stepping stone" theory was put forth. Along the way, defense lawyers began to claim that their clients suffered diminished responsibility due to cannabis dependence and men subject to the draft petitioned for exemption from military conscription on the same basis. The Boggs act, in particular, standardized penalties with other narcotics, which reinforced and stimulated "society's fear of drug dependence on the level of moral antipathy," thereby reflecting and enhancing a negative view of cannabis use (Bonnie & Whitebread, 1974).

It is not difficult to imagine how effective these alarming messages about cannabis dependence must have been in shaping public attitudes, particularly when delivered by putative experts:

- In the midst of the US Depression, a physician wrote in a medical journal of the dangers to the public order resulting from cannabis dependence: "Under the influence of cannabis indica, these human derelicts are quickly subjugated by the will of the master mind. The moral principles or training initiated in the mind from infancy deter from committing willful theft, murder or rape, but this inhibition from crime may be destroyed by the addiction to marihuana (Fossier, 1931)."
- A 1932 article in The Journal of Criminal Law and Criminology conveyed the opinions of law enforcement specialists. The authors wrote, "It is impossible to fix a definite time in which one becomes an addict.... After the chronic use of marihuana "cannabinomania" develops, which in

many persons, especially if psychopathic, leads to a loss of mental activity.... (E)ach [smoking] experience ends in the destruction of brain tissues and nerve center, and does irreparable damage...." (Hayes & Bowery, 1932).

- Mrs. Emily Murphy, a Canadian police magistrate, wrote, "The addict loses all sense of moral responsibility. Addicts to this drug, while under its influence, are immune to pain, become raving maniacs, and are likely to kill or indulge in any form of violence to other persons." She warned that marijuana users were public enemies who intended to destroy the white race (Murphy, 1973).

- Anslinger, in a March 1, 1935 letter to Rev. John J. Burke, wrote: "When an opium or cocaine habitué has been made, it is extremely difficult to effect a cure, although this has been done by scientific medical hospitalization. The case of Marihuana addicts is well nigh hopeless as the hasheesh or marihuana smoker becomes insane. Favorable action must be taken to prevent the spread of this pernicious weed because its evil consequences are irremediable (quoted in Bonnie & Whitebread, 1974, pp. 111–112)."

Periodically, voices were raised to offer alternative perspectives. The University of Indiana sociologist Alfred Lindesmith countered the stereotyped image of the dope fiend, arguing that drug use crossed class and racial lines and that dependence was more validly perceived as a medical or psychological condition. The federal narcotics bureaucracy reacted quite negatively to his ideas.

Marijuana's popularity grew substantially in the following decades, stimulated in part by written portrayals of personal drug-enhanced explorations by key figures in what came to be known as the beat generation (e.g., Allen Ginsburg, William Burroughs, and Jack Kerouac). Booth (2003) captures the impact of this literature in contesting societal mores of the time: "What the Beats did was not restricted to advertising drugs – more specifically if not intentionally, marijuana – and bringing them into the mainstream of cultural life. They created a climate of personal liberty, challenged traditional values, altered concepts of sexuality, countered hypocrisy, politicized literature, and undermined censorship (p. 204)."

As marijuana came into the mainstream and more Caucasian middle class individuals were subjected to the severe criminal penalties that had been enacted in the 1950s and 1960s, marijuana's addiction potential began to be questioned. King (1974) quotes from two presidential commissions in the 1960s where such assumptions about the drug's addiction liability were challenged.

From the 1963 President's Advisory Commission on Narcotics and Drug Abuse:

"An offender whose crime is sale of a marijuana reefer is subject to the same term of imprisonment as the peddler selling heroin. In most cases, the marijuana reefer is less harmful than any opiate. For one thing, while marijuana may provoke lawless behavior, it does not create physical dependence. This Commission makes a flat distinction between the two drugs and believes that the unlawful sale or possession of marijuana is a less serious offense than the unlawful sale or possession of an opiate."

From President Johnson's 1967 Commission on Law Enforcement and Administration of Justice:

"Marijuana is equated in law with the opiates, but the abuse characteristics of the two have almost nothing in common. The opiate produces physical dependence. Marijuana does not. A withdrawal sickness appears when use of the opiates is discontinued. No such symptoms are associated with marijuana. The desired dose of opiates tends to increase over time, but this is not true of marijuana. Both can lead to psychic dependence, but so can almost any substance that alters the state of consciousness." (King, 1974)

## The 1972 Report of the National Commission on Marihuana and Drug Abuse

Established by a provision of the US 1970 Comprehensive Drug Abuse Prevention and Control Act, what came to be known as The Shafer Commission produced the most thorough review of cannabis knowledge to date.

The Commission found that that marijuana does not induce physical dependence, although heavy long-term users may develop psychological dependence, and that cessation of use is not followed by a major withdrawal syndrome. The Commission's recommendation that personal possession of marijuana be decriminalized was based on its concluding that, "(f)rom what is known now about the effects of marihuana, its use at the present level does not constitute a major threat to public health (Marihuana: A Signal of Misunderstanding, 1972, pp. 90)" and "there is little proven danger of physical or psychological harm from the experimental or intermittent use of the natural preparations of cannabis (Marihuana: A Signal of Misunderstanding, pp. 65)." These conclusions signaled a turnabout in the credibility of beliefs about cannabis (e.g., the inevitability that use became abuse, its addiction liability, its classification as a narcotic, its role as a stepping stone to heroin addiction) that had underlain the heavily punitive sanctions imposed by state and federal laws in the preceding decades.

The decade of the 1970s in the US witnessed the emergence of an influential marijuana policy reform movement that saw well-organized efforts devoted to reducing penalties through state and federal legislation and the filing of law suits challenging such issues as the constitutionality of marijuana's classification as a narcotic. By 1978, 11 states had reduced cannabis use penalties to a misdemeanor level. Whether or not cannabis users risked becoming dependent on the drug remained an issue of debate, but the concern soon shifted from adults to children and from a debate about civil liberties to one of protecting youth.

The political tide had turned in the late 1970s in the USA as rapid growth of the paraphernalia industry and steep increases in marijuana experimentation by younger-aged children gave rise to what would become a powerful "parents movement" that opposed any tolerance of illicit drug use. The 1980s witnessed a retrenchment in the momentum in a number of states to reduce marijuana possession penalties, mandatory drug testing became more common, and liberalized policies were promulgated only with reference to marijuana's use for medical purposes.

As will be evident from the subsequent chapters in this volume, the pace of science in producing important new knowledge has quickened in the past 20 years. Emerging findings concerning cannabinoid neurochemistry, epidemiological data concerning how the drug has been used, enhancements to diagnostic approaches, and the findings of treatment studies targeting adults and adolescents with cannabis use disorders all have contributed to our current understanding of cannabis dependence.

## Understanding Cannabis Dependence and Withdrawal by Studying Cannabinoid Neurochemistry

As is discussed in the chapter by Aron Lichtman and Billy Martin, considerable evidence for a biological basis to marijuana dependence has accumulated since the identification of a specific cannabinoid receptor in the brain (Devane *et al.*, 1988) and the discovery of anandamide, a compound that binds to and activates the same receptor sites in the brain as delta-9-THC, the active ingredient in marijuana. (Devane *et al.*, 1992). Subsequently, researchers discovered a cannabinoid antagonist, a compound that blocks anandamide action in the brain (Huestis *et al.*, 2001; Rinaldi-Carmona *et al.*, 1994). Taken together, these discoveries have made it possible to systematically study the effects of chronic exposure to marijuana.

Relatedly, there is some evidence for the role of genetics in determining whether the marijuana user will become dependent. In a study of more than

8000 male twins, genes were shown to influence whether a person finds the effects of marijuana use pleasant (Lyons *et al.*, 1997). Kendler and Prescott reported that genetic risk factors in women contribute at a moderate level to the probability of ever use, and have strong impact on the liability for heavy use, abuse, and probably dependence on marijuana (1998). While factors in an individual's social environment clearly influence whether he or she ever tries marijuana, becoming a heavy user or abuser may be more determined by genetically transmitted individual differences, perhaps involving the brain's reward system. Research in this area may eventually identify individual risk factors for marijuana dependence that people can use in making decisions about their own use of this drug.

A mild syndrome of withdrawal from marijuana has been reported, with symptoms that may include: aggression, anger, restlessness, irritability, mild agitation, insomnia, decreased appetite, decreased body weight, sleep electroencephalography (EEG) disturbance, anxiety, stomach pain, nausea, runny nose, sweating, and cramping (Budney *et al.*, 1999, 2003; Crowley *et al.*, 1998; Haney *et al.*, 1999; Jones *et al.*, 1976). Commonly, these symptoms abate within a week to 14 days. Evidence from both animal and human research supporting the clinical importance of these symptoms *vis-à-vis* cannabis dependence is accumulating. Based on findings from their own lab as well as data from other inpatient, outpatient, clinical, and general population studies of cannabis abstinence effects, Budney and colleagues (2003) call for a cannabis withdrawal syndrome being included in the next revision of the Diagnostic and Statistical Manual of the American Psychiatric Association.

With greater understanding of the cannabinoid neurochemical system's physiology, the potential for a more detailed understanding of the nature of cannabis dependence and the development and testing of pharmacological interventions will be advanced. The US National Institute on Drug Abuse has expressed interest in developing a Medications Development for Cannabis Dependence Research Program, with likely emphases on examining the efficacy of cannabinoid agonists, antagonists, medications to alleviate withdrawal symptoms, and medications that facilitate overcoming dependence by effectively treating co-occurring psychiatric disorders such as depression.

## Specifying Cannabis Dependence through Classification and Diagnosis

As discussed earlier, fact-finding commissions in the 1960s and 1970s reported that cannabis had been misclassified in the law as a narcotic and as a consequence of the commonplace use of the term "addict" to refer to the drug's

users. Beginning in the late 1950s, the World Health Organization (WHO) contributed to the development of a nomenclature for the classification of drug-
and alcohol-related problems that was intended to resolve confusion emanating
from imprecise terms such as drug addiction, drug habituation, physical
dependence, psychic dependence, drug abuse, and drug misuse. A 1981 WHO
report called for a conceptualization of dependence that did not require either
tolerance or withdrawal for a diagnosis to be made, although both were among
the criteria that could comprise a drug dependence syndrome. Among the features of this syndrome (i.e., a clustering of cognitive, behavioral, and physiological phenomena) proposed by the WHO were: "a subjective awareness of
compulsion to use a drug or drugs, usually during attempts to stop or moderate
drug use; a desire to stop drug use in the face of continued use; a relatively
stereotyped drug-taking habit, that is a narrowing in the repertoire of drug-
taking behavior; evidence of neuroadaptation (tolerance and withdrawal symptoms); use of the drug to relieve or avoid withdrawal symptoms; the salience of
drug-taking behaviour relative to other important priorities; and rapid reinstatement of the syndrome after a period of abstinence (Edwards *et al.*, 1981)."

In his chapter on cannabis diagnosis, Tom Babor discusses diagnostic systems
and procedures that are based on current classification schemes in use in the US
and internationally.

## Determining the Prevalence of Cannabis Dependence through Epidemiological Research

Data concerning two subgroups, those who have used at least once in the past
year and those who have used at least once in the past month, can be used to
estimate the prevalence of problems associated with cannabis use. Two fairly
large longitudinal studies offer estimations concerning those who have used
one or more times in the previous year. Grant & Pickering (1998) found that
6% qualified for a diagnosis of cannabis dependence and 23% qualified for a
diagnosis of abuse. Another study, focusing on self-report of problems attributed to cannabis by respondents, found that 85% reported no problems, 15%
reported one, 8% reported at least two, and 4% reported at least three (National
Institute on Drug Abuse, 1991). When current users (i.e., used at least once in
the prior month) are considered, roughly 11–16% (1.6–2.3 million individuals)
qualify for the diagnosis of cannabis dependence. In summary, the risk for the
occurrence of three or more problems (a proxy indicator for dependence)
among those who have used at least once in the past year appears to be roughly
4–6%, and 11–16% for those who have used at least once in the past month.

The authors of a recent book that reviews the cannabis literature suggest the following rules of thumb for the risk of cannabis dependence: 1 in 10 for those who have ever used cannabis, between 1 and 5 and 1 and 3 for those who have used the drug more than a few times, and between 1 and 2 for daily users (Hall & Pacula, 2003).

Another approach to estimating problematic consequences involves time frame from initial use. Epidemiologists estimate that almost 2% of users develop cannabis dependence within the first 2 years of initiating use. Based on the estimate that 2.5 million individuals first used cannabis in 1999, 50,000 would be expected to have experienced cannabis dependence within 2 years of their initial use. Within roughly 10 years after first use of cannabis, an estimated 10% of cannabis users develop the cannabis dependence syndrome. (Anthony *et al.*, 1994; Wagner & Anthony, 2002).

Finally, the relative risk of becoming cannabis dependent if one uses this drug at least once can be examined in the context of risk levels for those who have used other substances at least once. Anthony and his colleagues (1994) identify the following relative risk levels for dependence: tobacco (31.9%), heroin (23.1%), cocaine (16.7%), alcohol (15.4%), stimulants (11.2%), and cannabis (9.1%).

Jim Anthony's chapter in this volume offers important data to further enhance how cannabis dependence can be understood.

**Addressing the Need for Cannabis Dependence Interventions**

As will be noted from many of this book's contributions, an emerging literature exists in which the findings of cannabis dependence counseling interventions are reported. Treatment approaches tested to date have been based on cognitive-behavioral and psychodynamic theory, with emphases on skills training, contingency management, and motivational enhancement. To date, the outcomes of tested interventions are modest in terms of their long-term successes, although the findings approximate those reported for other drug dependence interventions (Budney & Moore, 2002).

Data from treatment agencies in the US, Australia, and Europe point to an increasing demand for cannabis dependence counseling. In the US, agencies receiving state or federal funds reported that admissions for primary marijuana dependence rose from 92,518 (5.9% of all admissions) in 1992 to 286,189 (15.1% of all admissions) in 2002 (Substance Abuse and Mental Health Services Administration, 2003). Comparable figures from Australia for clients served for primary marijuana dependence reflect an increase from 4% in 1990 to 11% in 2000 (Copeland & Conroy, 2001). In 1998, treatment agencies in the European

Union saw between 2% and 16% of clients with cannabis as the primary drug problem (European Monitoring Centre for Drugs and Drug Addiction, 1998).

In interpreting the significance of treatment admissions data, one caveat that must be considered is the possibility that an unknown percentage of those seeking treatment may have done so solely to avoid criminal sanctions. Nonetheless, because cannabis has remained illegal in most of these jurisdictions during this period of increased treatment demand, the trend points to the importance of developing effective interventions for cannabis dependence.

## A Closing Note

In a 2004 report, the UN indicated that cannabis is the most widely used illicit drug worldwide, with an estimated 146.2 million people having consumed cannabis at least once in the previous 12-month period (United Nations Office on Drugs and Crime, 2004). Although this report suggested that the spread of drug abuse is losing momentum globally, the one notable exception was cannabis which was described as spreading at an accelerated pace.

## References

Abel, E. (1980). *Marijuana: the first twelve thousand years*. New York: Plenum.
Anthony, J. C., Warner, L. A., & Kessler, R. C. (1994). Comparative epidemiology of dependence on tobacco, alcohol, controlled substances, and inhalants: basic findings from the National Comorbidity Survey. *Experimental and Clinical Psychopharmacology, 2*, 244–268.
Bonnie, R. J., & Whitebread, C. H. (1974). *The marihuana conviction: a history of marihuana prohibition in the United States*. Charlottesville: University Press of Virginia.
Booth, M. (2003). *Cannabis: a history*. New York: St. Martin's Press.
Bromberg, W. (1939). Marihuana: a psychiatric study. *Journal of the American Medical Association, 113*, 4–12.
Bryant, A. T. (1970). The Zulu People, cited in T. James, Dagga: a review of fact and fancy. *Medical Journal, 44*, 575–580.
Budney, A. J., & Moore, B. A. (2002). Development and consequences of cannabis dependence. *Journal of Clinical Pharmacology, 42*, 28S–33S.
Budney, A. J., Moore, B. A., Vandrey, R. G., & Hughes, J. R. (2003). The time course and significance of cannabis withdrawal. *Journal of Abnormal Psychology, 112*, 393–402.
Budney, A. J., Novy, P. L., & Hughes, J. R. (1999). Marijuana withdrawal among adults seeking treatment for marijuana dependence. *Addiction, 94*, 1311–1322.
Copeland, J., & Conroy, A. (2001). Australian national minimum data set for clients of alcohol and other drug treatment services: findings of the national pilot and developments in implementation. *Drug and Alcohol Review, 20*, 295–298.

Crowley, T. J., Macdonald, M. J., Whitmore, E. A., & Mikulich, S. K. (1998). Cannabis dependence, withdrawal, and reinforcing effects among adolescents with conduct symptoms and substance use disorders. *Drug and Alcohol Dependence, 50*, 27–37.

Devane, W. A., Dysarz, F. A., Johnson, M. R., Melvin, L. S., & Howlett, A. C. (1988). Determination and characterization of a cannabinoid receptor in rat brain. *Molecular Pharmacology, 34*, 605–613.

Devane, W. A., Hanus, L., Breuer, A., Pertwee, R. G., Stevenson, L. A., Griffin, G., Gibson, D., Mandelbaum, A., Etinger, A., & Mechoulam, R. (1992). Isolation and structure of a brain constituent that binds to the cannabinoid receptor. *Science, 258*, 1946–1949.

Earleywine, M. (2002). *Understanding marijuana: a new look at the scientific evidence.* Oxford: Oxford University Press.

Edwards, G. (1968). The problem of cannabis dependence. *The Practitioner, 200*, 226–233.

Edwards, G., Arif, A., & Hodgson, R. (1981). Nomenclature and classification of drug- and alcohol-related problems: A WHO memorandum. *Bulletin of the World Health Organization, 59*, 225–242.

European Monitoring Centre for Drugs and Drug Addiction (1998). *Annual Report on the State of the Drugs Problem in the European Union, 1998.* Lisbon, Portugal: European Monitoring Centre for Drugs and Drug Addiction.

Fossier, A. E. (1931). The marihuana menace. *New Orleans Medical and Surgical Journal, 44*, 247.

Grant, P. F., & Pickering, R. (1998). The relationship between cannabis use and DSM-IV cannabis use and dependence: results from the national longitudinal alcohol epidemiology study. *Journal of Substance Abuse, 10*, 255–264.

Hall, W., & Pacula, R. L. (2003). *Cannabis use and dependence: public health and public policy.* Cambridge: Cambridge University Press.

Haney, M., Ward, A. S., Comer, S. D., Foltin, R. W., & Fischman, M. W. (1999). Abstinence symptoms following smoked marijuana in humans. *Psychopharmacology, 141*, 395–404.

Hayes, M. A., & Bowery, L. E. (1932). Marihuana. *Journal of Criminal Law and Criminology, 23*, 1086–1094.

Huestis, M. A., Gorelick, D. A., Heishman, S. J., Preston, K. L., Nelson, R. A., Moolchan, E. T., & Frank, R. A. (2001). Blockade of effects of smoked marijuana by the CB1-selective cannabinoid receptor antagonist SR141716. *Archives of General Psychiatry, 58*, 322–328.

Jones, R. T., Benowitz, N., & Bachman, J. (1976). Clinical studies of tolerance and dependence. *Annals of the New York Academy of Sciences, 282*, 221–239.

Kendler, K. S., & Prescott, C. A. (1998). Cannabis use, abuse, and dependence in a population-based sample of female twins. *American Journal of Psychiatry, 155*, 1016.

King, R. (1974). *The drug hang-up.* Springfield, Ill: Charles C. Thomas.

Ludlow, F. (1857). *The hasheesh eater: being passages from the life of a Pythagorean.* New York: Harper & Bros.

20                                                          *Roger A. Roffman* et al.

Lyons, M. J., Toomey, R., Meyer, J. M., Green, A. I., Eisen, S. A., Goldberg, J., True, W. R., & Tsuang, M. T. (1997). How do genes influence marijuana use? The role of subjective effects. *Addiction, 92*, 409–417.

Mandel, J. (1966). Hashish, assassins and the love of god. *Issues in Criminology, 2*, 149–156.

Marihuana: A signal of misunderstanding (1972). First Report of the National Commission on Marihuana and Drug Abuse. Washington, DC: Government Printing Office.

Indian Hemp Drugs Commission (1969). *Marijuana: report of the Indian Hemp Drugs Commission, 1893–1894*. Silver Spring, MD: Thomas Jefferson Co.

Mayor's Committee on Marihuana (1944). *The marihuana problem in the city of New York (LaGuardia Report)*. New York: Jaques Cattell.

Muggeridge, M. (1972). *Chronicles of wasted time: 1. The green stick*. London: Collins.

Murphy, E. (1973). *The black candle*. Toronto: Coles Publishing.

National Institute on Drug Abuse, Division of Epidemiology and Prevention Research (1991). *National household survey on drug abuse: main findings 1990*. Rockville, MD: Department of Health and Human Services.

Rinaldi-Carmona, M., Barth, F., Heaulme, M., Shire, D., Calandra, B., Congy, C., Martinez, S., Maruani, J., Neliat, G., Caput, D., Ferrara, P., Soubrie, P., Breliere, J. C., & LeFur, G. (1994). SR 141716A, a potent and selective antagonist of the brain cannabinoid receptor. Federation of European Biochemical Societies *FEBS Letters, 350*, 240–244.

Rosenthal, F. (1971). *The herb*. Leiden: E.J. Brill.

Schultes, R. E., Klein, W. M., Plowman, T., & Lockwood, T. E. (1975). Cannabis: an example of taxonomic neglect. In V. Rubin (Ed.), *Cannabis and culture* (pp. 21–38). The Hague: Mouton.

Substance Abuse and Mental Health Services Administration, Office of Applied Studies (2003). *Treatment Episode Data Set (TEDS); 1992–2002. National Admissions to Substance Abuse Treatment Services. DASIS Series: S-20, DHHS Publication No. (SMA) 03-3778*. Rockville, MD: Department of Health and Human Services, Substance Abuse and Mental Health Services Administration, Office of Applied Studies.

Thompson, G. (1967). *Travels and adventures in Southern Africa*. Cape Town: Van Riebeeck Society.

United Nations Office on Drugs and Crime (2004). *2004 World Drug Report*. United Nations Publication Sales No. E.04.XI.16.

Wagner, F. A., & Anthony, J. C. (2002). From first drug use to drug dependence: developmental periods of risk for dependence upon marijuana, cocaine, and alcohol. *Neuropsychopharmacology, 26*, 479–488.

# 2

# The Diagnosis of Cannabis Dependence

THOMAS F. BABOR

## Introduction

Classification and diagnosis of psychiatric disorders are critical steps in the development of effective methods for their treatment and prevention. This chapter considers the classification and diagnosis of cannabis dependence from several perspectives. First, the nature of the cannabis dependence syndrome is reviewed in terms of its theoretical basis in addiction psychiatry (Edwards *et al.*, 1981). Next, the nature and purpose of psychiatric classification are described in relation to cannabis-related disorders, and this is followed by a review of standard diagnostic procedures recommended by the major classification systems used in the USA and in other parts of the world. The chapter also reviews the scientific evidence for the syndrome, its etiology, course and natural history and closes with a summary of new developments in the measurement of cannabis dependence.

## Nature of the Syndrome

Central to current attempts to characterize, classify and diagnose cannabis dependence is the concept of a dependence syndrome that is distinguished from problems or disabilities caused by substance use. A psychiatric syndrome is a cluster of symptoms that co-occur in a way that signals the presence of an underlying disorder. According to an influential position paper developed for the World Health Organization (WHO) (Edwards *et al.*, 1981), the drug dependence syndrome is seen as an interrelated cluster of elements that may be present for a specific substance (e.g., tobacco, alcohol or cannabis), for a class of substances (e.g., opioid drugs) or for a wider range of pharmacologically different substances. The main elements of drug dependence are psychological symptoms (e.g., a strong desire to use cannabis), physiological signs (e.g., tolerance

and withdrawal) and behavioral symptoms (e.g., use of cannabis in inappropriate times and places). Although drug dependence may be conceived and classified in binary terms as either present or absent, this practical distinction does not
contradict the fact that dependence tends to vary along a continuum of severity.

According to this formulation, neuroadaptation in the form of tolerance or
withdrawal is neither necessary nor sufficient for the diagnosis of dependence.
Cannabis users, for example, may develop a dependence syndrome without
experiencing withdrawal symptoms during periods of abstinence. What ties
together the syndrome elements and accounts for their interrelationships is an
often unstated set of assumptions about the learning mechanisms and neurobiological processes behind the acquisition and maintenance of addictive behavior (Babor, 1992). Theories of alcohol and drug use suggest that dependence is
a complex neurobiological phenomenon that results from social reinforcement
of the initiation of substance use, neurochemical reinforcement of substance-
taking behavior and cognitive mediation of substance-related cues that are
interpreted as "cravings" (Gardner & David, 1999). The scope of the elements
included in the dependence syndrome concept suggests that both positive and
negative reinforcements are strongly involved in the initiation and maintenance
of dependence. Many patients with a history of drug dependence experience
rapid reinstatement of the features of the syndrome following resumption of
substance use after a period of abstinence. Rapid reinstatement is a powerful
diagnostic indicator of dependence because it points to the likelihood that
neuroadaptation and consequent impairment of control over substance use
have already developed. The adaptation of this generic syndrome concept to
the diagnosis of cannabis dependence is the subject of the remainder of this
chapter.

## Classification

As used in medicine, classification refers to the naming and categorization of
medical and psychiatric disorders. The goal of classification is to allow clinicians and scientists to communicate more effectively by using a convenient and
economical method to describe the most likely characteristics and course of a
disorder. As knowledge about different substance-related conditions has advanced,
so too has the classification of these conditions. Classification is a prerequisite
to diagnosis, which is the use of signs, symptoms and decision rules to determine whether a specific disorder is present and should be classified as such.
This section describes the classification of cannabis dependence within the two
standard nomenclatures used both in the USA and worldwide.

The first is the WHO International Classification of Diseases (ICD). The tenth revision of this classification system (WHO, 1993) includes a separate chapter on Mental and Behavioral Disorders, among which are the Disorders due to Psychoactive Substance Use. For more than half a century the ICD has been the primary system used throughout the world to classify and record medical and psychiatric conditions for statistical purposes. With the tenth revision of ICD (WHO, 1993), which now includes detailed diagnostic guidelines (WHO, 1992), the system has become a very useful way to guide clinical diagnosis as well as psychiatric research.

The second standard nomenclature useful for the classification of cannabis use disorders is the Diagnostic and Statistical Manual (DSM) of the American Psychiatric Association (APA). This system was designed for clinical use by psychiatrists and related professionals. The fourth edition of DSM (APA, 1994) consists of a comprehensive listing of psychiatric disorders that are organized into two primary axes: (1) clinical disorders and (2) personality disorders.

Cannabis dependence in DSM-IV is classified as one of the clinical disorders, within the broader category of substance-related disorders that describes psychiatric conditions associated with 11 psychoactive substances: alcohol; amphetamines; caffeine; cannabis; cocaine; hallucinogens; inhalants; nicotine; opioids; phencyclidine; and sedatives, hypnotics or anxiolytics. Like these other substance-related disorders, cannabis-related disorders are divided into two categories: (1) cannabis-induced disorders, and (2) cannabis use disorders. Cannabis-induced disorders, such as cannabis intoxication, are conditions that are caused by the direct toxic and psychoactive properties of cannabis.

The cannabis use disorders, abuse and dependence, are partially overlapping categories that are defined by criteria sets common to all of the substance-related disorders. Cannabis abuse is a residual category that applies primarily to the consequences of periodic cannabis use and intoxication, such as legal problems, interference with performance at work or school, or elevated risk of accidents or injuries. When the symptoms of cannabis abuse are associated with compulsive use and tolerance, then the diagnosis of cannabis dependence takes precedence.

Another aspect of classification, covered only tangentially in the standard diagnostic systems, is the issue of polydrug abuse or dependence. Many alcohol and drug users report cannabis as a secondary or tertiary drug, whereas others use it as their primary drug. Both patterns are commonly found in clinical settings. Using the public domain version of the Treatment Episode Data Set (TEDS, Office of Applied Studies, 2002), it is possible to describe the kinds of primary and secondary cannabis users presenting for treatment within the US public treatment system. Primary marijuana abuse accounted for 15% of TEDS admissions in the year 2000. Among those being treated for other drugs, marijuana was the most frequent secondary substance reported by alcohol admissions (61%), methamphetamine/amphetamine admissions (44%) and persons admitted for hallucinogens (56%). Moreover, marijuana was the third most frequently reported problem substance by those admitted for opiates other than heroin (14%), cocaine (32%), tranquilizers (20%), sedatives (20%), inhalants (33%) and phencyclidine (36%). These data indicate that cannabis is one of the most frequently reported substances among persons admitted for treatment of alcohol and drug problems, both as a primary drug of abuse and as a secondary drug involved in a pattern of polydrug use.

### Diagnosis

Diagnosis typically involves a systematic evaluation of signs, symptoms and laboratory data as these relate to the history of the patient's present illness or condition. The purpose of diagnosis is to provide the clinician with a logical basis for planning treatment and estimating prognosis. Diagnosis also may serve a variety of administrative, statistical and scientific purposes. When a patient is suspected of having a substance use disorder, diagnostic procedures are needed to exclude false positives and borderline cases. Health-care reimbursement policies often require that a formal diagnosis be confirmed according to standard procedures or criteria. The need for uniform reporting of statistical data, as well as the generation of prevalence estimates for epidemiological research, often requires a diagnostic classification of the patient. Finally, research on substance use disorders can be enhanced considerably when subjects or cases included in a study sample meet standard criteria for having a particular diagnosis.

Diagnosis provides patients with an explanation of the condition that may be responsible for their illness and disease. It gives clinicians a clear idea of the nature, natural history and future course of the problems being experienced by the patient. But formal clinical diagnosis, applied mechanically, may have disadvantages, especially with regard to cannabis users who have mild or moderate levels of dependence. Despite its convenience, the use of a binary (present, absent) categorical decision rule may result in misclassification errors and inappropriate treatment recommendations for individuals who may not require intensive treatment. Another risk is stigma, which may result from the diagnostic labeling process. There is little evidence, however, that either stigma or over diagnosis result from the use of the formal diagnostic systems discussed in this chapter.

Diagnosis of a cannabis-related disorder should be accompanied by a detailed history to determine whether cannabis use is impairing the patient's physical and psychological functioning. It is particularly important to inquire about the patient's pattern of substance use, including tobacco, alcohol and other substances. How often does the person use cannabis? Daily or almost daily use is an indication of impaired control over use. Is cannabis used in conjunction with tobacco and alcohol? If so, these substances may provide reciprocal cues that might impede cessation and precipitate relapse. Is cannabis part of a broader pattern of psychoactive drug use that involves substances with a higher dependence potential like heroin or cocaine? The frequency and duration of cannabis use should also be documented, as well as any periods of infrequent use or cessation. Most people who present for treatment of cannabis dependence are daily or near daily users. However, general population data concerning the co-occurrence of dependence and daily or near daily use are not available.

Urine toxicology screening for drugs of abuse is a reliable way to verify cannabis use and to identify other substances that are part of the clinical picture. The approximate duration of detectability of cannabinoids in urine varies from 3 days for a single use to as much as 10 days for heavy use, and similar variability exists for other substances (Wolff *et al.*, 1999). But this information may have limited usefulness for diagnostic purposes because it merely indicates that the substance has been used in the past few days.

Based on the two dominant and somewhat similar classification systems described above, the diagnosis of cannabis dependence has now become a central feature of psychiatric nosology. The procedures and contents of these systems, which have been revised and expanded approximately every 10 years, are now described in more detail.

## *ICD-10*

Within the ICD, cannabis dependence is described as a syndrome consisting of a cluster of physiological, behavioral and cognitive phenomena in which the use of cannabis or a class of cannabis-like substances takes on a much higher priority for a given individual than other behaviors that once had greater value (WHO, 1993). According to the ICD-10 *Guidelines for Mental and Behavioural Disorders* (WHO, 1992), the subjective awareness of compulsion to use cannabis (reported as a strong desire or craving by the patient) is a central characteristic of the dependence syndrome. It is most commonly seen during attempts to stop or control cannabis use. A definite diagnosis of dependence is usually made only if

Table 2.1. *ICD-10 diagnostic guidelines for cannabis dependence syndrome**

1. A strong desire or sense of compulsion to use cannabis
2. Difficulties in controlling cannabis-taking behavior in terms of its onset, termination, or levels of use
3. A physiological withdrawal state when cannabis use has ceased or been reduced, as evidenced by: a characteristic withdrawal syndrome for the substance; or use of the same (or a closely related) substance with the intention of relieving or avoiding withdrawal symptoms
4. Evidence of tolerance, such that increased doses of cannabis are required in order to achieve effects originally produced by lower doses
5. Progressive neglect of alternative pleasures or interests because of cannabis use, increased amount of time necessary to obtain or use cannabis or to recover from its effects
6. Persisting with cannabis use despite clear evidence of overtly harmful consequences, such as depressive mood states consequent to periods of heavy use, or cannabis-related impairment of cognitive functioning; efforts should be made to determine that the user was actually, or could be expected to be, aware of the nature and extent of the harm

* Adapted from ICD-10 (WHO, 1992).

three or more of the six symptoms shown in Table 2.1 have been experienced or exhibited at some time during the previous year.

In addition to the diagnostic criteria listed in Table 2.1, there are several other features that are useful to provide accurate classification and to estimate the severity of the syndrome. The first is the narrowing of the personal repertoire of cannabis use patterns. With the development of dependence, the pattern of cannabis use becomes less variable and more stereotyped in terms of times and places of use. With severe dependence cannabis is used multiple times throughout the day, every day of the week. Another feature of the clinical picture is rapid reinstatement of the syndrome after a period of abstinence. Once substance use recommences, dependence symptoms re-appear much more quickly than it took for their initial development.

In its broad outlines as well as its theoretical underpinnings, the cannabis dependence syndrome in ICD-10 is a direct adaptation of the drug dependence syndrome concept described by Edwards *et al.* (1981). As ICD-10 was developed several years before the fourth revision of DSM, the concept was also influential in the process of writing the DSM-IV criteria for substance dependence (Babor, 1995). The need to maintain consistency on an international level between the DSM system used in the USA and the ICD system used in the rest of the world was also an important consideration.

## DSM-IV

Whereas ICD-10 was designed for use by general medical practitioners, DSM-IV was designed for psychiatrists. Diagnosis within DSM-IV is more complicated and comprehensive than ICD-10, requiring diagnostic training and skilled clinical judgment in order to evaluate the patient according to its "multiaxial" system. The multiaxial approach requires that important diagnostic information be noted on each of five different axes. Axis I includes the more florid psychiatric disorders such as schizophrenia and the mood disorders as well as the developmental disorders and substance-related disorders. Axis II is reserved for personality disorders. Axis III provides a means to note clinically relevant general medical conditions. Axis IV is used to record clinically relevant psychosocial and environmental problems (e.g., homelessness). Finally, Axis V consists of a Global Assessment of Functioning Scale, which takes into account psychological, social and occupational functioning on a hypothetical continuum ranging from mental health to mental illness.

The generic aspects of dependence under the Axis I substance use disorders in DSM-IV are defined by a common set of criteria that apply to all dependence-producing psychoactive substances. As applied to cannabis, dependence is defined as a maladaptive pattern of cannabis use, leading to clinically significant impairment or distress, as manifested by three (or more) of the seven symptoms listed in Table 2.2 occurring at any time in the same 12-month period. According to the DSM-IV (APA, 1994, p. 216), "individuals with cannabis dependence have compulsive use and do not generally develop physiological dependence." Although tolerance to most of the effects of cannabis is considered common in those who use cannabis chronically, withdrawal symptoms "have not yet been reliably shown to be clinically significant." As noted below, empirical research concerning cannabis withdrawal has called this conclusion into question.

### Evidence for Cannabis Dependence, Including Tolerance and Withdrawal

Recent research has examined the validity and coherence of the marijuana dependence diagnosis, and whether regular use of *Cannabis sativa* can lead to a drug dependence syndrome characterized by impaired control over cannabis use, preoccupation with cannabis, tolerance to its effects and a set of recognizable withdrawal symptoms following abrupt discontinuation of use. The evidence comes from at least four lines of investigation:

1. Animal research on the neurobiological basis of cannabis reinforcement.

Table 2.2. *DSM-IV criteria for cannabis dependence*\*

1. Tolerance, as defined by either:
   (a) a need for markedly increased amounts of cannabis to achieve intoxication or desired effect
   (b) markedly diminished effect with continued use of the same amount of cannabis
2. Withdrawal, as manifested by either of the following:
   (a) the characteristic withdrawal syndrome for cannabis
   (b) cannabis, or a cannabis-like substance is taken to relieve or avoid withdrawal symptoms
3. Cannabis is often taken in larger amounts or over a longer period than was intended
4. There is a persistent desire or unsuccessful efforts to cut down or control cannabis use
5. A great deal of time is spent in activities necessary to obtain cannabis (e.g., driving long distances), use cannabis (e.g., socializing with cannabis using friends), or recover from its effects
6. Important social, occupational, or recreational activities are given up or reduced because of substance use
7. Cannabis use is continued despite knowledge of having a persistent or recurrent physical or psychological problem that is likely to have been caused or exacerbated by cannabis (e.g., chronic cough related to smoking; excessive sedation resulting from repeated use of high doses)

Specify if:
(a) With Physiological Dependence: evidence of tolerance or withdrawal (i.e., either Item 1 or 2 is present), or
(b) Without Physiological Dependence: no evidence of tolerance or withdrawal (i.e., neither Item 1 or 2 is present)

\* Adapted from APA (1994).

2. Laboratory investigations of human subjects using moderate to large doses of delta-9 THC.
3. Research on clinical samples of treatment-seeking cannabis users, including adolescents.
4. Epidemiological research on dependence symptoms reported by cannabis users in the general population.

As is discussed in Chapter 3 by Lichtman and Martin in this volume, considerable evidence for a biological basis to marijuana dependence has accumulated since the identification of a specific cannabinoid receptor in the brain and the discovery of anandamide, a compound that activates the same receptor sites in the brain as delta-9-tetrahydrocannabinol (THC), the active ingredient in marijuana

Table 2.3. *Marijuana dependence symptoms reported in a sample of*
*450 chronic marijuana users presenting for treatment\**

| Symptom | % of total n = 450 |
|---|---|
| Unsuccessful attempts to quit or cut down | 96.0 |
| Using despite persistent or recurrent psychological or physical problems | 95.1 |
| Considerable time spent buying, using, or recovering from the effects | 83.3 |
| Withdrawal | 77.6 |
| Using for a longer period of time or more than intended | 76.9 |
| Tolerance | 68.2 |
| Using takes up the time normally spent on other important activities | 64.2 |

\* This table is reprinted (with permission) from an article by Stephens, Babor, Kadden, Miller and the Marijuana Treatment Project (2002).

(Devane *et al.*, 1992). Researchers have also discovered a cannabinoid antagonist. This compound blocks anandamide action in the brain (Rinaldi-Carmona *et al.*, 1994). With greater understanding of the neurochemical basis of cannabis' reinforcing effects on brain systems, the reasons for the persistence of marijuana use have become more apparent.

The symptoms of marijuana dependence, as defined in DSM and ICD, are often reported by chronic marijuana smokers who are evaluated in treatment outcome studies or treatment settings. Typically, these individuals have difficulty controlling the amount, timing and frequency of marijuana use. Marijuana users recruited into treatment outcome studies averaged over 10 years of near-daily use and over six serious attempts at quitting in the past (Stephens *et al.*, 1994, 2000). Their use had persisted in the face of multiple social, psychological and medical problems, and most perceived themselves as unable to stop.

Table 2.3 shows the prevalence of marijuana dependence symptoms reported by a sample of 450 chronic cannabis users seeking treatment as part of a large multisite intervention trial (Marijuana Treatment Project Research Group, 2004). Each of the seven DSM-IV dependence symptoms was rated as present for more than 69% of the sample. Symptoms measuring the salience of marijuana were reported most frequently. Almost all participants (96%) had unsuccessful attempts to quit or cut down; 95% said they continued to use marijuana despite recurrent psychological or physical problems; and 83% reported that large amounts of their time were spent using or recovering from marijuana use. Withdrawal symptoms were reportedly 77.6% of the sample and impaired control by 76.9%.

Physiological withdrawal symptoms resulting from marijuana use were once believed to be of relatively low intensity. For this reason marijuana was not viewed in the same way as other dependence-producing substances. However, recent studies have found that chronic heavy users develop both physiological and psychological dependence on cannabis, and that cessation from use may produce a withdrawal syndrome broadly characterized by restlessness, irritability, mild agitation, insomnia, decreased appetite, sleep disturbance, anxiety, stomach pain, nausea, runny nose, sweating and cramping (Budney *et al.*, 1999; Crowley *et al.*, 1998; Haney *et al.*, 1999; Weisbeck *et al.*, 1996). These symptoms commonly abate within a week to 10 days of abstinence from cannabis products. Findings from studies of clinical samples are consistent with laboratory studies of human marijuana users exposed to high doses of THC (Jones *et al.*, 1976; Mendelson *et al.*, 1984). Laboratory studies have also documented the development of tolerance to marijuana's subjective and physiological effects when large doses are ingested on a regular basis (Babor *et al.*, 1975).

Although there has not been much research on the coherence of the cannabis syndrome elements and psychometric properties of its diagnostic procedures, one study (Rounsaville *et al.*, 1993b) found strong evidence that the marijuana dependence symptoms included in both ICD and DSM formed a single factor with high loadings, similar to what has been found for a variety of other psychoactive substances. Another study (Kranzler *et al.*, 1997) compared DSM-III-R cannabis dependence diagnoses (which share most of the DSM-IV symptoms) with a more systematic longitudinal evaluation of cannabis users in treatment, concluding that the dependence syndrome diagnosis had good concurrent, discriminative and predictive validity. Test-retest reliability for past year and lifetime diagnoses of cannabis dependence has also been found to be good (Easton *et al.*, 1997). In general, the drug syndrome concept seems to apply well to the symptoms of dependence specified in ICD and DSM.

## Etiology, Course and Natural History

The etiology of cannabis dependence is at present poorly understood. It shares many of the same predisposing factors that characterize other substance use disorders. The amount of exposure to the substance, personality traits, peer support and a variety of other factors have been implicated (see chapter by James Anthony, in this volume). Cannabis dependence typically develops gradually following a period of initial experimentation that evolves into a pattern of regular and then more compulsive use (Gruber & Pope, 1997).

For those who have used marijuana at least once, the relative probability of ever becoming dependent on the substance was estimated to be 9% (Anthony *et al.*, 1994). This level of risk is considerably lower than risk estimates of dependence for those who have used tobacco (32%), heroin (23%), cocaine (17%) or alcohol (15%). The risk of developing marijuana dependence is higher among individuals who have smoked marijuana more frequently. Among those who have used marijuana five or more times, the risk of dependence is 17% (Hall *et al.*, 1999). For daily or near daily users, the risk increases to one in three (Kandel & Davies, 1992).

One way to investigate natural history is to study the time sequencing of clinical features that emerge during a relatively long period of exposure. Two types of studies have been reported, one using community samples, the other using clinical samples. In a prospective, longitudinal study of a population sample of relatively young marijuana users, Rosenberg and Anthony (2001) found that when clinical features of cannabis dependence were observed, the onset of the first symptoms tended to occur within the first 10 years of use. Loss of control (using larger amounts than intended) emerged early, followed by increased salience (i.e., a great deal of time spent getting, using, recovering from cannabis) and tolerance. Withdrawal symptoms were reported at an average age later than all other symptoms, and were reported by the smallest number of users.

Stephens *et al.* (1993) interviewed a sample of 290 male and 92 female adult marijuana users who were screened for participation in a treatment study. The average age of initiation to marijuana use was 16 years. The average subject had begun daily or near daily use by the age of 20 years. By the time they had reached their 30s, these chronic smokers had experienced substantial dysfunction as a consequence of marijuana use and most had expressed a desire to reduce or discontinue use. The average number of previous attempts at quitting or cutting down was seven. While these data show the use trajectory of a subset of users who sought treatment, it is not clear whether they characterize all cannabis users.

## Measurement of Cannabis Dependence

Concurrent with by the growing amount of diagnostic research on cannabis use disorders, a variety of self-report instruments have been developed for the purposes of classification and diagnosis of cannabis dependence. Perhaps the most common way to measure cannabis dependence in clinical and community settings is to use a fully structured psychiatric diagnostic interview. These interviews have highly specified questions and response categories. They can be administered by trained interviewers in person or by telephone. They cover a variety of psychiatric disorders, including the substance use disorders in DSM and ICD.

The Composite International Diagnostic Interview (CIDI) is one such instrument that has been used extensively in psychiatric epidemiology research throughout the world. Its content and structure are based on the Diagnostic Interview Schedule, modified for international use (Robins *et al.*, 1988). The CIDI is sufficiently comprehensive to provide ICD-10 and DSM-IV diagnoses. Several studies have used the University of Michigan adaptation of the Composite International Diagnostic Interview (UM-CIDI) (Kessler *et al.*, 1994; Rosenberg & Anthony, 2001). The UM-CIDI, like its parent interview, the WHO CIDI (Robins *et al.*, 1988), includes questions specifically designed to measure both ICD-10 and DSM-IV dependence symptoms for a variety of psychoactive substances, including cannabis products. The questions also assesses amount and history of cannabis use, age of onset, as well as recency of individual symptoms.

A second type of diagnostic interview, referred to as "semistructured," does not require strict adherence to written questions. It does, however, rely heavily on the clinical experience of the interviewer and the interviewer's knowledge of psychiatric symptoms and syndromes. Two interviews of this genre are the Structured Clinical Interview for DSM (SCID) (Spitzer *et al.*, 1988) and the Schedules for Clinical Assessment in Neuropsychiatry (SCAN) (Wing *et al.*, 1990). The SCID produces an accurate classification of patients with marijuana dependence (Kranzler *et al.*, 1996). SCAN, developed by WHO, is designed to meet the need for a comprehensive procedure for clinical examination that is also capable of generating ICD and DSM diagnoses, including substance use disorders. The interview is based on clinical "cross examination," with the aim of discovering whether each symptom is present and, if so, with what degree of severity. For most symptoms, a prescribed form of questioning is suggested, although the interviewer is free to depart from this if clinical judgment is preferred. SCAN diagnoses of cannabis dependence have been found to be reliable across a variety of national and cultural groups (Easton *et al.*, 1997).

The reader is referred to the comprehensive reviews and compendia listed in the bibliography (Inciardi, 1994; Rounsaville *et al.*, 1993a). These sources give evidence of the tremendous array of assessment instruments that are currently available for program administrators and providers of clinical care. In most cases, these instruments are easy to use, and provide useful standardized information for the purpose of diagnosis and clinical assessment of persons with cannabis use disorders. A study of several brief cannabis symptom measures (Swift *et al.*, 1998), including the CIDI, indicated that they were able to diagnose cannabis dependence at levels substantially better than chance and were generally robust in terms of the optimal diagnostic cut-offs within different contexts. Despite advances in the classification and assessment of cannabis dependence, there has been considerably less progress in the development of valid and reliable instruments to measure cannabis-related problems. An exception is the 19-item Marijuana Problems Scale (Marijuana Treatment Project Research Group, 2004; Stephens *et al.*, 2000). In summary, these instruments may be useful for both diagnostic evaluation and for research designed to understand the patterns of use that lead to dependence.

## Conclusion

As this chapter has shown, developments in the classification, diagnosis and measurement of cannabis dependence have progressed in conjunction with research on the epidemiology, neurobiology and treatment of cannabis-related disorders. Unlike the historical portrayal of marijuana as a benign drug, recent research suggests that individuals can develop a dependence syndrome. The syndrome typically develops over the course of years rather than months, with daily, chronic marijuana smoking being the hallmark indicator.

With the development of standard nomenclatures and classification systems, such as ICD and DSM, there has been a concomitant move to develop operational criteria that permit reliable and valid diagnostic classification. These criteria have made it possible to design better research tools, such as structured psychiatric interviews, that have improved the reliability and accuracy of diagnostic classification. With these tools it becomes possible to characterize participants in clinical research, to obtain population estimates of cannabis use disorders and to provide better treatment to individuals who develop cannabis-related disorders.

## References

American Psychiatric Association (1994). *Diagnostic and Statistical Manual of Mental Disorders* (4th ed.). Washington, DC: American Psychiatric Association.

Anthony, J. C., Warner, L. A., & Kessler, R. C. (1994). Comparative epidemiology of dependence on tobacco, alcohol, controlled substances, and inhalants: basic findings from the National Comorbidity Survey. *Experimental and Clinical Psychopharmacology, 2*, 244–268.

Babor, T. F. (1992). Nosological considerations in the diagnosis of substance use disorders. In M. Glantz, & R. Pickens (Eds.), *Vulnerability to drug abuse* (pp. 53–73). Washington, DC: American Psychological Association.

Babor, T. F. (1995). The road to DSM-IV: confessions of an erstwhile nosologist. *Drug and Alcohol Dependence, 38*, 75–79.

Babor, T. F., Mendelson, J. H., Greenberg, I., & Kuehnle, J. C. (1975). Marihuana consumption and tolerance to physiological and subjective effects. *Archives of General Psychiatry, 32,* 1548–1552.

Budney, A. J., Novy, P. L., & Hughes, J. R. (1999). Marijuana withdrawal among adults seeking treatment for marijuana dependence. *Addiction, 94,* 1311–1321.

Crowley, T. J., Macdonald, M. J., Whitmore, E. A., & Mikulich, S. K. (1998). Cannabis dependence, withdrawal, and reinforcing effects among adolescents with conduct symptoms and substance use disorders. *Drug and Alcohol Dependence, 50,* 27–37.

Devane, W. A., Hanus, L., Breuer, A., Pertwee, R. G., Stevenson, L. A., Griffin, G., *et al.* (1992). Isolation and structure of a brain constituent that binds to the cannabinoid receptor. *Science, 258,* 1946–1949.

Easton, C., Meza, E., Mager, D., Ulug, B., Kilic, C., Gogus, A., *et al.* (1997). Test-retest reliability of the alcohol and drug use disorder sections of the schedules for clinical assessment in neuropsychiatry (SCAN). *Drug and Alcohol Dependence, 47,* 187–194.

Edwards, G., Arif, A., & Hodgson, R. (1981). Nomenclature and classification of drug- and alcohol-related problems: a WHO memorandum. *Bulletin of the World Health Organization, 59,* 225–242.

Gardner, E., & David, J. (1999). The neurobiology of chemical addiction. In J. Elster, & O. J. Skog (Eds.), *Getting hooked: rationality and addiction* (pp. 93–136). Cambridge, UK: Cambridge University Press.

Gruber, A. J., & Pope, H. G. (1997). Cannabis-related disorders. In A. Tasman, J. Kay, & J. A. Liberman (Eds.), *Psychiatry* (Vol. 1, pp. 795–806). Philadelphia, PA: WB Saunders Company.

Hall, W., Johnston, L., & Donnelly, N. (1999). Epidemiology of cannabis use and its consequences. In H. Kalant, W. A. Corrigal, W. A. Hall, & R. Smart (Eds.), *The health effects of cannabis* (pp. 71–125). Toronto, Ont. Addiction Research Foundation.

Haney, M., Ward, A. S., Comer, S. D., Foltin, R. W., & Fischman, M. W. (1999). Abstinence symptoms following smoked marijuana in humans. *Psychopharmacology, 141,* 395–404.

Inciardi, J. A. (1994). Screening and assessment for alcohol and other drug abuse among adults in the criminal justice system. *Treatment improvement protocol (TIP) series 7,* DHHS Publication No. (SMA) 94B2076. Rockville, MD: Center for Substance Abuse Treatment of the Substance Abuse and Mental Health Services Administration.

Jones, R. T., Benowitz, N., & Bachman, J. (1976). Clinical studies of tolerance and dependence. *Annals of the New York Academy of Sciences, 282,* 221–239.

Kandel, D. C., & Davies, M. (1992). Progression to regular marijuana involvement: phenomenology and risk factors for near daily use. In M. Glantz, & R. Pickents (Eds.), *Vulnerability to drug abuse* (pp. 211–253). Washington, DC: American Psychological Association.

Kessler, R. C., McGonagle, K. A., Zhao, S., Nelson, C. B., Hughes, M., Eshleman, S., *et al.* (1994). Lifetime and 12-month prevalence of DSM-III-R psychiatric disorders in the United States: results from the National Comorbidity Survey. *Archives of General Psychiatry, 51*, 8–19.

Kranzler, H. R., Kadden, R. M., Babor, T. F., Tennen, H., & Rounsaville, B. J. (1996). Validity of the SCID in substance abuse patients. *Addiction, 91*, 859–868.

Kranzler, H. R., Tennen, H., Babor, T. F., Kadden, R. M., & Rounsaville, B. J. (1997). Validity of the longitudinal, expert, all data procedure for psychiatric diagnosis in patients with psychoactive substance use disorders. *Drug and Alcohol Dependence, 45*, 93–104.

Marijuana Treatment Project Research Group (2004). Brief treatments for cannabis dependence: findings from a randomized multi-site trial. *Journal of Consulting and Clinical Psychology, 72*, 455–466.

Mendelson, J., Mello, N., Lex, B., & Bavli, S. (1984). Marijuana withdrawal syndrome in a woman. *American Journal of Psychiatry, 141*, 1289–1290.

Rinaldi-Carmona, M., Barth, F., Heaulme, M., Shire, D., Calandra, B., Congy, C., *et al.* (1994). SR 141716A, a potent and selective antagonist of the brain cannabinoid receptor. *Federation of European Biochemical Societies Letters, 350*, 240–244.

Robins, L. N., Wing, J., Wittchen, H. U., Helzer, J. E., Babor, T. F., & Burke, J. (1988). The Composite International Diagnostic Interview: an epidemiological instrument suitable for use in conjunction with different diagnostic systems and in different cultures. *Archives of General Psychiatry, 45*, 1069–1077.

Rosenberg, M. F., & Anthony, J. C. (2001). Early clinical manifestations of cannabis dependence in a community sample. *Drug and Alcohol Dependence, 64*, 123–131.

Rounsaville, B. J., Tims, F. M., Horton Jr., A. M., & Sowder, B. J. (Eds.) (1993a) *Diagnostic source book on drug abuse research and treatment.* Rockville, MD: National Institute on Drug Abuse.

Rounsaville, B. J., Bryant, K., Babor, T., Kranzler, H., & Kadden, R. (1993b). Cross system agreement for substance use disorders: DSM-II-R, DSM-IV and ICD-10. *Addiction, 88*, 337–348.

Spitzer, R. L., Williams, J. B., Gibbon, M., & First, M. B. (1988). *Instruction manual for the structural clinical interview for DSM-III-R.* New York: Biometrics Research.

Stephens, R. S., Roffman, R. A., & Simpson, E. E. (1993). Adult marijuana users seeking treatment. *Journal of Consulting and Clinical Psychology, 61*, 1100–1104.

Stephens, R. S., Roffman, R. A., & Simpson, E. E. (1994). Treating adult marijuana dependence: a test of the relapse prevention model. *Journal of Consulting and Clinical Psychology, 62*, 92–99.

Stephens, R. S., Roffman, R. A., & Curtin, L. (2000). Comparison of extended versus brief treatments for marijuana use. *Journal of Consulting and Clinical Psychology, 68*, 898–908.

Stephens, R. S., Babor, T. F., Kadden, R., Miller, M., & the Marijuana Treatment Project Research Group (2002). The Marijuana Treatment Project: rationale, design and participant characteristics. *Addiction, 97* (Suppl. 1), 109–124.

Substance Abuse and Mental Health Services Administration, Office of Applied Studies (2002). Treatment Episode Data Set (TEDS): 1992–2000. National admissions to substance abuse treatment services, DASIS Series: S-17, DHHS publication No. (SMA) 02-3727. Rockville, MD: Office of Applied Studies.

Swift, W., Copeland, J., & Hall, W. (1998). Choosing a diagnostic cut-off for cannabis dependence. *Addiction*, *93*, 1681–1692.

Weisbeck, G. A., Schuckit, M. A., Kalmijn, J. A., Tipp, J. E., Bucholz, K. K., & Smith, T. L., *et al.* (1996). An evaluation of the history of marijuana withdrawal syndrome in a large population. *Addiction*, *91*, 1469–1478.

Wing, J. K., Babor, T., Brugha, T., Burke, J., Cooper, J. E., Giel, R., *et al.* (1990). SCAN – Schedules for clinical assessment in neuropsychiatry. *Archives of General Psychiatry*, *47*, 589–593.

Wolff, K., Farrell, M., Marsden, J., Monteiro, M. G., Ali, R., Welch, S., *et al.* (1999). A review of biological indicators of illicit drug use, practical considerations and clinical usefulness. *Addiction*, *94*, 1279–1298.

World Health Organization (1992). *The ICD-10 classification of mental and behavioral disorders: clinical descriptions and diagnostic guidelines*. Geneva, Switzerland: World Health Organization.

World Health Organization (1993). *The ICD-10 classification of mental and behavioral disorders: diagnostic criteria for research*. Geneva, Switzerland: World Health Organisation.

# 3

# Understanding the Pharmacology and Physiology of Cannabis Dependence

ARON H. LICHTMAN AND BILLY R. MARTIN

Growing evidence from rodent, dog, monkey, and human studies indicates that prolonged administration of cannabis results in physical dependence. The goal of this chapter is to present an overview of this research and highlight several important advances that have been made in both characterizing and delineating the molecular mechanisms underlying this dependence. We will first provide a brief summary of several important advances that have been made in the basic understanding of the actions of cannabis and its interaction with an endogenous cannabinoid system. In addition, the results from both animal and *in vitro* studies that have enhanced our understanding of cannabinoid dependence will be described. Of considerable interest is the proposed reciprocal relationship between cannabinoid and opioid systems in drug dependence.

## Basic Neuropharmacology of Cannabis Effects and the Existence of an Endocannabinoid System

The pharmacological effects and potential medicinal uses of cannabis have been known since antiquity, thousands of years before the elucidation of the structure of $\Delta^9$-tetrahydrocannabinol ($\Delta^9$-THC), the primary psychoactive constituent of this plant (Gaoni & Mechoulam, 1964). In addition to $\Delta^9$-THC, cannabis contains over 400 chemical constituents, 66 of which have been classified as cannabinoids (Turner *et al.*, 1980). Moreover, hundreds of cannabinoid agonists have also been synthesized in the laboratory. For decades the pharmacological activity of these highly hydrophobic drugs was attributed to a non-specific mechanism of general membrane perturbation. However, results from structure–activity relationship studies demonstrating stereoselectivity in which subtle changes in structure could lead to dramatic increases or decreases in pharmacological potency led to the postulation of a specific cannabinoid receptor mechanism of action (Razdan, 1986). The subsequent discovery of cannabinoid binding sites (Devane *et al.*, 1988) and the cloning of two cannabinoid receptor subtypes (Matsuda *et al.*, 1990; Munro *et al.*, 1993) provided definitive support for the existence of cannabinoid receptors. The $CB_1$ receptor is located primarily in the central nervous system (Matsuda *et al.*, 1990) and is believed to mediate the subjective effects of marijuana intoxication. On the other hand, the $CB_2$ receptor has only been found in the periphery (Munro *et al.*, 1993), is predominantly associated with the immune system, and may play a role in inflammatory pain. Both receptor subtypes belong to a family of G-protein related receptors (Mountjoy *et al.*, 1992). Cannabinoid agonists stimulate inhibitory G-proteins that inhibit both cyclic AMP (cAMP) activity (Howlett *et al.*, 1988) and N-type calcium channels (Mackie & Hille, 1992). A selective $CB_1$ receptor antagonist SR 141716A, has been found to block the centrally mediated effects of cannabinoids in rodents (Rinaldi-Carmona *et al.*, 1994) as well as both tachycardia and the subjective effects of smoked marijuana in humans (Huestis *et al.*, 2001). This drug has also been particularly useful tool in characterizing cannabinoid dependence syndromes in laboratory animals (Aceto *et al.*, 1995; Tsou *et al.*, 1995). Finally, attempts to identify endogenous cannabinoid ligands have resulted in the isolation of the fatty acid amide arachidonoylethanolamide (i.e., anandamide) and the mono-acylglycerol 2-arachidonoylglycerol (2-AG) (Devane *et al.*, 1992; Sugiura *et al.*, 1995). The existence of an endocannabinoid system in the central nervous system has gained general acceptance as a result of the discovery of both endogenous cannabinoids and cannabinoid receptors. This system has been proposed to serve several physiological functions including the modulation of pain (Calignano *et al.*, 1998; Richardson *et al.*, 1998; Walker *et al.*, 1999), feeding (Di Marzo *et al.*, 2001), cognition (Lichtman, 2000; Terranova *et al.*, 1996), and drug dependence (Ledent *et al.*, 1999; Lichtman *et al.*, 2001b).

## Characterization of Cannabis Dependence

### Overview

Two general procedures that induce states of withdrawal in drug-dependent organisms are abstinence withdrawal and precipitated withdrawal. Abstinence withdrawal occurs when drug administration is abruptly discontinued or reduced, following prolonged exposure to the drug. As the agent is metabolized and/or excreted, physiological symptoms ranging from mild rebound to severe life-threatening effects can emerge. The pharmacokinetic (i.e., factors related to distribution and metabolism) and pharmacodynamic (i.e., factors related to sites of action) characteristics of the drug, as well as dosing regimen, influence the specific withdrawal syndrome, its intensity, and the onset of withdrawal responses. In contrast, a second procedure used to induce withdrawal is a receptor antagonist that precipitates withdrawal in a drug-dependent organism. The antagonist displaces the agonist from the receptor, immediately eliciting withdrawal effects. A common clinical example of precipitated withdrawal is naloxone treatment or other opioid receptor antagonist for an opioid overdose. Upon near instantaneous reversal of respiratory depression and other overdose symptoms, an opioid-dependent individual will present with opioid withdrawal effects. The precipitated withdrawal procedure has been particularly useful in investigating cannabinoid withdrawal symptoms in laboratory animals.

### Clinical Significance of Cannabis Withdrawal Symptoms

For more than 50 years, there have been anecdotal and case reports describing physical withdrawal symptoms in chronic cannabis users (Fraser, 1949; Wikler, 1976). More recently, chronic marijuana use has been associated with an increased risk of cannabis dependence (Chen *et al.*, 1997; Swift *et al.*, 2000). However, the issue of whether or not a withdrawal syndrome occurs upon marijuana cessation has been a controversial topic. According to the Diagnostic and Statistical Manual of Mental Disorders (DSM-IV) (American Psychiatric Association, 1994), cannabis withdrawal symptoms are not considered clinically significant. The delayed onset of withdrawal, most likely due to $\Delta^9$-THC's long half-life, combined with the relatively mildness of its symptoms compared to various other substances (e.g., cocaine, alcohol, and opioids) may contribute to the doubts regarding the clinical relevance of cannabinoid withdrawal. On the other hand, a growing body of research from laboratory, retrospective, and outpatient studies indicates that cannabis-dependent individuals experience a clinically significant physical withdrawal syndrome following the cessation of marijuana smoking. Resolving this issue has important implications for treatment because the occurrence of, or fears related to, physical withdrawal effects upon abstinence could be a contributing factor to the continued use of this drug by cannabis-dependent individuals.

Human laboratory studies have demonstrated the occurrence of a cannabinoid withdrawal syndrome following abrupt discontinuation from chronic $\Delta^9$-THC (Jones & Benowitz, 1976; Jones *et al.*, 1976). These symptoms included disturbed sleep, decreased appetite, restlessness, irritability, sweating, chills, and nausea. Recent studies have also demonstrated similar abstinence symptoms that included subjective effects of anxiety, irritability, and stomach pain, as well as

decreases in food intake, following abrupt withdrawal from continued administration of either oral $\Delta^9$-THC (Haney *et al.*, 1999a) or marijuana smoke inhalation (Haney *et al.*, 1999b). One potential implication of these findings is that
regular marijuana use may be continued, in part, to alleviate or avoid abstinence
symptoms.

Although a cannabis withdrawal syndrome can be obtained in a controlled
laboratory setting, these findings do not address whether a cannabis withdrawal
syndrome represents a clinically significant malady. The results of both retrospective and outpatient studies addressing this issue argue that a cannabis withdrawal syndrome is indeed clinically significant. Frequent marijuana users
identified from a population of alcohol-dependent subjects, their family members, and non-alcoholic controls recalled a variety of symptoms from when they
had previously abstained from marijuana smoking that included nervousness,
sleep disturbances, and changes in appetite (Wiesbeck *et al.*, 1996). Despite the
inherent limitations associated with retrospective self-reports in polysubstance
abuse subjects, the pattern of withdrawal symptoms was similar to those
described in the laboratory studies investigating cannabis and $\Delta^9$-THC and distinct from those associated with other drugs. In another retrospective study,
adults seeking treatment for marijuana dependence recalled similar symptoms
upon their most recent period of abstinence that included craving for marijuana,
irritability, nervousness, restlessness, depressed mood, increased anger, sleep
difficulties, strange dreams, decreased appetite, and headaches (Budney *et al.*,
1999). In addition, the amount of marijuana smoked per day yielded a positive
correlation with withdrawal severity. Finally, the results of an outpatient study
of regular marijuana smokers corroborated the findings of the retrospective and
laboratory studies (Budney *et al.*, 2001). In this study, subjects were instructed
to smoke marijuana as usual during a 5-day baseline period, followed by a 3-day
marijuana abstinence period, a second 5-day baseline period, and a final 3-day
marijuana abstinence period. During each abstinence period, withdrawal symptoms included significant increases in craving for marijuana, decreased appetite,
sleep difficulty, and a global withdrawal discomfort score that consisted of the
other three measures as well as anger, depressed mood, headaches, irritability,
nervousness, restlessness, and strange dreams. Additionally, the subjects lost a
significant amount of weight during each abstinence phase. The fact that the
withdrawal symptoms increased during abstinence from marijuana smoking,
returned to baseline when smoking was reinitiated, and increased again during
the second abstinence period suggests that the effects were caused by cessation
of marijuana use. Collectively, these studies indicate that cannabis withdrawal
is clinically significant.

*Abrupt Cannabinoid Withdrawal in Laboratory Animals*

Unlike humans in whom subjective withdrawal effects can be verbally obtained, the observation of withdrawal in laboratory animals presents more of a challenge. The long half-life of $\Delta^9$-THC and consequent delay of effects further contribute to the difficulty in studying withdrawal in non-human animals. Not surprisingly, the investigation of abstinence withdrawal following prolonged cannabinoid administration in laboratory animals has led to mixed results. A variety of unconditional behavioral effects including hyperirritability, tremors, and anorexia have been reported (Kaymakcalan & Deneau, 1972), though other studies failed to observe abrupt withdrawal effects following chronic $\Delta^9$-THC administration in dogs (McMillan *et al.*, 1971) or rats (Aceto *et al.*, 1996; Leite & Carlini, 1974). However, rats have been observed to exhibit mild withdrawal effects upon discontinuation of chronic infusion of the aminoalkylindole WIN 55,212-2, a potent cannabinoid analog (Aceto *et al.*, 2001). Operant procedures in which animals are trained to press a lever for food reinforcement may be more sensitive to detect withdrawal than observing unconditional withdrawal responses. The animal is inferred to be physically dependent to a substance if response rates are suppressed following discontinuation of a chronic drug regimen and re-administration of the drug returns response rates return to normal. Response rates of rhesus monkeys that were given chronic $\Delta^9$-THC and trained to press a lever for food reinforcement were suppressed during abstinence and returned to normal upon re-administration of drug (Beardsley *et al.*, 1986). Taken together, these studies indicate that abrupt cannabinoid withdrawal occurs in laboratory animals, but several factors including the time at which withdrawal is assessed and the particular withdrawal measures that are scored present difficulties in using this procedure to study cannabinoid withdrawal.

*Precipitated Cannabinoid Withdrawal in Cannabinoid-Dependent Animals*

*Characterization of SR 141716A Precipitated Withdrawal in*
*Cannabinoid-Dependent Animals*

The development of SR 141716A, a selective $CB_1$ receptor antagonist, represented a major breakthrough for cannabinoid research and this drug has been found to block many pharmacological effects of the cannabinoids in rodents (Compton *et al.*, 1996; Rinaldi-Carmona *et al.*, 1994), dogs (Lichtman *et al.*, 1998), rhesus monkeys (Vivian *et al.*, 1998), and humans (Huestis *et al.*, 2001). SR 141716A has also been a particularly useful tool in precipitating cannabinoid withdrawal symptoms in laboratory animals (Aceto *et al.*, 1995; Tsou *et al.*, 1995). In contrast to the challenge of observing abrupt withdrawal in laboratory animals, SR 141716A elicits immediate and quantifiable withdrawal reactions in a variety of species including mice, rats, and dogs that had repeatedly been given cannabinoid agonists.

Rats exhibit a variety of somatic cannabinoid withdrawal signs that include wet dog shakes, facial rubs, horizontal and vertical activity, forepaw fluttering, chewing, tongue rolling, paw shakes and head shakes, retropulsion, myoclonic spasms, front paw treading, and eyelid ptosis (Aceto *et al.*, 1995; Tsou *et al.*, 1995). SR 141716A also reliably precipitates withdrawal in cannabinoid-dependent mice, though the specific responses appear to vary according to mouse strain and dosing regimen. Whereas paw tremors and head shakes were found to be the most reliable cannabinoid withdrawal signs in some studies (Cook *et al.*, 1998; Lichtman *et al.*, 2001b), others found these signs as well as hunched position, mastication, sniffing, and piloerection (Hutcheson *et al.*, 1998; Ledent *et al.*, 1999; Tzavara *et al.*, 2000; Valverde *et al.*, 2000b). On the other hand, precipitated scratching has been observed in $\Delta^9$-THC-dependent Swiss Webster mice, but not in other strains (Lichtman *et al.*, 2001b). Writhing and ptosis only occurred sporadically, and diarrhea and jumping, which are salient symptoms in morphine-dependent mice undergoing withdrawal, are not part of the precipitated cannabinoid withdrawal syndrome. In $\Delta^9$-THC-dependent dogs, SR 141716A precipitated another unique pattern of withdrawal signs that included excessive salivation, vomiting, diarrhea, restless behavior, trembling, and decreases in social behavior (Lichtman *et al.*, 1998). Interestingly, several symptoms similar to these, including restlessness, nausea, and loose stools have been reported in humans undergoing abrupt $\Delta^9$-THC withdrawal (Jones *et al.*, 1981), lending credence to the validity of the precipitated cannabinoid withdrawal dog model. Notwithstanding the influence that species and strain differences may influence the specific withdrawal effects that are observed, the utility of the animal models is verified by the fact that SR 141716A reliably precipitates withdrawal in cannabinoid-dependent animals.

The effects of SR 141716A precipitated withdrawal have been evaluated following repeated administration of several other cannabinoid agonists, in addition to $\Delta^9$-THC, including WIN 55,212-2, CP 55,940, HU-210, anandamide, and a stable anandamide analog 2-methyl-flouro-anandamide (2-Me-F-AN). While it is clear that SR 141716A precipitated withdrawal responses following administration of most cannabinoid analogs, the anandamide results are less definitive. SR 141716A failed to precipitate withdrawal in rats that were infused constantly with anandamide (25–100 mg/kg/day) for 4 days (Aceto *et al.*, 1998).

Although it is not surprising that anandamide lacked dependence liability given its short half-life (Willoughby *et al.*, 1997), the fact that SR 141716A also failed to precipitated withdrawal in rats that were infused with the stable anandamide analog, 2-Me-F-AN (5–20 mg/kg), for 4 days suggests that metabolism may not be the only factor. On the other hand, a regimen of 15 days of daily intraperitoneal (IP) injections of anandamide (20 mg/kg) was reported to elicit both abstinence and SR 141716A precipitated withdrawal (Costa *et al.*, 2000). In future replications of this work it will be important to assess whether re-administration of anandamide will reverse the abstinence signs. The use of mice lacking fatty acid amide hydrolase (FAAH), the primary enzyme responsible for anandamide metabolism (Cravatt *et al.*, 2001), will be of value to investigate further the role that anandamide plays in cannabinoid dependence. One implication of developing a cannabinoid agonist that lacks abuse liability would be for medicinal uses.

Taken together these studies indicate that a variety of species can become physically dependent to cannabinoids, though the actual withdrawal responses that are manifested are species specific. Within each respective species tested to date, SR 141716A precipitates a multitude of behavioral responses that can be quantitatively assessed by using global abstinence scores in which different signs are scored and given a weight depending on the frequency or magnitude of the response. These scores distinguish severity of withdrawal in dogs (Lichtman *et al.*, 1998), rats (Rodriguez de Fonseca *et al.*, 1997), and mice (Hutcheson *et al.*, 1998). Similarly, a global abstinence score has also been used to quantify degree of withdrawal in cannabis-dependent humans undergoing abstinence withdrawal (Budney *et al.*, 2001).

*Intrinsic Effects of SR 141716A*

SR 141716A was initially believed to act as a pure $CB_1$ receptor antagonist in that it merely displaced cannabinoid agonists from the receptors and did not directly affect cell signaling. However, the results of *in vitro* studies suggest that SR 141716A is not inert at the receptor but can produce biochemical responses opposite that of the agonists, an action that has been termed inverse agonism. Whereas cannabinoid agonists have been reliably found to stimulate Gi/o-protein activity as assessed in the $[^{35}S]$GTPgammaS binding assay (Burkey *et al.*, 1997; Sim *et al.*, 1996), SR 141716A can decrease G-protein activity in a variety of cell types (Landsman *et al.*, 1997; Pan *et al.*, 1998). However, the relevancy of this inverse agonist effect in the whole animal has not yet been established. Moreover, SR 141716A was greater than 7000-fold more potent as a $CB_1$ receptor antagonist than as an inverse agonist (Sim-Selley *et al.*, 2001), suggesting that it is substantially more selective as a receptor antagonist than as an inverse agonist.

Nonetheless, SR 141716A given alone has been found to elicit behavioral effects that resemble a mild form of withdrawal (Aceto *et al.*, 1995, 1996; Rodriguez de Fonseca *et al.*, 1997). These effects include scratching of the face and body (Aceto *et al.*, 1996; Rubino *et al.*, 1998), head shakes (Cook *et al.*, 1998; Lichtman *et al.*, 2001a), and forepaw fluttering (Rubino *et al.*, 1998). It should be noted that the magnitude of SR 141716A-induced head shakes and paw tremors is generally significantly less than that found in cannabinoid-dependent animals (Aceto *et al.*, 1996, 1998; Cook *et al.*, 1998). The fact that SR 141716A possesses intrinsic activity on its own underscores the importance of including appropriate control groups to ensure that the behavioral effects are indeed a withdrawal response.

## Cannabinoid Self-Administration

The high prevalence of cannabis use in young adults and adolescents indicates that this drug is a positive reinforcer. According to a recent Monitoring the Future Survey of Adolescents in the USA on behaviors and attitudes regarding drug use, 49% of all high school graduates in the class of 2001 have used marijuana and more than 10% of this age group use it on a regular basis (Johnston *et al.*, 2002). It is not surprising that the nucleus accumbens, a cortical region strongly associated with the rewarding effects of drugs, contains a high concentration of cannabinoid receptors (Herkenham *et al.*, 1991). Moreover, administration of $\Delta^9$-THC was found to increase dopamine efflux in this brain area of rats (Chen *et al.*, 1990), an effect that is similar to other drugs that are reported to have positive hedonic effects in humans.

Studies of drug self-administration in animals have proved valuable in elucidating the mechanisms of action underlying drug-reinforced behavior as well as predicting the abuse liability of new drugs. In contrast to the majority of drugs abused by humans, early studies failed to establish cannabinoid self-administration in animals. In these self-administration tasks, an operant procedure is typically employed in which a subject is required to press a lever, under different schedules of reinforcement, for an infusion of drug. Whereas the psychomotor stimulants, opioids, barbiturates, phencyclidine, and other drugs are readily self-administered, in early studies $\Delta^9$-THC was an ineffective reinforcer in both monkeys and rats (Carney *et al.*, 1977; Harris *et al.*, 1974; Mansbach *et al.*, 1994; van Ree *et al.*, 1978).

However, a recent study found that squirrel monkeys pressed a lever for infusions of low doses of $\Delta^9$-THC (Tanda *et al.*, 2000). Importantly, operant responding extinguished following substitution with vehicle and lever pressing was reinstated when the monkeys were again given access to drug. Pretreatment with SR 141716A led to decreases in $\Delta^9$-THC self-administration, but had no effect on cocaine self-administration, suggesting that the effect was mediated via a $CB_1$ receptor mechanism of action. It was suggested that the dose of drug given per infusion and/or other procedural differences such as the choice of vehicle accounts for the apparent discrepancy of $\Delta^9$-THC's reinforcing effects between this and previous studies. In particular, the doses of $\Delta^9$-THC that were reinforcing were far lower than those used in the other experiments. In contrast to previous studies in which the doses ranged from 7.5 to 300 μg of $\Delta^9$-THC per infusion (Mansbach *et al.*, 1994; van Ree *et al.*, 1978), Tanda *et al.* (2000) found that 2.0 and 4.0 μg, but not higher doses, of $\Delta^9$-THC per infusion were self-administered. Cannabinoids have been documented to elicit various aversive effects, particularly at higher doses. Consequently, these apparent negative hedonic properties may have masked the appetitive properties and thus account for their failure to serve as positive reinforcers at higher doses.

In addition to the classic operant approaches in which animals press a lever under various schedules of reinforcement for drug, another operant method to investigate drug self-administration is the "nose-poke" procedure. In this paradigm, a mouse or a rat is placed in a restraining cage in which the tail extends outside of the cage and an injecting needled is inserted into a lateral tail vein. In the front of the cage is a hole with an infrared detector so that when the animal pokes its nose an infusion of vehicle or drug is delivered intravenously. Both rats and mice were found to self-administer the synthetic cannabinoid analog WIN 55,212-2 (Fattore *et al.*, 2001; Martellotta *et al.*, 1998). Nose-poke behavior extinguished when either vehicle was substituted for drug or animals were pretreated with SR 141716A. The demonstration that at least three non-human species will self-administer cannabinoids indicates the utility of animal models for drug dependence and drug seeking behavior.

**Neurochemical Mechanisms Underlying Cannabis Dependence**

*CB₁ Cannabinoid Receptor Mechanisms of Action*

The use of genetically altered mice is becoming an increasingly important tool in investigating the molecular mechanisms underlying drug dependence. Molecular biological techniques have been used to develop lines of mice in which the $CB_1$ receptor has been deleted or knocked out (Ledent *et al.*, 1999; Zimmer *et al.*, 1999). In these studies, $CB_1$ heterozygous ($CB_1^{+/-}$) breeding pairs are used to derive the $CB_1$ knockout ($CB_1^{-/-}$) mice and $CB_1$ wild type ($CB_1^{+/+}$) control mice, as well as $CB_1^{+/-}$ mice. Whereas cannabinoid agonists elicit the full spectrum of pharmacological effects in the $CB_1^{+/+}$ mice, the $CB_1^{-/-}$ mice are generally impervious to these drugs. In contrast, non-cannabinoid agents such as opioids continue to elicit acute pharmacological effects in $CB_1^{-/-}$ mice (Valverde *et al.*, 2000a).

The use of $CB_1^{-/-}$ mice has provided important confirmatory information demonstrating that cannabinoid agonists elicit dependence through a $CB_1$ receptor mechanism of action. A dosing regimen of $\Delta^9$-THC sufficient to produce cannabinoid dependence in $CB_1^{+/+}$ mice was without affect in the $CB_1^{-/-}$ mice (Ledent *et al.*, 1999; Lichtman *et al.*, 2001b). SR 141716A precipitated rearing, sniffing, wet dog shakes, paw tremors, piloerection, penile licking, mastication, hunched posture, and body tremors in the $CB_1^{+/+}$ mice, but not in the $CB_1^{-/-}$ mice, on a CD1 background strain (Ledent *et al.*, 1999). A similar pattern of findings was found in $CB_1^{-/-}$ mice on a C57BL/6 background. In this group, SR 141716A precipitated head shakes and paw tremors following repeated $\Delta^9$-THC administration in $CB_1^{+/+}$ mice, but not in $CB_1^{-/-}$ mice (Lichtman *et al.*, 2001b). Finally, $CB_1^{+/+}$, but not $CB_1^{-/-}$, mice self-administered the potent cannabinoid analog WIN 55,212-2 (Ledent *et al.*, 1999). The findings that $CB_1^{-/-}$ mice on two different background strains failed to exhibit SR 141716A precipitated withdrawal and that $CB_1^{-/-}$ mice would not self-administer cannabinoids indicates that the $CB_1$ receptor is necessary for cannabinoid dependence.

### *Neuroadaptive Changes Underlying Cannabinoid Dependence*

Repeated stimulation of $CB_1$ receptors by cannabinoid agonists is necessary for the development of cannabinoid dependence; however, the underlying cellular mechanisms of action as well as brain regions that mediate this phenomenon remain elusive. Most of this research has been *in vitro* and has focused on characterizing changes of $CB_1$ receptor binding, $CB_1$ receptor mRNA, cannabinoid-stimulated G-protein activity, and cAMP activity in brains following repeated administration of cannabinoids or vehicle.

Repeated administration of a cannabinoid agonist generally results in decreases in $CB_1$ receptor density in a variety of brain regions as measured by radioligand binding (Breivogel *et al.*, 1999; Romero *et al.*, 1998). At the level of the G-protein, a daily injection of $\Delta^9$-THC for 21 days produced significant decreases of $CB_1$ receptor-stimulated G-protein activity in various brain regions, including hippocampus, cerebellum, caudate-putamen, globus pallidus, substantia nigra, septum and various regions of cortex. In addition to being region-dependent, this desensitization was time dependent and appeared to be specific for $CB_1$ receptors and not other G-protein coupled receptors (Breivogel *et al.*, 1999). However, it is unclear whether these biochemical correlates play a causal role in tolerance and dependence or are merely associated with prolonged cannabinoid treatment.

Recent studies have linked alterations in the cAMP second messenger cascade with cannabinoid withdrawal. SR 141716A administered to $\Delta^9$-THC-dependent mice resulted in significant increases of both basal and forskolin-stimulated adenylyl cyclase activity in the cerebellum, but not in other brain regions including the cortex, hippocampus, striatum, and periaqueductal gray (Hutcheson *et al.*, 1998). Similarly, significantly higher levels of calcium-calmodulin stimulated adenylyl cyclase were found in the cerebella of $\Delta^9$-THC-dependent rats undergoing withdrawal than in non-dependent rats treated with SR 141716A. In another well-controlled study (Rubino *et al.*, 2000b), G-protein, adenylyl cyclase, and protein kinase A (PKA) (another important second messenger involved in cell signaling) activity were assessed in cerebral cortex, striatum, hippocampus, and cerebellum of rats undergoing precipitated withdrawal. Significant increases of adenylyl cyclase and PKA activity, but not receptor density or G-protein activity, in the cerebella of these animals were found, further implicating the involvement of this brain region in dependence. Functional evidence also suggests that the adenylyl cyclase second messenger cascade in the cerebellum may be involved in cannabinoid withdrawal. An intracerebellar infusion of the cAMP blocker Rp-8Br-cAMPs reduced several behavioral signs of withdrawal including tremors, ataxia, mastication, front paw tremors, ptosis, piloerection, and wet dog shakes in $\Delta^9$-THC-dependent mice following SR 141716A challenge (Tzavara *et al.*, 2000). Interestingly, Sp-8Br-cAMPs, a cAMP analog, actually induced each of these behavioral effects in vehicle-treated mice. Taken together with the biochemical data, these intriguing findings suggest that up-regulation of cAMP signal transduction in the cerebellum may represent a biochemical event underlying precipitated withdrawal.

### Interrelationships with Other Neurochemical Systems

Dopamine is well known to play an important role in drug reward and consequently there has also been interest in assessing its role in cannabinoid withdrawal. Rats undergoing either abrupt withdrawal or SR 141716A precipitated withdrawal following 6 days of repeated $\Delta^9$-THC administration exhibited decreases in dopaminergic functioning of the mesolimbic system (Diana *et al.*, 1998) compared to the increased dopaminergic functioning of control animals that had been treated acutely with $\Delta^9$-THC (Gessa *et al.*, 1998). Although both D1 and D2 antagonists failed to alter SR 141716A precipitated withdrawal in $\Delta^9$-THC-dependent rats (Sanudo-Pena *et al.*, 1999), it is unknown whether dopaminergic agonists would ameliorate cannabinoid withdrawal responses.

There is also evidence suggesting that corticotropin-releasing factor (CRF) and other hormones associated with stress may play a role in cannabinoid dependence. Plasma corticosterone levels were significantly higher in cannabinoid-dependent rats challenged with SR 141716A than in either SR 141716A-treated non-dependent rats or dependent rats not going through precipitated withdrawal (Rodriguez de Fonseca *et al.*, 1997). Moreover, SR 141716A challenge to cannabinoid-dependent rats led to significant concomitant increases in CRF and Fos-immunopositive cell activity in the central nucleus of the amygdala. Similar alterations in amygdaloid CRF function have also been found following ethanol, cocaine, and opioid withdrawal. The increase of Fos-immunopositive activity in SR 141716A-treated cannabinoid-dependent animals was not limited to the central nucleus of the amygdala. Other regions included the accumbens shell, piriform cortex, hippocampus, caudate-putamen, ventral pallidum, ventral tegmental area, locus coeruleus solitary tract, and area postrema. Once again, it remains to be established whether these biochemical changes represent an underlying mechanism of action for cannabinoid tolerance and dependence or are merely correlated with these phenomena.

It has been well established that clonidine, as well as other alpha$_2$-agonists, abrogates many of the withdrawal effects in morphine-dependent animals (Fielding *et al.*, 1978) and can even alleviate some withdrawal symptoms in moderately dependent human opioid addicts (Gold *et al.*, 1978). Similarly, clonidine also ameliorated SR 141716A-precipitated paw tremors in $\Delta^9$-THC-dependent mice independently of motor depressive or motor impairment effects (Lichtman *et al.*, 2001a). Although clonidine may hold some promise for treating withdrawal, its hypotensive side effects (Gossop, 1988) must be considered before any potential development for its use in alleviating drug withdrawal.

### Reciprocal Roles of the Cannabinoid and Opioid Systems in Dependence

#### *Cannabinoid Systems Modulate Opioid Dependence*

Substantial evidence is mounting that the antinociceptive effects, drug reinforcing actions, and dependence liability of morphine and $\Delta^9$-THC may share common neuroanatomical sites. Consistent with this notion is that the $CB_1$ receptor and $\mu$-opioid receptor mRNA are co-localized in brain limbic areas associated with dependence (Navarro *et al.*, 1998). It has long been known that $\Delta^9$-THC produces a moderate amelioration of naloxone-precipitated withdrawal in morphine-dependent mice (Bhargava, 1976, 1978) and rats (Frederickson *et al.*, 1976; Hine *et al.*, 1975). Similarly, the endogenous cannabinoids anandamide (Vela *et al.*, 1995) and 2-AG (Yamaguchi *et al.*, 2001) have both been reported to decrease naloxone-induced morphine withdrawal.

Curiously, $CB_1^{-/-}$ mice exhibited substantial decreases in naloxone-precipitated morphine withdrawal as well a failure to self-administer morphine (Ledent *et al.*, 1999). Consistent with this finding, SR 141716A blocked heroin self-administration in rats and morphine self-administration in mice (Navarro *et al.*, 2001). SR 141716A also reduced the rewarding responses of morphine in the conditioned place preference paradigm and led to decreases in naloxone-precipitated wet dog shakes and jumping but had no effects on other indices of opioid withdrawal including paw tremors, ptosis, sniffing, and body tremors (Mas-Nieto *et al.*, 2001). Repeated administration of SR 141716A in rats implanted with morphine pellets reduced some, but not all, naloxone-precipitated withdrawal effects (Rubino *et al.*, 2000a). SR 141716A reduced teeth chattering, digging, and penile licking, as well as a slight decrease in the incidence of diarrhea in morphine-dependent rats undergoing precipitated withdrawal. Conversely, jumping and ptosis were not reduced, and salivation was actually increased by SR 141716A (Rubino *et al.*, 2000a). Although it is presently unclear why deleting or blocking $CB_1$ signaling would have the same effect in reducing opioid withdrawal as administering cannabinoid agonists, these apparently paradoxical effects may be related to the different roles that the endocannabinoid system plays on the acquisition, maintenance, and expression of opioid dependence.

### *Opioid Systems Modulate Cannabinoid Dependence*

Evidence is also beginning to emerge suggesting that opioid receptors may play a modulatory role on cannabinoid dependence. The finding that SR 141716A-precipitated $\Delta^9$-THC withdrawal symptoms were significantly diminished in pre-proenkephalin-deficient mice compared to the wild type mice indicates the potential importance of endogenous opioids (Valverde *et al.*, 2000b). Similarly, mice lacking the $\mu$-opioid receptor exhibited a significant attenuation of SR 141716A-precipitated withdrawal paw tremors and head shakes compared to the wild type controls (Lichtman *et al.*, 2001b). However, both of these withdrawal indices were completely blocked in a dose-dependent fashion by an acute injection of morphine in wild type mice (Lichtman *et al.*, 2001b). The observations that cannabinoid withdrawal is ameliorated by the acute administration of opioid agonists as well as by deletion of either μ-opioid receptors or endogenous opioids parallels the results of alterations of the endocannabinoid system on opioid dependence. Consequently, further research is needed to investigate the role that endogenous opioids play on the acquisition, maintenance, and expression of cannabinoid dependence. Moreover, additional research is needed to determine whether endogenous opioids modulate cannabinoid self-administration. However, the present data suggest that the association between cannabinoids and opioids on dependence is bi-directional.

### Implications of Animal Studies for Understanding Human Dependence

Although some doubts may persist in the medical community, the results of retrospective, inpatient, and outpatient studies strongly support the assertion that a cannabis withdrawal syndrome is clinically significant. These symptoms include significant increases in craving for marijuana, decreased appetite, sleep difficulty, anger, depressed mood, headaches, irritability, nervousness, restlessness, and strange dreams. The availability of laboratory animal models of dependence and self-administration has been of great value in both characterizing and beginning to understand the underlying mechanisms of cannabis dependence. Administration of the $CB_1$ receptor antagonist SR 141716A to animals repeatedly given $\Delta^9$-THC or other cannabinoids has been shown to precipitate withdrawal effects in a variety of laboratory animals. Although these withdrawal syndromes appear to be species specific, they will be of value in developing pharmacotherapies for the treatment of cannabis dependence. In addition, the recent availability of both rodent and non-human primate cannabinoid self-administration procedures can be used to investigate the drug reinforcing effects of this class of drugs. The molecular mechanisms that underlie cannabinoid dependence appear to involve the cAMP second messenger system. Moreover, growing evidence indicates the existence of a reciprocal relationship between the endocannabinoid and opioid systems in dependence. A multidisciplinary approach using *in vitro*, laboratory animal, and human studies will undoubtedly further our basic understanding of the endocannabinoid system as it relates to drug dependence as well as develop treatments.

### References

Aceto, M., Scates, S., Lowe, J., & Martin, B. (1995). Cannabinoid precipitated withdrawal by the selective cannabinoid receptor antagonist, SR 141716A. *European Journal of Pharmacology, 282*, R1–R2.

Aceto, M., Scates, S., Lowe, J., & Martin, B. (1996). Dependence on $\Delta^9$-tetrahydro-cannabinol: studies on precipitated and abrupt withdrawal. *The Journal of Pharmacology and Experimental Therapeutics, 278,* 1290–1295.

Aceto, M. D., Scates, S. M., Razdan, R. K., & Martin, B. R. (1998). Anandamide, an endogenous cannabinoid, has a very low physical dependence potential. *The Journal of Pharmacology and Experimental Therapeutics, 287,* 598–605.

Aceto, M. D., Scates, S. M., & Martin, B. B. (2001). Spontaneous and precipitated withdrawal with a synthetic cannabinoid, WIN 55212-2. *European Journal of Pharmacology, 416,* 75–81.

American Psychiatric Association (1994). *Diagnostic and statistical manual of mental disorders: DSM-IV.* Washington, DC: American Psychiatric Association.

Beardsley, P. M., Balster, R. L., & Harris, L. S. (1986). Dependence on tetrahydrocannabinol in rhesus monkeys. *The Journal of Pharmacology and Experimental Therapeutics, 239,* 311–319.

Bhargava, H. N. (1976). Effect of some cannabinoids on naloxone-precipitated abstinence in morphine-dependent mice. *Psychopharmacology, 49,* 267–270.

Bhargava, H. N. (1978). Time course of the effects of naturally occurring cannabinoids on morphine abstinence syndrome. *Pharmacology, Biochemistry, and Behavior, 8,* 7–11.

Breivogel, C. S., Childers, S. R., Deadwyler, S. A., Hampson, R. E., Vogt, L. J., & Sim-Selley, L. J. (1999). Chronic delta9-tetrahydrocannabinol treatment produces a time-dependent loss of cannabinoid receptors and cannabinoid receptor-activated G proteins in rat brain. *Journal of Neurochemistry, 73,* 2447–2459.

Budney, A. J., Novy, P. L., & Hughes, J. R. (1999). Marijuana withdrawal among adults seeking treatment for marijuana dependence. *Addiction, 94,* 1311–1322.

Budney, A. J., Hughes, J. R., Moore, B. A., & Novy, P. L. (2001). Marijuana abstinence effects in marijuana smokers maintained in their home environment. *Archives of General Psychiatry, 58,* 917–924.

Burkey, T. H., Quock, R. M., Consroe, P., Roeske, W. R., & Yamamura, H. I. (1997). $\Delta^9$-Tetrahydrocannabinol is a partial agonist of cannabinoid receptors in mouse brain. *European Journal of Pharmacology, 323,* R3–R4.

Calignano, A., La Rana, G., Giuffrida, A., & Piomelli, D. (1998). Control of pain initiation by endogenous cannabinoids. *Nature, 394,* 277–281.

Carney, J. M., Uwayday, I. M., & Balster, R. L. (1977). Evaluation of a suspension system for intravenous self-administration studies with water-insoluble compounds in the Rhesus monkey. *Pharmacology, Biochemistry, and Behavior, 7,* 357–364.

Chen, J., Paredes, W., Lowinson, J. H., & Gardner, E. L. (1990). Delta 9-tetrahydrocannabinol enhances presynaptic dopamine efflux in medial prefrontal cortex. *European Journal of Pharmacology, 190,* 259–262.

Chen, K., Kandel, D. B., & Davies, M. (1997). Relationships between frequency and quantity of marijuana use and last year proxy dependence among adolescents and adults in the United States. *Drug and Alcohol Dependence, 46,* 53–67.

Compton, D., Aceto, M., Lowe, J., & Martin, B. (1996). *In vivo* characterization of a specific cannabinoid receptor antagonist (SR141716A): inhibition of $\Delta^9$-tetrahydrocannabinol-induced responses and apparent agonist activity. *The Journal of Pharmacology and Experimental Therapeutics, 277*, 586–594.

Cook, S. A., Lowe, J. A., & Martin, B. R. (1998). CB1 receptor antagonist precipitates withdrawal in mice exposed to Delta9-tetrahydrocannabinol. *The Journal of Pharmacology and Experimental Therapeutics, 285*, 1150–1156.

Costa, B., Giagnoni, G., & Colleoni, M. (2000). Precipitated and spontaneous withdrawal in rats tolerant to anandamide. *Psychopharmacology (Berlin), 149*, 121–128.

Cravatt, B. F., Demarest, K., Patricelli, M. P., Bracey, M. H., Giang, D. K., Martin, B. R., *et al.* (2001). Supersensitivity to anandamide and enhanced endogenous cannabinoid signaling in mice lacking fatty acid amide hydrolase. *Proceedings of the National Academy of Sciences of the United States of America, 98*, 9371–9376.

Devane, W. A., Dysarz, F. A., Johnson, M. R., Melvin, L. S., & Howlett, A. C. (1988). Determination and characterization of a cannabinoid receptor in rat brain. *Molecular Pharmacology, 34*, 605–613.

Devane, W. A., Hanus, L., Breuer, A., Pertwee, R. G., Stevenson, L. A., Griffin, G., *et al.* (1992). Isolation and structure of a brain constituent that binds to the cannabinoid receptor. *Science, 258*, 1946–1949.

Di Marzo, V., Goparaju, S. K., Wang, L., Liu, J., Batkai, S., Jarai, Z., *et al.* (2001). Leptin-regulated endocannabinoids are involved in maintaining food intake. *Nature, 410*, 822–825.

Diana, M., Melis, M., Muntoni, A. L., & Gessa, G. L. (1998). Mesolimbic dopaminergic decline after cannabinoid withdrawal. *Proceedings of the National Academy of Sciences of the United States of America, 95*, 10269–10273.

Fattore, L., Cossu, G., Martellotta, C. M., & Fratta, W. (2001). Intravenous self-administration of the cannabinoid CB1 receptor agonist WIN 55,212-2 in rats. *Psychopharmacology (Berlin), 156*, 410–416.

Fielding, S., Wilker, J., Hynes, M., Szewczak, M., Novick Jr., W. J., & Lal, H. (1978). A comparison of clonidine with morphine for antinociceptive and antiwithdrawal actions. *The Journal of Pharmacology and Experimental Therapeutics, 207*, 899–905.

Fraser, J. D. (1949). Withdrawal symptoms in cannabis-indica addicts. *Lancet, 257*, 747–748.

Frederickson, R. C., Hewes, C. R., & Aiken, J. W. (1976). Correlation between the *in vivo* and an *in vitro* expression of opiate withdrawal precipitated by naloxone: their antagonism by 1-(-)-$\Delta^9$-tetrahydrocannabinol. *The Journal of Pharmacology and Experimental Therapeutics, 199*, 375–384.

Gaoni, Y., & Mechoulam, R. (1964). Isolation, structure, and partial synthesis of an active constituent of hashish. *Journal of the American Chemical Society, 86*, 1646–1647.

Gessa, G. L., Melis, M., Muntoni, A. L., & Diana, M. (1998). Cannabinoids activate mesolimbic dopamine neurons by an action on cannabinoid CB1 receptors. *European Journal of Pharmacology, 341*, 39–44.

Gold, M. S., Redmond Jr., D. E., & Kleber, H. D. (1978). Clonidine blocks acute opiate-withdrawal symptoms. *Lancet*, *2*, 599–602.

Gossop, M. (1988). Clonidine and the treatment of the opiate withdrawal syndrome. *Drug and Alcohol Dependence*, *21*, 253–259.

Haney, M., Ward, A. S., Comer, S. D., Foltin, R. W., & Fischman, M. W. (1999a). Abstinence symptoms following oral THC administration to humans. *Psychopharmacology (Berlin)*, *141*, 385–394.

Haney, M., Ward, A. S., Comer, S. D., Foltin, R. W., & Fischman, M. W. (1999b). Abstinence symptoms following smoked marijuana in humans. *Psychopharmacology (Berlin)*, *141*, 395–404.

Harris, R. T., Waters, W., & McLendon, D. (1974). Evaluation of reinforcing capability of $\Delta^9$-tetrahydrocannabinol in rhesus monkeys. *Psychopharmacologia*, *37*, 23–29.

Herkenham, M., Lynn, A. B., Johnson, M., Ross, M., Lawrence, S., de Costa, B. R., et al. (1991). Characterization and localization of cannabinoid receptors in rat brain: a quantitative *in vitro* autoradiographic study. *Journal of Neuroscience*, *11*, 563–583.

Hine, B., Friedman, E., Torellio, M., & Gershon, S. (1975). Morphine-dependent rats: blockade of precipitated abstinence by tetrahydrocannabinol. *Science*, *187*, 443–445.

Howlett, A. C., Johnson, M. R., Melvin, L. S., & Milne, G. M. (1988). Nonclassical cannabinoid analgetics inhibit adenylate cyclase: development of a cannabinoid receptor model. *Molecular Pharmacology*, *33*, 297–302.

Huestis, M. A., Gorelick, D. A., Heishman, S. J., Preston, K. L., Nelson, R. A., Moolchan, E. T., et al. (2001). Blockade of effects of smoked marijuana by the CB1-selective cannabinoid receptor antagonist SR141716. *Archives of General Psychiatry*, *58*, 322–328.

Hutcheson, D. M., Tzavara, E. T., Smadja, C., Valjent, E., Roques, B. P., Hanoune, J., et al. (1998). Behavioural and biochemical evidence for signs of abstinence in mice chronically treated with delta-9-tetrahydrocannabinol. *British Journal of Pharmacology*, *125*, 1567–1577.

Johnston, L. D., O'Malley, P. M., & Bachman, J. G. (2002). *Monitoring the future. National results on adolescent drug use: overview of key findings 2001*. Bethdesda, MD: National Institute on Drug Abuse.

Jones, R. T., & Benowitz, N. (1976). The 30-day trip – clinical studies of cannabis tolerance and dependence. In M. C. Braude, & S. Szara (Eds.), *Pharmacology of marihuana* (pp. 627–642). New York: Raven Press.

Jones, R. T., Benowitz, N., & Bachman, J. (1976). Clinical studies of cannabis tolerance and dependence. *Annals of the New York Academy of Sciences*, *282*, 221–239.

Jones, R. T., Benowitz, N. L. & Herning, R. I. (1981). Clinical relevance of cannabis tolerance and dependence. *Journal of Clinical Pharmacology*, *21*, 143S–152S.

Kaymakcalan, S., & Deneau, G. A. (1972). Some pharmacologic properties of synthetic $\Delta^9$-tetrahydrocannabinol. *Acta Medica Turcica, Supplementum 1*, 5.

Landsman, R. S., Burkey, T. H., Consroe, P., Roeske, W. R., & Yamamura, H. I. (1997). SR141716A is an inverse agonist at the human cannabinoid CB1 receptor. *European Journal of Pharmacology, 334*, R1–R2.

Ledent, C., Valverde, O., Cossu, G., Petitet, F., Aubert, J. F., Beslot, F., *et al.* (1999). Unresponsiveness to cannabinoids and reduced addictive effects of opiates in CB1 receptor knockout mice. *Science, 28*(3), 401–404.

Leite, J. R., & Carlini, E. A. (1974). Failure to obtain "cannabis-directed behavior" and abstinence syndrome in rats chronically treated with cannabis sativa extracts. *Psychopharmacologia, 36*, 133–145.

Lichtman, A. H. (2000). SR 141716A enhances spatial memory as assessed in a radial-arm maze task in rats. *European Journal of Pharmacology, 404*, 175–179.

Lichtman, A. H., Wiley, J. L., LaVecchia, K. L., Neviaser, S. T., Arthrur, D. B., Wilson, D. M., *et al.* (1998). Acute and chronic cannabinoid effects: characterization of precipitated withdrawal in dogs. *European Journal of Pharmacology, 357*, 139–148.

Lichtman, A. H., Fisher, J., & Martin, B. R. (2001a). Precipitated cannabinoid withdrawal is reversed by Delta(9)- tetrahydrocannabinol or clonidine. *Pharmacology, Biochemistry, and Behavior, 69*, 181–188.

Lichtman, A. H., Sheikh, S. M., Loh, H. H., & Martin, B. R. (2001b). Opioid and cannabinoid modulation of precipitated withdrawal in delta(9)-tetrahydrocannabinol and morphine-dependent mice. *The Journal of Pharmacology and Experimental Therapeutics, 298*, 1007–1014.

Mackie, K., & Hille, B. (1992). Cannabinoids inhibit N-type calcium channels in neurobalstoma-glioma cells. *Proceedings of the National Academy of Sciences of the United States of America, 89*, 3825–3829.

Mansbach, R. S., Nicholson, K. L., Martin, B. R., & Balster, R. L. (1994). Failure of Delta(9)-tetrahydrocannabinol and CP 55,940 to maintain intravenous self-administration under a fixed-interval schedule in rhesus monkeys. *Behavioural Pharmacology, 5*, 219–225.

Martellotta, M. C., Cossu, G., Fattore, L., Gessa, G. L., & Fratta, W. (1998). Self-administrarion of the cannabinoid receptor agonist WIN 55,212-2 in drug-naive mice. *Neuroscience, 85*, 327–330.

Mas-Nieto, M., Pommier, B., Tzavara, E. T., Caneparo, A., Da Nascimento, S., Le Fur, G., *et al.* (2001). Reduction of opioid dependence by the CB(1) antagonist SR141716A in mice: evaluation of the interest in pharmacotherapy of opioid addiction. *British Journal of Pharmacology, 132*, 1809–1816.

Matsuda, L. A., Lolait, S. J., Brownstein, M. J., Young, A. C., & Bonner, T. I. (1990). Structure of a cannabinoid receptor and functional expression of the cloned cDNA. *Nature, 346*, 561–564.

McMillan, D. E., Dewey, W. L., & Harris, L. S. (1971). Characteristics of tetrahydrocannabinol tolerance. *Annnals of the New York Academy of Sciences, 191*, 83–99.

Mountjoy, K. G., Robbins, L. S., Mortrud, M. T., & Cone, R. D. (1992). The cloning of a family of genes that encode the melanocortin receptors. *Science, 257*, 1248–1251.

Munro, S., Thomas, K. L., & Abu-Shaar, M. (1993). Molecular characterization of a peripheral receptor for cannabinoids. *Nature, 365*, 61–64.

Navarro, M., Chowen, J., Carrera, M., Rocio, A., del Arco, I., Vallanua, M. A., *et al.* (1998). CB1 cannabiniod receptor antagonist-induced opiate withdrawal in morphine-dependent rats. *Neuroreport, 9*, 3397–3402.

Navarro, M., Carrera, M. R., Fratta, W., Valverde, O., Cossu, G., Fattore, L., *et al.* (2001). Functional interaction between opioid and cannabinoid receptors in drug self-administration. *Journal of Neuroscience, 21*, 5344–5350.

Pan, X., Ikeda, S. R., & Lewis, D. L. (1998). SR 141716A acts as an inverse agonist to increase neuronal voltage-dependent $Ca^{2+}$ currents by reversal of tonic CB1 cannabinoid receptor activity. *The American Society for Pharmacology and Experimental Therapeutics, 54*, 1064–1072.

Razdan, R. K. (1986). Structure-activity relationships in cannabinoids. *Pharmacological Reviews, 38*, 75–149.

Richardson, J. D., Aanonsen, L., & Hargreaves, K. M. (1998). Hypoactivity of the spinal cannabinoid system results in NMDA-dependent hyperalgesia. *Journal of Neuroscience, 18*, 451–457.

Rinaldi-Carmona, M., Barth, F., Héaulme, M., Shire, D., Calandra, B., Congy, C., *et al.* (1994). SR141716A, a potent and selective antagonist of the brain cannabinoid receptor. *FEBS Letters, 350*, 240–244.

Rodriguez de Fonseca, F., Carrera, M., Navarro, M., Koob, K., & Weiss, F. (1997). Activitation of corticotropin-releasing factor in the limbic system during cannabinoid withdrawal. *Science, 276*, 2050–2054.

Romero, J., Berrendero, F., Garcia-Gil, L., De La Cruz, P., Ramos, A., & Fernandez-Ruiz, J. J. (1998). Loss of cannabinoid receptor binding and messenger RNA levels and cannabinoid agonist-stimulated [35s]guanylyl-5'-O-(thio)-triphosphate binding in the basal ganglia of rats. *Neuroscience, 84*, 1075–1083.

Rubino, T., Patrini, G., Massi, P., Fuzio, D., Vigano, D., Giagnoni, G., *et al.* (1998). Cannabinoid-precipitated withdrawal: a time-course study of the behavioral aspect and its correlation with cannabinoid receptors and G protein expression. *The Journal of Pharmacology and Experimental Therapeutics, 285*, 813–819.

Rubino, T., Massi, P., Vigano, D., Fuzio, D., & Parolaro, D. (2000a). Long-term treatment with SR141716A, the CB1 receptor antagonist, influences morphine withdrawal syndrome. *Life Sciences, 66*, 2213–2219.

Rubino, T., Vigano, D., Zagato, E., Sala, M., & Parolaro, D. (2000b). *In vivo* characterization of the specific cannabinoid receptor antagonist, SR141716A: behavioral and cellular responses after acute and chronic treatments. *Synapse, 35*, 8–14.

Sanudo-Pena, M. C., Force, M., Tsou, K., McLemore, G., Roberts, L., & Walker, J. M. (1999). Dopaminergic system does not play a major role in the precipitated cannabinoid withdrawal syndrome. *Zhongguo Yao Li Xue Bao, 20*, 1121–1124.

Sim, L. J., Selley, D. E., Xiao, R., & Childers, S. R. (1996). Differences in G-protein activation by μ- and δ-opioid, and cannabinoid, receptors in rat striatum. *European Journal of Pharmacology, 307*, 97–105.

Sim-Selley, L. J., Brunk, L. K., & Selley, D. E. (2001). Inhibitory effects of SR141716A on G-protein activation in rat brain. *European Journal of Pharmacology, 414*, 135–143.

Sugiura, T., Kondo, S., Sukagawa, A., Nakane, S., Shinoda, A., Itoh, K., *et al.* (1995). 2-Arachidonoyglycerol: a possible endogenous cannabinoid receptor ligand in brain. *Biochemical and Biophysical Research Communications, 215*, 89–97.

Swift, W., Hall, W., & Copeland, J. (2000). One year follow-up of cannabis dependence among long-term users in Sydney, Australia. *Drug and Alcohol Dependence, 59*, 309–318.

Tanda, G., Munzar, P., & Goldberg, S. R. (2000). Self-administration behavior is maintained by the psychoactive ingredient of marijuana in squirrel monkeys. *Natural Neuroscience, 3*, 1073–1074.

Terranova, J. P., Storme, J. J., Lafon, N., Perio, A., Rinaldi-Carmona, M., Le Fur, G., *et al.* (1996). Improvement of memory in rodents by the selective CB1 cannabinoid receptor antagonist, SR 141716. *Psychopharmacology, 126*, 165–172.

Tsou, K., Patrick, S., & Walker, J. M. (1995). Physical withdrawal in rats tolerant to $\Delta^9$-tetrahydrocannabinol precipitated by a cannabinoid receptor antagonist. *European Journal of Pharmacology, 280*, R13–R15.

Turner, C. E., Bouwsma, O. J., Billets, S., & Elsohly, M. A. (1980). Constituents of Cannabis sativa L. XVIII – Electron voltage selected ion monitoring study of cannabinoids. *Biomedical Mass Spectrometry, 7*, 247–256.

Tzavara, E. T., Valjent, E., Firmo, C., Mas, M., Beslot, F., Defer, N., *et al.* (2000). Cannabinoid withdrawal is dependent upon PKA activation in the cerebellum. *European Journal of Neuroscience, 12*, 1038–1046.

Valverde, O., Ledent, C., Beslot, F., Parmentier, M., & Roques, B. P. (2000a). Reduction of stress-induced analgesia but not of exogenous opioid effects in mice lacking CB1 receptors. *European Journal of Neuroscience, 12*, 533–539.

Valverde, O., Maldonado, R., Valjent, E., Zimmer, A. M., & Zimmer, A. (2000b). Cannabinoid withdrawal syndrome is reduced in pre-proenkephalin knock-out mice. *Journal of Neuroscience, 20*, 9284–9289.

van Ree, J. M., Slangen, J. L., & de Wied, D. (1978). Intravenous self-administration of drugs in rats. *The Journal of Pharmacology and Experimental Therapeutics, 204*, 547–557.

Vela, G., Ruiz-Gayo, M., & Fuentes, J. (1995). Anandamide decreases naloxone-precipitated withdrawal signs in mice chronically treated with morphine. *Neuropharmacology, 34*, 665–668.

Vivian, J. A., Kishioka, S., Butelman, E. R., Broadbear, J., Lee, K. O., & Woods, J. H. (1998). Analgesic, respiratory and heart rate effects of cannabinoid and opioid agonists in rhesus monkeys: antagonist effects of SR 141716A. *The Journal of Pharmacology and Experimental Therapeutics, 286*, 697–703.

Walker, J. M., Huang, S. M., Strangman, N. M., Tsou, K., & Sanudo-Pena, M. C. (1999). Pain modulation by release of the endogenous cannabinoid anandamide. *Proceedings of the National Academy of Sciences of the United States of America, 96,* 12198–12203.

Wiesbeck, G. A., Schuckit, M. A., Kalmijn, J. A., Tipp, J. E., Bucholz, K. K., & Smith, T. L. (1996). An evaluation of the history of a marijuana withdrawal syndrome in a large population. *Addiction, 91,* 1469–1478.

Wikler, A. (1976). Aspects of tolerance to and dependence on cannabis. *Annals of the New York Academy of Science, 282,* 126–147.

Willoughby, K. A., Moore, S. F., Martin, B. R., & Ellis, E. F. (1997). The biodisposition and metabolism of anandamide in mice. *The Journal of Pharmacology and Experimental Therapeutics, 282,* 243–247.

Yamaguchi, T., Hagiwara, Y., Tanaka, H., Sugiura, T., Waku, K., Shoyama, Y., et al. (2001). Endogenous cannabinoid, 2-arachidonoylglycerol, attenuates naloxone-precipitated withdrawal signs in morphine-dependent mice. *Brain Research, 909,* 121–126.

Zimmer, A., Zimmer, A. M., Hohmann, A. G., Herkenham, M., & Bonner, T. I. (1999). Increased mortality, hypoactivity, and hypoalgesia in cannabinoid CB1 receptor knockout mice. *Proceedings of the National Academy of Sciences of the United States of America, 96,* 5780–5785.

# 4

# The Epidemiology of Cannabis Dependence

JAMES C. ANTHONY

## Introduction

This chapter describes selected features of cannabis epidemiology, with a focus upon recent evidence from field studies of cannabis dependence. An epidemiologist's interest in cannabis can be motivated by an appreciation that cannabis smoking represents the most common illegal drug use behavior in the world, with a roughly estimated 140–150 million cannabis users, as compared to rough estimates of 14–15 million for cocaine and 13–14 million for opium, heroin, and other opioid drugs (United Nations, 2002). Based upon recent estimates, projections, and averages for the USA, an estimated 7000–8000 individuals start using cannabis every day and there are 95 million US community residents who have tried cannabis on at least one occasion (Substance Abuse and Mental Health Services Administration, Office of Applied Studies (SAMHSA), 2002c, d). As will be documented later in this chapter, our rough averaged estimate is that some 50–80 recent-onset cannabis users develop a cannabis dependence syndrome each day during the year; some substantial fraction of these cases appear to require clinical intervention services.

It is generally possible to dissect epidemiological research in relation to five general rubrics or sub-headings. The first rubric concerns quantification of disease burden, including the burdens associated with mental and behavioral disturbances that do not qualify as formal diseases, as well as the population-averaged "incidence" and individual-level risk of becoming a cannabis user, and the separately estimated population-averaged "prevalence" and individual-level likelihood of being an active or former cannabis user (e.g., see Anthony & Van Etten, 1998, Wu, *et al.*, 2003, for detailed discussions of the distinctions between incidence and prevalence). The second rubric concerns localization of domains of population experience where these behaviors, diseases and disturbances are more or less likely to occur and to persist. The third rubric addresses causes, and represents epidemiology's participation in tests of etiological hypotheses and theories. The distinction between the second and the third rubric is congruent with the distinction between descriptive or predictive models versus causal or explanatory models in various domains of science. The fourth rubric is concerned with pathogenesis and natural history, including co-occurring conditions, as well as disabilities and other adverse consequences that may befall cases when there has been no effective intervention to remediate disturbances of health. The distinction between the third and fourth rubric is congruent with a distinction between etiology versus studies of pathogenesis and natural history, with the former more oriented toward identification of root causes, and the latter more oriented toward processes leading to a disease and its complications. In general, epidemiological studies under the fourth rubric require longitudinal designs, with repeated measurements or observations of a designated sample, or with careful attention to temporal sequencing of events and processes in cross-section. In contrast, many etiological studies under the third rubric are single-measurement and retrospective case-control studies, designs based upon cross-sectional surveys, ambidirectional surveys, or prospective cohort studies with no attempt to link from one endogenous response variable to another. The fifth and final rubric concerns epidemiology's contributions to studies of prevention, intervention, and control – studies that generally are large sample population-based randomized trials to test the efficacy or effectiveness of preventive or curative interventions, or population-based studies of a non-experimental character, where the goal is evaluation of a policy change or programmatic difference (Anthony & Van Etten, 1998).

The present chapter covers epidemiology's contributions to nosologic studies of cannabis dependence as well as the first two rubrics of epidemiological research. Working under the first rubric of epidemiology, epidemiologists have tried to answer questions about how many individuals in the population are becoming affected by cannabis dependence each year, with implications for development of clinical intervention services, and have studied the probability of becoming cannabis-dependent among cannabis users. Working under the second rubric of epidemiology, we have examined cross-national and within-country variations in the frequency and occurrence of cannabis use and dependence, as well as variations in relation to time, features of individual and social life (e.g., age, sex, ethnicity), and local area conditions (e.g., urban–rural differences).

## Epidemiology's Contribution to Nosological Studies of Cannabis Dependence

One pertinent starting point for this chapter on the epidemiology of cannabis dependence is the question of whether there is such a thing. Until about 35 years ago, the answer to this question generally was a resounding negative. Most observers judged that the evidence was unconvincing with respect to cannabis withdrawal, presumed to be a necessary feature of any cannabis dependence syndrome if "opiate dependence" were to serve as a "model" disturbance for comparison.

Thereafter, in the mid-1960s, a World Health Organization expert committee unshackled the concept of drug dependence from its original links in a conceptual chain with the opioid withdrawal syndrome. A more behaviorally-oriented concept of drug dependence gained sway (e.g., see Pickens & Meisch, 1973).

As alcohol and illegal drug problems often co-occur within the same individuals (e.g., see Anthony, 1991; Anthony & Helzer, 1991; Russell *et al.*, 1994), it is understandable that the general form and contents of a fledgling "alcohol dependence syndrome" were borrowed when clinicians sought to understand the experiences of users who came to them for help with problems associated with illegal drug use, often involving cannabis, less often involving cocaine. The psychiatric community's general consensus about a cannabis dependence syndrome was shaped into a case definition for the third edition of the American Psychiatric Association's (APA) *Diagnostic and Statistical Manual* (DSM), published in 1980. Nevertheless, general consensus about the cocaine dependence syndrome did not emerge until the revised third edition of the DSM, published in 1987 (APA, 1980, 1987). A concurrent international consensus process led to a general drug dependence case definition resembling the DSM approach in some respects, now specified within the tenth revision of the *International Classification of Diseases* (ICD) and its accompanying glossary for mental and behavioral disturbances (World Health Organization, 1992).

In other chapters of this book, readers will find authoritative descriptions of the DSM case definitions, insofar as the recognizable clinical features of the cannabis dependence syndrome have been recorded and codified in careful observations by members of APA expert panels, and the ICD-10 experts, including the most recent revisions made by DSM-IV task panels. In general, cannabis dependence is conceptualized as a true *syndrome*, a "running together" of distinctive clinical features with greater than chance co-occurrence. The main elements of these clinical features encompass:

(a) disturbances of the mental life, such as obsession-like ruminations and recurrent thoughts or cravings about cannabis and cannabis involvement;
(b) disturbances of behavior, sometimes expressed in the form of compulsion-like repetitions of cannabis-involved behavior;
(c) manifestations of neuroadaptation secondary to cannabis exposures, which might be experienced as a subjective feeling that the same dose of cannabis

is less efficacious, or which might be observable in the form of clinical features of a cannabis withdrawal syndrome after long-sustained daily or near-daily cannabis consumption.

The syndrome definition does not require presence of all of these clinical features and manifestations. Typically, three distinguishable clinical features are required to be present if a clinical diagnosis of cannabis dependence is to be made. There is debate about where to set this cutting point for diagnosis, and some investigators and clinicians prefer to examine cannabis dependence as a dimensional response to cannabis exposure. Others are skeptical about the existence of cannabis dependence (and other categorical psychiatric disorders), particularly when the patients have not reached adulthood (e.g., see Coffey *et al.*, 2002; Compton *et al.*, 1990; Farrell 1999; Zoccolillo *et al.*, 1999); some observers are extremely enthusiastic about this clinical concept (e.g., see Dennis *et al.*, 2002). Chen *et al.* (1997) responded to the contentious nature of case definition and case ascertainment, and described their work as pertaining to "proxy dependence" on cannabis, due to uncertainty about the diagnostic validity of what they were studying.

Whereas some investigators have studied the syndrome character of cannabis dependence using samples of help-seeking drug users (e.g., Nelson *et al.*, 1999), epidemiology functions as a lens that allows clinicians and clinical scientists to look beyond the thresholds of their clinical practices, out into the community experience of individuals whose ailments never have come to the attention of a doctor, helping professional, or counselor (Anthony & Van Etten, 1998). Consistent with the seven "uses of epidemiology" outlined by Morris almost 50 years ago (Morris, 1957), one of the aims of epidemiological studies of cannabis users in the community has been to seek evidence on whether cannabis dependence has cogency as a biomedical construct, even when cannabis users never have come into contact with clinicians or other authorities. By working to secure representative probability samples of cannabis users in the community, epidemiologists can reach out to users who never have sought help for cannabis problems and who may be almost completely isolated from clinical or academic environments where there are opportunities to learn the DSM and ICD concepts of cannabis dependence. In our epidemiological community samples, no more than a small minority of the cannabis users have talked to a doctor or other counselor about cannabis problems (estimated as fewer than one in six active drug dependence cases, and fewer than one in 14 drug dependence cases in remission), and very few illegal drug users ($<$10%) have been arrested and booked for cannabis-related offenses (e.g., see Anthony & Helzer, 1991; SAMHSA, 2002c, d). In more recent national survey estimates, the fraction of recent cannabis users receiving treatment for drug problems has been estimated at values under 5%; among daily or almost daily users, the estimate was under 10% (SAMHSA, 2002b). Hence, our best evidence is that the vast majority of cannabis users are not in treatment and never have received clinical interventions; for more than 90% of recent users there has been no recent contact with criminal justice systems, as indicated by arrests and bookings for drug-associated offenses.

In the epidemiological context, without medicalizing the assessment, we can use highly standardized assessments, sometimes computerized self-interviews, to ask whether the reported experiences with cannabis have the character of a syndrome, even in the absence of clinical contact (i.e., do these experiences run together with greater than chance co-occurrence?). In order to augment the rigor of the scientific challenge, we recently have started to focus our work on cannabis users in the earliest stages of their cannabis experiences (i.e., recent-onset cannabis users who started to use cannabis within the 24 months prior to the time of the epidemiological assessments).

A recent study by Chen & Anthony (2003) illustrates our epidemiological approach. The sample of almost 1000 recent-onset cannabis users originated with national probability surveys of household residents living within the USA, ages ranging from early adolescence upward. As participants in recent US National Household Surveys on Drug Abuse (NHSDA, now called "National Surveys on Drug Use and Health," NSDUH), each individual self-designated cannabis user in the sample was asked standardized survey questions about age of onset of cannabis use and occurrence of cannabis-related experiences in the year prior to assessment. There were seven items on cannabis-related experiences, all framed in relation to clinical features discussed in the DSM and ICD manuals, of the type listed in Table 2.2.

The design of these standardized survey items followed the cannabis dependence theory grounded in clinical experience, as described above. There were questions about the subjectively felt experience of what might be neuroadaptational changes subsequent to repeated occasions of cannabis use (needing larger amounts to obtain effects previously felt with smaller amounts). There were questions about disturbances of the mental life such as the feeling that it is difficult to stop or cut back on cannabis use even when the user desired to cut back, and behavioral disturbances such as using more than had been intended during an occasion of cannabis use, or for longer periods than had been intended. Other questions in this study pertained to emotional disturbances and health problems that the users themselves attributed to their cannabis use, or other features of the cannabis dependence syndrome as defined in the DSM and ICD.

Whereas all survey-identified cannabis users have been asked questions as part of the NHSDA and NSDUH, the work of our research group has been focused on the experiences of recent-onset cannabis users. In this subset of the NHSDA community probability sample of illegal drug users, none had accumulated more than 24 months of cannabis use experience since onset of first cannabis use. Within the subset, the age of onset of cannabis use was equal to the participant's age at the time of assessment or was within 1 year of that age.

In this context of very recent onset of cannabis use, we were able to confirm an internal coherence of reported experiences that users connect with their cannabis use, even though no more than a miniscule number of the users ever had received clinical services or counseling for cannabis problems. Within the framework of latent trait analyses, the best-fitting statistical model is one that expresses occurrence of these problems as a function of an underlying single dimension of cannabis involvement, which we chose to label as "level of cannabis dependence." That is, there is sufficient co-occurrence of these cannabis-related experiences to say that each experience can function as an observable manifestation of an underlying dimension of cannabis problems or difficulties (Chen & Anthony, 2003). Notwithstanding limited exceptions such as those that might arise when samples are limited to patients seeking treatment (e.g., Nelson *et al.*, 1999), similar conclusions about the unidimensionality of the cannabis dependence constructs have been described by others studying epidemiological samples in the USA, Australia, and elsewhere (e.g., see Morgenstern *et al.*, 1994; Swift *et al.*, 2001a, as well as a pertinent discussion of "diagnostic orphans" in Degenhardt *et al.*, 2002).

Our research group recently has re-approached the same NHSDA data with a different statistical model – one that posits underlying classes of cannabis users, which is more consistent with the DSM's discrete categorical approach to case definition, less consistent with the ICD-10 dimensional approach. In this context, we have considered the possibility that there are three classes of recent-onset cannabis users:

1. those users who have experienced little in the way of the above-mentioned difficulties with cannabis use (a class of cannabis users with essentially "no problems");
2. those users who have started to experience difficulties but who have not progressed beyond the experience of one or two difficulties (a "prodrome" class);
3. those users who have progressed and for whom the probability of experiencing any given difficulty is greater than 50% and most have experienced three or more problems (a "dependent" class).

When we examine the data on recent-onset cannabis users with this specification, we find that roughly 70–80% of the recent-onset cannabis users fall into the "no problem" class (no significant cannabis-related difficulties experienced within the first 24 months of cannabis use), about 17–27% of the recent-onset cannabis users fall into the second "prodrome" class (at least one cannabis-related difficulty occurring, but none with substantial frequency), and under 5% (closer to 2–3%) fall into the third "cannabis dependence" class, within which the seven cannabis-related difficulties have occurred at a class-specific mean probability of 60% or greater. For example, virtually all of the recent-onset cannabis users in this third and more difficulty-laden "dependence" class have experienced emotional or psychological problems which they attribute to cannabis, and 80% report that they have felt tolerant and needed more cannabis in order to achieve effects previously obtained with smaller amounts. Within this third "cannabis dependence" class, the least commonly reported cannabis-related difficulties involved health problems; however, even so, a total of 60% of the cannabis users in our "cannabis dependence" class self-identified health problems that they themselves attribute to their use of cannabis (Anthony *et al.*, unpublished manuscript).

Epidemiological evidence of this quality will not set to rest all concerns or post-DSM critiques about the categorical approach to cannabis dependence. Nonetheless, in our epidemiological evidence from a community sample of recent-onset cannabis users, there is a much-constrained possibility for forces and biases that affect studies of help-seeking cannabis users. Without prompting, special pleading, coaching, or social learning processes such as can occur when patients come into contact with clinicians and counselors, an estimated 2–3% of the recent-onset cannabis users in the NHSDA community sample have progressed to the point that they have a high likelihood of reporting each and every clinical feature of cannabis dependence included in the survey assessment. Given the large numbers of individuals who start to use cannabis in any given year, a value of 2% can translate into many individuals who might need clinical attention for their cannabis related difficulties early in the cannabis dependence process.

## How Many Are Becoming Affected, with Focus on the USA?

Recent epidemiological evidence from the USA also speaks to the question of how many individuals might need clinical services early in the cannabis dependence process (i.e., the question involves how many are becoming affected for the first time each year). For this purpose in this chapter, we have been able to harness data reported by Gfroerer *et al.* (2002), who have estimated the annual incidence rates for initiation of cannabis use for the span from 1965 to the present.

Annual incidence estimates derived by Gfroerer *et al.* (2002) are depicted in Figure 4.1 for the pool of potential users ("at risk" individuals) who were living in US households and were 12–17 years old in each year, and for the separate pool of potential users who were 18–25 years old.

Estimates of this type convey the dynamic epidemiological character of cannabis use experiences in the USA during the past 30–40 years, may help us to understand underlying population processes that govern recent increases in treatment admissions for cannabis problems, and by themselves clarify several important issues that are impossible to resolve in other ways (e.g., by studying prevalence of cannabis use among school-attending youths or arrestees). Namely, for adolescents in this country, recent years may have corresponded with an unprecedented high level of risk of starting to use marijuana, as large and possibly substantially larger than levels estimated for the years of the Vietnam conflict and the "flower power" heyday, and as high or higher than the peak values observed during the late 1970s. (The uncertainty expressed in the prior statement mainly is due to concerns about the completeness of recall and reporting of each survey respondent's age of first cannabis use. Some observers believe that there is more under-reporting when adults are asked about their adolescent cannabis experiences; other observers speculate that the greatest under-reporting occurs among those who have just started to use cannabis and who continue to be active cannabis users. At present, there is no definitive evidence on this methodological topic.)

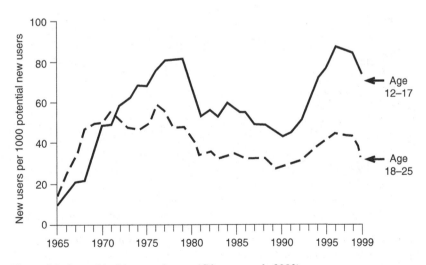

Figure 4.1 Annual incidence estimates (Gfroerer *et al.*, 2002).

Based upon these survey estimates, the estimated risk of starting to use cannabis in the US has been more stable for 18–25-year olds, and adolescent risk estimates have been larger than young adult risk estimates for more than two decades. As noted above, parenthetically, here is some concern about methodology in the backward projection approach – namely, it is possible that these risk estimates are downwardly biased (i.e., decay with passing time). However, Gfroerer *et al.* (2002) provide data to suggest that the size of downward bias might be small, and there is convergent evidence of increases in cannabis use from surveillance of more selected population segments such as school-attending youths and arrestees between 1990 and 1996. Monitoring The Future estimates, year by year, indicate that about 60% of high school seniors in the USA had tried cannabis in 1980, as compared to values of about 50–55% across the span from 1996 through 2002 (e.g., see Golub & Johnson, 2001; Johnston *et al.*, 2001; SAMHSA, 2002b; Figure 10.1).

The same backward projection method can be used to convey the actual number of new initiates by year, as shown for all persons age 12 years and older in Figure 4.2. The actual numbers backward-projected by Gfroerer *et al.* (2002) are shown as circles; our own regression-based smoothed estimates

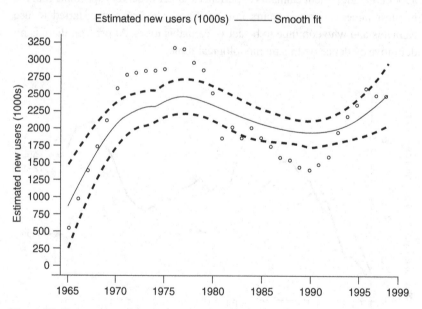

Figure 4.2 Estimated number of new users each year for the span 1965–1999. Adapted by J. C. Anthony from data in Gfroerer *et al.* (2002). May be reproduced without permission.

based on numbers provided in the Gfroerer report are plotted along a solid line, and approximate error bars based on the smoothed estimates are plotted as dashed lines above and below the smoothed point estimates.

With calendar year 1999 taken as an example, the smoothed point estimate indicates roughly 2,500,000 new cannabis users in that year. Projecting from our epidemiological evidence presented in the first section of this chapter (entitled "Epidemiology's contribution to nosological studies of cannabis dependence"), and estimating that 2% of the recent-onset cannabis users have entered the "cannabis dependence" class, we can derive an estimate that 50,000 recent-onset cannabis users might have become newly in need of clinical intervention services in that year (i.e., $2,500,000 \times 0.02 = 50,000$). These are the individuals in our "cannabis dependence" class, each of whom has cannabis problems, most with multiple problems, and each reporting each one of the problems with a probability of 60% or greater.

To be especially conservative, we cut the 2% value in half, leading us to a range of 20,000–30,000 individuals with apparent newly developed needs for these services, based upon what they themselves described and attributed as problems due to their use of cannabis. Based on this rough averaged estimate for the USA, it may be said that some 50–80 recent-onset cannabis users develop the cannabis dependence syndrome each day of the year; a substantial proportion may be expected to require clinical intervention services.

The same type of projection method can be applied to more recent estimates of the number of newly incident cannabis users, and to more recent estimates for the population-averaged risk of becoming cannabis dependent within the first 24 months after onset of cannabis use. For example, the US government estimated that in calendar year 2000 there were 2,604,000 new cannabis users, including about 2,000,000 adolescents who started using cannabis for the first time (SAMHSA, 2002c, d). Studying the cannabis dependence experiences of those who had started to use cannabis during the years 2000–2001, and applying the NHSDA's DSM-IV algorithm, we have estimated that roughly 3.9% developed the cannabis dependence syndrome during a span of 0–24 months after onset of use (Chen *et al.*, 2005). Note that the DSM-IV approach yields a slightly larger risk estimate than the 2–3% estimate derived via our latent class approach. In consequence, the projection for these more recent years of the 21st century continues to be consistent with a value of at least 50 new cases of cannabis dependence each day in the USA.

To be sure, as noted above, there also may be an under-reporting of recent-onset cannabis use within these most recent national samples (e.g., due to concerns about whether there will be total confidentiality of the anonymous survey data, as discussed by Anthony *et al.*, 2000). If we were to make a correction for under-reporting, it would tend to counterbalance any over-estimation of the occurrence of cannabis dependence in the population.

Of course, our estimates based on these "newly incident" users of cannabis do not take into account the "prevalent" cannabis users (i.e., those whose cannabis dependence problems developed after the first 12–24 months of cannabis use and who are excluded during estimation of annual incidence). To clarify what may be an accumulation of cannabis dependence cases during the passing years after first cannabis use, we drew upon data from the nationally representative probability sample secured for the US National Comorbidity Survey (NCS), first gathered in 1990–1992. In the NCS, a detailed assessment of the DSM-IIIR cannabis dependence syndrome was included as part of the University of Michigan version of the Composite International Diagnostic Interview (CIDI) (e.g., see Anthony *et al.*, 1994; Wagner & Anthony 2002a). Based on these NCS data with the CIDI diagnosis of cannabis dependence, we found that the cumulative occurrence of cannabis dependence among cannabis users increased across the first 4 years after the start of cannabis use, and then grew less rapidly. Within roughly 10 years after first use of cannabis, an estimated 10% of cannabis users had developed the DSM-IIIR cannabis dependence syndrome; almost 2% developed DSM-IIIR cannabis dependence within the first 2 years of cannabis use, consistent with but slightly lower than the separately derived estimate for recent-onset cannabis users we reported earlier in this chapter (Anthony *et al.*, unpublished manuscript; Wagner & Anthony, 2002a).

Once error bars are taken into account, the NCS estimates indicate that there is roughly one case of cannabis dependence for every 9–11 persons who used cannabis on at least one occasion, with a point estimate of about 10% (Anthony *et al.*, 1994; Wagner & Anthony, 2002a). A different estimation procedure yields current prevalence of active cannabis dependence among currently active cannabis users – which is a more useful statistic for planning of new clinical intervention services, but a less useful statistic for research on the causes of cannabis dependence (e.g., see Anthony & Van Etten, 1998). When prevalence of active cannabis dependence among active cannabis users has been estimated, the results have tended to be somewhat larger than the 10% value reported above. A reason to expect a larger value is that the development of a cannabis dependence process is one of the reasons that cannabis users continue to be active users. That is, if cannabis dependence has developed, the user is more likely to remain an active user, and if cannabis dependence has not developed, the user is more likely to have stopped using or to have cut back to infrequent use (almost by definition). Hence, among currently active cannabis users, we should find an accumulated concentration of individuals who have become cannabis dependent.

Estimates of the number of currently active cannabis dependence cases can be derived from statistics provided by the Office of Applied Statistics at SAMHSA in the USA based on the most recent National Household Surveys (active cannabis dependence prevalence from SAMHSA, 2001; number of active cannabis users from Gfroerer *et al.*, 2002). These estimates, from calendar year 1999 and 2000 survey data, are for individuals age 12 years and older who have used cannabis within 1 month of assessment, totaling roughly 14 million currently active users, or an estimated 6.3% of the US population in this age range.

Among the 14 million current users, roughly 1.6–2.3 million users qualified as a recently active DSM-IV cannabis dependence case according to the National Survey field assessment methods and DSM-IV diagnostic algorithm (i.e., with three or more active clinical features in the year prior to assessment). Converted to a prevalence proportion, these values indicate that some 11–16% of current cannabis users are active cannabis dependence cases. (Chen *et al.*, 1997, have reported similar estimates from prior NHSDA surveys from earlier in the 1990s.)

Projected back to the total US population age 12 years and older, and with attention to precision of the survey estimate, it is possible to estimate a prevalence value of some 5–15 cases per 1000 persons in the total surveyed population. Converting this prevalence estimate to a percentage, we can say that among all population members age 12 and older, non-users as well as cannabis users, about 0.5–1.5% of these persons now qualifies as a recently active case of cannabis dependence, representing individuals who might be in need of clinical intervention services.

## Where Are We More or Less Likely to Find Cases of Cannabis Dependence?

In order to identify where we are most likely to find cases and where we might look for clues about pathogenesis, etiology, and intervention, epidemiologists generally study variation in frequency and occurrence of health and disease for segments of populations or population experience as subdivided in relation to characteristics of place (e.g., country to country variation), time (e.g., secular time trends), and person (e.g., age, sex, race-ethnicity, social class). For example, the estimates of the second section of the chapter (entitled "How Many Are Becoming Affected, with Focus on the USA?") suggest that roughly 1% of the US population age 12 years and older is a currently active case of cannabis dependence. Among recent-onset cannabis users, this estimate is 2%, and among currently active users (new users plus persisting users), the corresponding value could be as large as 11–16%. We should expect such values to vary across countries or local areas, across periods of time, and across subgroups of the population characterized by individual or social features (e.g., ethnicity), and by conditions of local environment (e.g., urban–rural, local area policies toward illegal drug use).

## Variation In Relation to Geography and Geopolitical Location

As noted in the introduction to this chapter, the United Nations has estimated that 140–150 million world citizens use cannabis. There is general concern about increased prominence of cannabis use in most regions of the world, including the USA (e.g., Chen *et al.*, 2004a, b; Dormitzer *et al.*, 2004; El-Guebaly, 2002; Fergusson & Horwood, 2000; Kokkevi *et al.*, 2000; Krausz *et al.*, 2002; Perkonigg *et al.*, 1998; Swift *et al.*, 2001a, b; von Sydow *et al.*, 2001; Wallace *et al.*, 1999). Up to this point in time, it has been necessary to rely upon standardized questionnaire surveys of school-aged youths in order to make virtually all of our cross-national comparisons of cannabis involvement, and these comparisons generally are focused upon the prevalence of cannabis use, rather than dependence upon cannabis (e.g., see Plant & Miller, 2001).

As an illustration of cross-national comparison with respect to cannabis dependence, Furr-Holden and Anthony (2003) found evidence that active drug dependence (mainly cannabis dependence) was occurring slightly less often in a United Kingdom adult survey population assessed in the early 1990s, when compared to an otherwise generally equivalent NHSDA sample from the USA assessed at the same time. Surprisingly, despite the US-associated excess prevalence of cannabis dependence observed in this study, UK cannabis users were more likely than US users to have become daily or near-daily smokers.

Studying adult community residents in Australia, Swift *et al.* (2001b) reported that about 1.5% of the adult Australia population were active cases of DSM-IV cannabis dependence (95% confidence interval (CI) = 1.2–1.8%). More than 30% of the active cannabis users in Australia qualified as active cases of cannabis dependence. These values are not too distant from the US–UK comparative prevalence estimates reported in the Furr-Holden and Anthony study, but are somewhat larger than the corresponding US values of 1% and 11–16% reported above. Indeed, in the US survey data, in order to find a group of cannabis users with such a high cannabis dependence prevalence estimate (i.e., above 30%), it is necessary to restrict the analysis of the NHSDA data to adolescents using cannabis on a daily or near-daily basis within the past year. In this sub-segment of the US population, it is found that roughly 35% of cannabis users qualify as recent active cases of cannabis dependence, and the corresponding value for adult daily or near-daily users is only 18% (Chen *et al.*, 1997).

Independently, also within Australia, Lynskey *et al.* (2002) studied a large epidemiology sample of twins born between 1964 and 1971, finding that 11% of the sample had become dependent upon cannabis (15% for men, 8% for women). This is a quite large value. However, this assessment of cannabis dependence was based upon a report of at least two clinical features of cannabis dependence, whereas most studies have specified a requirement for three or more reported clinical features.

In a series of publications on a Christchurch (New Zealand) birth cohort studied to age 26 years, a research group led by David M. Fergusson and others has plotted the cumulative occurrence of cannabis use, and later risk of cannabis dependence, and have studied suspected consequences and antecedents of these experiences. In one of the earlier publications, Fergusson *et al.* (1993) found that by age 14–15 years, about 10% of the birth cohort of almost 949 Christchurch-born children had already started to use cannabis, and 75% of the users reported positive reactions to cannabis use while only 30–31% reported adverse reactions.

In the Christchurch cohort, by age 21, the cumulative occurrence of cannabis use was almost 70%. Nearly 10% had developed cannabis dependence (Fergusson & Horwood, 2000). In a separate cohort maintained by the Dunedin Multidisciplinary Health and Development Study, the cumulative occurrence of cannabis use to age 26 was about 75%, and just under 10% had developed cannabis dependence (Poulton *et al.*, 1997). By implication, one in seven or 7.5 cannabis users in these NZ samples had developed cannabis dependence by the time of follow-up in young adulthood.

Coffey *et al.* (2002) have produced interesting comparative estimates on the basis of repeated longitudinal survey assessments of a large Australian representative population sample (though not a birth cohort sample). Surveyed at mean age 20.7 years, an estimated 59% of this Australian sample had started cannabis use (*cf.* 70% of the Christchurch NZ sample) and an estimated 7% met criteria for cannabis dependence (*cf.* 10% of the Christchurch NZ sample). By implication, one in six cannabis users had developed cannabis dependence by the time of this follow-up in Australia.

A prospective study of adolescents and young adults in Germany offers useful but not completely comparable data with respect to the American and New Zealand research on cannabis. As reported by Perkonigg *et al.* (1999) and by von Sydow *et al.* (2001), about one-third of the surveyed adolescents and young adults (age 14–24 years) initiated cannabis use within 2 years of baseline assessment (mean follow-up, 19.7 months), and a cumulative total of about one-half had started to use cannabis within 3–4 years after baseline. By the 3–4 year follow-up assessment, slightly more than 2% (2.2%) had developed cannabis dependence. By implication, about one in 20–25 of the cannabis users had developed cannabis dependence by the time of the young adult follow-up in Germany, based on values reported by von Sydow *et al.* (2001).

Published data from the just-cited US, New Zealand, Australia, and Germany studies permit some crude epidemiological comparisons of substantive note. Among community respondents studied in the USA during the NCS national probability sample survey, an estimated one in 6–7 adolescent and young adult cannabis users (age 15–24 years) had become dependent by the time of assessment (16%, as reported by Anthony *et al.*, 1994). Corresponding values by young adulthood for the New Zealand, Australia, and German studies can be projected, respectively, as one cannabis dependence case per seven or 7.5 cannabis users (NZ, 14%, 13.3%), one cannabis dependence case per six cannabis users (Australia, 16.7%), and one cannabis dependence case per 20–25 users (Germany, 4–5%). It may be pertinent to note that one US-based study of female twins has reported one cannabis dependence case per 20–25 cannabis users in the sample, but it is possible that this study had under-ascertainment of cannabis dependence due to the method of diagnostic assessment (Kendler & Prescott, 1998). Otherwise, there seems to be some replicability of the "1 in 6–7" value observed for 15–24-year olds in the NCS research, at least for cannabis users in Australia and New Zealand. The reason for a smaller transition probability from cannabis use to cannabis dependence in Germany is unknown.

Interpretation of these crude cross-national epidemiological contrasts is compromised by differences between the samples (e.g., birth cohort follow-up in NZ versus cross-sectional sampling in the USA, as well as age structure differences). In order to facilitate a more direct and refined comparison between these studies, it will be necessary to conduct new analyses of the original data, with derivation of statistical approximations based upon survival analysis methods, with an opportunity for covariate adjustments, and with greater attention to the value of direct cross-national comparisons, age by age (e.g., see Wagner & Anthony, 2002a). Through these survival analysis methods, it will be possible to estimate the cumulative occurrence of cannabis use by any given age (e.g., by age 18 and 21 years), and also to estimate the cumulative occurrence of cannabis dependence by that same age. It is not yet possible to derive these more directly comparative estimates using published data from these several independent studies.

Some other limited cross-national comparisons of cannabis dependence prevalence now are possible, with publication of Epidemiologic Catchment Area (ECA)- and NCS-like surveys in multiple countries. For example, Russell *et al.* (1994) found an estimated 5.9% of Edmonton (Canada) residents to qualify as cases of DSM-III cannabis use disorders, a value slightly larger than corresponding estimate of 4.4% from the ECA surveys in the USA (e.g., see Anthony & Helzer, 1991). A new set of cross-national prevalence comparisons of this type will become possible with completion of a new multi-national program of representative probability sample studies, entitled the "World Mental Health Surveys," which includes modules and standardized assessments of cannabis use and dependence. These epidemiological surveys, now being completed in more than 32 countries of the world, are following a common protocol. This approach will reduce methodological sources of variation that otherwise complicate cross-national comparisons of the type described in the first part of this section (e.g., see Vega *et al.*, 2002).

## *Variation In Relation to Time*

It might be useful to compare and contrast secular trends in the occurrence of cannabis dependence while we are comparing and contrasting cross-national findings as observed in studies conducted during the late 20th century. However, we actually have no readily interpretable time trends in the rates of cannabis dependence, with a recent comparative exception that involved two points in time. This comparison was presented by Compton *et al.* (2004), who argued that prevalence of active cannabis use in the USA was the same in 2001–2002 as in 1991–1992, but prevalence of cannabis use disorders increased from 1.2% to 1.5%, a small but apparently statistically robust increase. Available time trends with respect to incidence of cannabis *use* (such as the trends depicted above) generally must suffice unless we wish to turn to historical data or to official administrative statistics subject to special biases.

With respect to historical data within the USA, we can find survey-based evidence of temporal trends in a 30-year old report from a presidentially sponsored Commission on Marihuana and Drug Abuse in the USA (e.g., United States, National Commission on Marihuana and Drug Abuse, 1972). On the basis of a national survey undertaken by the President's Commission in the early 1970s, the following estimates were obtained:

On the basis of the Commission-sponsored National Survey, we [the Commission members] have concluded that contemporary marihuana use is pervasive, involving all segments of the U.S. population. The Survey estimated that about 24 million Americans over the age of 11 years (15% of the adults 18 and over, and 14% of the 12–17 year olds) have used marihuana at least once, referred to in this Report as ever-users.

...

Twenty-nine percent of the adult [ever-users] and 43% of the youth [ever-users] reported that they are still using marihuana. When asked why they had terminated use, the overwhelming majority of adults (61%) specified, among other reasons, that they had simply lost interest in the drug.

... 2% of the adults and 4% of the youth who have ever used marihuana are heavy users: they use the drug several times daily. A very small fraction of these heavy users may be very heavy users, who are intoxicated most of their waking hours and probably use very potent preparations of the drug.

...

... the United States is at the present time in a fortunate position. All of the studies available to the Commission have indicated that only a minute number of Americans can be designated as very heavy marihuana users. These studies uniformly indicate that chronic, constant intoxication with very potent cannabis preparations is exceedingly rare in this country (United States, National Commission on Marihuana and Drug Abuse, 1972, Chapter II).

To make a comparison of cannabis consumption across the years from the Commission's survey in the early 1970s to a more recent date, we can turn to data based upon recent survey procedures roughly comparable to those used by the Presidential Commission – namely, data from the CY1999 and CY2000 NHSDA. These surveys found that by the end of CY2000 an estimated 76–77 million individuals in the survey population had tried cannabis at least once, representing 34–35% of the population over the age of 11 years, 18–19% of 12–17-year olds, 45–47% of 18–25-year olds, and 34–35% of persons age 26 years and older – substantially larger values than those observed by the commission. A total of 24–25% of the "ever-users" in the total population were still using cannabis, as defined by use in the year prior to assessment. Corresponding values for persons in the 12–17, 18–25, and 26+ age ranges were estimated, respectively, as 73%, 52%, and 14–15% – also substantially larger than the commission's estimates.

With respect to the "heavy use" category designated by the National Commission, it is possible to identify a roughly comparable but somewhat more broadly encompassing "heavy use" segment of the cannabis user group within the CY2000 NHSDA survey population – namely, individuals who used cannabis on 20 or more days during the month prior to assessment. In CY2000, an estimated 1.6% of the "ever-users" qualified for this broader category of heavy use; corresponding values for those aged 12–17 years, 18–25 years, and 26+ years were, respectively, 3%, 4%, and 1% – values not too distant from the Commission-observed values from the early 1970s, despite the slightly broader CY2000 specification for "heavy use" (SAMHSA, 2001).

These "heavy use" categories reflect a degree of cannabis involvement that is daily or weekly, neither of which are required for DSM-III, DSM-IIIR, or DSM-IV diagnostic criteria for cannabis dependence. Accordingly, ECA survey estimates, obtained during the interval between 1980 and 1984, indicated that some 4–5% of adults had developed into cases of DSM-III cannabis use disorders; about 2.5% had developed cannabis dependence (DSM-III criteria; DIS assessment), and an estimated two-thirds of the cannabis dependence cases remained recent users of cannabis (Anthony & Helzer, 1991). The NCS estimate, obtained between 1990 and 1992, indicated that 4–5% of 15–54-year olds had become cannabis dependent (DSM-IIIR criteria; CIDI assessment), also with about 60% remaining recent cannabis users (Anthony *et al.*, 1994; Warner *et al.*, 1995). Drawing upon data from the National Longitudinal Alcohol Epidemiology Study conducted in the USA during the early 1990s, Grant (1996) reports values for overall drug dependence that are substantially lower than these cannabis dependence estimates from the ECA and NCS surveys. The same research team has produced a more recent survey with somewhat larger estimates for prevalence of active cannabis use disorders (e.g., see Compton *et al.*, 2004).

As backdrop to the Commission recommendation in favor of "partial prohibition" policy with respect to simple possession and use of cannabis, the President's Commission members noted with concern an upsurge in the number of federal cannabis arrests, from 523 arrests in 1965 to 3323 arrests in 1971 (US, 1972). The number of federal prison inmates due to prosecution and sentencing under federal cannabis laws continued to grow and crossed the 100,000 mark some years after release of the commission report in 1974. During the three decades since 1970, the annual number of marijuana arrests in the USA has grown to just under 500,000. During the same span, cannabis has become much more prominent among admissions to drug treatment programs. National level drug treatment statistics for the USA in 1999 show 220,000 cases admitted to publicly funded treatment, with cannabis listed as the case's primary drug of abuse, 57% counted as originating in a criminal justice referral (e.g., from a drug court). The value observed in 1999 was almost double the value from 1993. Expressed epidemiologically as a treatment admission rate, in 1993 the rate of admission to treatment for a primary cannabis problem was 55 cases per 100,000 US residents 12 years or older, and in 1999, the rate was 103 per 100,000 residents (DASIS Report, SAMHSA, 2002a).

Trying to explain the previously mentioned apparent increases in the numbers of officially recognized cases with cannabis problems, one might note a trend of increased THC content of cannabis, with the idea that the greater THC of smoked cannabis might now be placing cannabis users at greater risk of becoming dependent (e.g., see Hall & Swift, 2000, for a pertinent discussion, as well as Compton *et al.*, 2004). Indeed, some observers have commented that these increases might account for the observed increases in the number of cases admitted to treatment with a primary diagnosis of cannabis problems. However, if we look back to estimates from the National Commission's survey in the early 1970s and to estimate from the more recent surveys, we generally see no substantial increases in the occurrence of cannabis dependence or heavy cannabis use in the community populations under study within the USA, with one noteworthy exception (Compton *et al.*, 2004). Something other than the prevalence of cannabis dependence and heavy use must explain the substantially increased numbers of arrests and admissions to treatment. One viable explanation is an increasing judicial use of treatment as an alternative to incarceration in criminal justice facilities during a renaissance of interest in the "partial prohibition" position of the earlier President's Commission on Marihuana and Drug Abuse. This possibility could be intensified by an increased social sentiment that the consequences of a criminal record and jail time may be more harmful than the consequences of cannabis use.

### Variation In Relation to Characteristics of Individuals: Sociodemographics

As reported recently in several papers, age is the most striking sociodemographic characteristic associated with the occurrence of first-time cannabis use (Chen & Kandel, 1995; Gfroerer *et al.*, 2002; Wagner & Anthony, 2002a). Onset of cannabis dependence also shows a strong age dependence, with more than 90% of cases in the USA arising between age 15 and age 35, and an extremely low probability of becoming cannabis dependent after age 40. If cannabis dependence is going to develop, it typically surfaces within the first 10 years after cannabis use, which tends to occur before age 30 (Wagner & Anthony, 2002a). Evidence from other countries seems congruent (e.g., see DeWit *et al.*, 1997; Perkonnig *et al.*, 1998, 1999; Swift *et al.*, 2001b). For a very large proportion of cannabis users, the duration of smoking is quite limited, with high quit rates in the first years after onset of use when cessation generally occurs without clinical or other intervention (e.g., see Chen & Kandel, 1995; DeWit *et al.*, 1997; Kandel & Raveis, 1989; von Sydow *et al.*, 2001). Labouvie *et al.* (1997) regard cannabis and other illegal drug use as an adolescent-limited phenomenon; they urge focus on the following:

(a) delaying onset of illegal drug use to late adolescence or beyond;
(b) intervening with active young adult drug users to reduce levels of use.

With respect to sex/gender, a male excess generally is noted, but there is recent evidence of convergence in risk of starting cannabis use among females and males (e.g., see Gfroerer *et al.*, 2002). Lynskey *et al.* (2002) found cannabis dependence to have occurred among 15% of the male twins and among only 8% of the female twins. Based on the NCS in the USA, some 6–7% of men had developed cannabis dependence versus 2.3% of women (Anthony *et al.*, 1994).

With respect to race-ethnicity, minority status may confer excess risk, perhaps due to associated social disadvantage. In the USA, estimates of persistent cannabis use have tended to be larger for Native American/American Indian heritage members of the population, and in New Zealand, Fergusson and Horwood (2000) describe excess risk for people of Maori heritage. The recent report from Compton *et al.* (2004) suggests that men and women of African heritage have experienced marked increases in prevalence of cannabis use disorders, but does not explain whether this is due to an increase in risk of becoming a case or in a possibly increased duration of cannabis use disorders.

### *Variation In Relation to Other Characteristics of Individuals*

As the causes and pathogenesis of cannabis dependence are being highlighted in other sections of this chapter and other chapters of this book, this subsection draws attention only to a few emerging new issues in epidemiological research on cannabis use and dependence, each of which merits some attention in new research.

With respect to educational attainment and social status, there may have been a change in relationships since the early 1970s when cannabis use was overrepresented among college-attenders. In recent estimates, there are no strong education or social status differences (e.g., see Anthony *et al.*, 1994; Furr-Holden & Anthony, 2003; O'Malley & Johnston, 2002).

### *Personality Traits*

Brook and colleagues (e.g., D. W. Brook *et al.*, 2002; J. S. Brook *et al.*, 1999a, 2002) focus on early conventionality as a predictor of onset and later progression of cannabis involvement. Masse and Tremblay (1997) seek to explain early onset of drug use, including cannabis, in relation to high novelty seeking and low harm avoidance, but not reward dependence. Rios-Bedoya *et al.* (2004) held constant early aggression, rule-breaking, and unconventionality and found that risk of starting cannabis use by age 20–24 was greater in relation to an early childhood measure of risk-taking propensities.

*Psychiatric Disturbances*

Clinical case reports and anecdotes link cannabis dependence with psychiatric disturbances such as mood disorders, but epidemiological evidence is mixed, in part because most studies have been cross-sectional without the resolving power of fine-grained time-to-event data required to check for reciprocities, and in part because most cannabis dependence cases use other drugs as well. Degenhardt *et al.* (2001a, b) found that cannabis use was not associated with presence of affective or anxiety disorders once neuroticism, demographics, and other drug use were taken into account. Chen *et al.* (2003) found a modestly excess risk of major depressive episode (MDE) in association with cannabis use, within the context of a statistical model that held constant many alternative explanatory variables, including tobacco use.

*Pubertal Timing*

Lanza and Collins (2002) report on novel longitudinal latent transition analyses; they find that adolescent girls with more advanced pubertal development are more likely to become cannabis users and to transition to higher levels of cannabis involvement. To the extent that early-onset cannabis use is linked to greater risk of cannabis dependence, puberty timing may deserve more detailed investigation.

*Frequent Geographic Relocation*

Recently, DeWit (1998) expressed occurrence of cannabis problems as a function of frequent geographic relocation of residence during the years of one's youth and found a noteworthy association, especially for males in their prospective study sample. Once confirmed by replication, this association and others just noted can be probed for causal significance and possible preventative importance.

## Variation In Relation to Socially Shared Characteristics of Individuals or Environments

Several new issues and studies merit attention in relation to this category of predictors. For example, a profile of mental health and behavioral disturbances is being studied as possible consequences of socially shared exposure to traumatic events such as the September 11th terrorist attacks, as well as individually-experienced events such as child neglect or abuse (e.g., see Lynskey *et al.*, 2002). In a recent report, Vlahov *et al.* (2002) present evidence consistent with a possible increase in cannabis use among New York city area residents who suffered clinical features resembling post-traumatic stress disorder in the aftermath of the terrorist attack. The increases in cannabis use do not appear to be as pronounced as the increases in other drug use. Nevertheless, this source of variation in cannabis involvement creates some new opportunities for research on social contagion or diffusion processes that might tend to promote cannabis use in communities or social groups more generally.

### Diffusion Processes

Seeking evidence on diffusion processes that influence community incidence and prevalence of cannabis involvement, Bobashev and Anthony (1998, 2000) applied a novel contextualizing multi-level "alternating logistic regressions" approach in research on community-level clustering of cannabis involvement. They discovered that the degree of clustering of cannabis involvement within US neighborhoods is on the same order of magnitude as clustering of diarrheal diseases within villages of the developing world. There is neighborhood-level clustering in the early stages of cannabis involvement (e.g., opportunities to try cannabis) and in the later stages (e.g., daily cannabis use). In addition, within neighborhoods, the magnitude of clustering of daily cannabis use among male residents is greater than the magnitude of clustering of daily cannabis use among female residents. These new observations are consistent with diffusion processes at work within US neighborhoods, and within peer groups of the neighborhoods. They are also consistent with hypothesized in-migration of cannabis users to some neighborhoods and not to others for example, differential migration into neighborhoods where cannabis smoking is more tolerated, where there is less police presence, or where there are higher levels of availability of cannabis for sale. These uncertainties should help to motivate new longitudinal research on these diffusion processes and alternative explanations for the now-documented clustering.

*The Context of Military Environments*

Enlistment and service in the US Army and National Guard appear to be inversely associated with cannabis use and dependence. Between 1997 and 2000, only 0.51% of thousands of Army urinalysis results tested positive for cannabinoids; the corresponding value for the National Guard was 1.7%. The expected value based on civilian urinalysis programs during that period was 6.3% (Bruins *et al.*, 2002). This descriptive or predictive relationship may actually be attributable to the program of periodic urinalysis screening for drugs within the military; it may be a consequence of anticipatory screening or other selection processes that would combine to foster low cannabis prevalence within the military. Or, it may be due to other factors, such as an attenuation of the just-described diffusion processes by which cannabis can spread from person to person within and between social groups.

*Antidrug Advertising*

With limited experimental control of error, Block *et al.* (2002) have found that recall of anti-drug advertising has an inverse association with occurrence of cannabis use. As with the previously mentioned lead for new research on unconventionality and cannabis involvement, this study merits close inspection and systematic replication, especially with randomization designs and sustained longitudinal follow-up to bring into balance some of the possible confounding variables, and to clarify whether it is the recall of advertising that is suppressing the cannabis use, or vice versa. If confirmed, this association may have important implications for future prevention efforts via mass media campaigns. However, advertising has a spotty record of success in this domain, and definitive evidence on the effectiveness of these campaigns is scarce (e.g., see Palmgreen *et al.*, 2001).

## Why Do Some People Become Cannabis Dependent When Others Do Not?

The advantages of epidemiology's attention to community samples already has been discussed within the introductory sections of this chapter, where it can be seen that epidemiological samples have advantages over samples of help-seeking or arrested cannabis users in studies of nosology and classification. Similar advantages accrue when epidemiologically informed community samples are drawn for research in the domains of pathogenesis and etiology of cannabis dependence, where clinical samples may be subject to special selection biases (e.g., those that distinguish help-seekers or treated cases from the majority of cases who remain untreated). Pandina and Johnson (1990) have included a discussion of this methodological challenge for etiological research in their report of empirical research on serious drug problems experienced by adolescents with and without a family history of alcoholism.

Once there is an appreciation of the value of epidemiological concepts, principles, and methods in the context of etiological research, it is possible to generate a long list of covariates that might be investigated as contributing causes of cannabis use and dependence in particular and illegal drug use and dependence in general (e.g., see Petraitis *et al.*, 1998; West, 2001). For many years of the 20th century, sociologically and social psychologically oriented theories held sway. During the final decades of the 20th century, the pendulum started to swing in the direction of field studies within behavior genetics and genetic epidemiology, as well as continuing progress in the bench sciences of molecular biology, molecular genetics, and neuroscience. Selected examples of each type will be discussed in this chapter.

## *A History of Other Forms of Drug Dependence*

The ECA program within the USA included follow-up assessments that produced prospectively gathered data on the risk of becoming a case of drug use disorders, as defined by DSM-III criteria. Chen and Anthony (1991) identified incident (newly onset) cases of drug use disorders within the ECA sample and matched them to non-cases who lived in the same local area neighborhoods in order to constrain the influences of socially shared local characteristics (e.g., street level availability of drugs). They then used the method of conditional logistic regression to study antecedent antisocial personality (ASP) disorder, antecedent alcohol dependence and related problems, and other suspected causes of drug dependence. In the process, they found that adult community residents with a baseline history of DSM-III alcohol use disorder were 4.8 times more likely to become incident cases of DSM-III drug use disorder (mainly cannabis dependence) during the 1-year span of the ECA follow-up study, even with statistical adjustment for multiple alternative sources of variation in risk of drug dependence; the association was statistically significant by conventional standards ($p < 0.001$). In a sub-analysis, they restricted the sample to individuals who had started to use illegal drugs before the baseline assessment so as to focus on the transition from use to dependence. In this sub-analysis, there remained an excess risk of drug dependence among drug users with a history of alcohol use disorders; the relative risk (RR) estimate from conditional logistic regression was 4.01 (also with $p < 0.001$). This type of evidence has helped to build a case that a history of other forms of drug dependence in general or alcohol dependence specifically might qualify as an important contributing cause of cannabis dependence. That is, effective treatment of the alcohol use disorders found at baseline assessment during the ECA study might have resulted in a reduced risk of cannabis dependence in that sample during the follow-up interval (Chen & Anthony, 1991).

A more recent investigation, the Harvard Twin Study (HTS), has strengthened the epidemiological evidence about associations linking cannabis dependence with other forms of drug dependence, with a discovery that may challenge the just-mentioned possibility for preventive intervention. What has been discovered is that the associations among alcohol and other drug use disorders may be traced back, in part, to a common vulnerability influenced by both genetic and environmental factors (Tsuang *et al.*, 1998, 2001). More specifically, analyzing HTS data, True *et al.* (1999) found that the genetic liability for clinical features of cannabis dependence was due to a 36% specific contribution (i.e., specific to cannabis dependence) and an 8% contribution from genetic influence common with clinical features of alcohol dependence. Common family environmental sources of variation were found for conduct problems, alcohol dependence, and cannabis dependence. Nonetheless, each category of drug except psychedelics had genetic influences unique to itself, in addition to common underlying vulnerability traits of a genetic–environmental character. A subsequent analysis of data from a separate sample of female twins, conducted by Kendler and colleagues, has led to a somewhat different conclusion, with evidence balanced more in favor of a common vulnerability with respect to a profile of illegal drug use, and against any specific genetic or familial environmental factors (see Karkowski *et al.*, 2000).

The existence of common vulnerability traits that lead to associations between alcohol dependence and cannabis dependence does not eliminate the possibility of interventions to reduce risk of cannabis dependence by intervening in the earlier alcohol dependence process. Indeed, both chickenpox and shingles share a common vulnerability in the form of infection by the varicella-zoster virus (VZV), which is the root cause of both chickenpox in childhood or adolescence (for most people) and shingles decades later in adulthood (for most people). Nonetheless, antiviral intervention when a child has a severe case of chickenpox might prevent or reduce the later risk of shingles for that child (e.g., see discussion by Anthony, 2002).

## ASP Disorder

Robins (1998) has reviewed evidence linking ASP disorder and related conduct problems to later risk of drug dependence. As noted above, Chen and Anthony (1991) studied ASP as a suspected cause of drug dependence in their prospective study based on neighborhood-matched ECA residents. Their multiple logistic regression model showed an excess risk of drug dependence among individuals with a baseline ASP history, even with statistical adjustment for alcohol use disorders and the other covariates mentioned above (RR = 5.25; $p = 0.009$). But in the case of ASP, there was some moderate attenuation of an RR estimate when the analysis was focused on the transition from illegal drug use to onset of drug dependence (RR = 3.41; $p = 0.066$). Hence, the evidence may be interpreted as being consistent with an ASP influence on risk of becoming drug dependent in adulthood (again mainly cannabis dependence), but the influence may be in relation to onset of illegal drug use on the way to drug dependence, as opposed to an influence on the transition from use to dependence. (Here, the $p$-value of 0.066 may make some observers concerned that actually there is no ASP-drug dependence association in these prospective study data.) In this context, it is also worth noting that the HTS has produced pertinent evidence on this topic. True *et al.* (1999) also studied conduct disorder (part of the ASP prodrome) in their work, and found a common vulnerability that accounts for at least some of the observed association between conduct disorder and marijuana dependence. In this instance, True and colleagues reported that the common vulnerability may be due largely to shared environmental influences (True *et al.*, 1999).

## Primary Socialization Theory

There is some evidence that cannabis involvement might depend upon a social psychological process of bonding with primary socialization sources and the transmission of norms through those sources. This idea falls under the heading of a "primary socialization theory" developed by Oetting and colleagues (e.g., see Oetting, 1999), but has been incorporated within many of the conceptual models of illegal drug use investigated by National Institute on Drug Abuse (NIDA) supported research teams. For example, the research team led by Brook and Brook has stressed the importance of parent–child bonding in this respect. Their team offers a suggestion that parent–child bonding can be cultivated deliberately as a protective or buffering process to reduce risk of cannabis involvement when children are growing up within environments characterized by high levels of violence or when fathers have histories of active or recent illegal drug use (e.g., see J. S. Brook *et al.*, 1998, 1999a, b, 2002; D. W. Brook *et al.*, 2002).

Of course, social bonding can occur within the context of deviant peer groups as well. For example, research on the New Zealand sample studied by Lynskey *et al.* (1998) shows links between earlier affiliation with delinquent and drug-using peers and later excess risk of cannabis involvement. In the Christchurch birth cohort, Fergusson *et al.* (2002b) found affiliation with deviant peers to be more strongly associated with cannabis problems in the earlier adolescent years as compared with the later years in adolescence and in young adulthood. As for the research of Hofler *et al.* (1999) and von Sydow *et al.* (2002), with its longitudinal study of adolescents followed to young adulthood in Germany, higher levels of affilation with drug-using peers predicted onset of cannabis use and regular cannabis use, but not cannabis dependence, which depended more strongly upon parental death before age 15 years, deprived socioeconomic status, and baseline use of illegal drugs other than cannabis.

*Religion, Religiosity, Spirituality*

Another form of social bond links individuals to religion, promotes church attendance and is promoted by church attendance, and fosters religiosity or spirituality. Recently analyzing NCS data on a variety of drugs in order to clarify relationships observed within the USA, Miller *et al.* (2000) found that cannabis use and cannabis dependence were inversely associated with personal devotion (a personal relationship with the divine); there was also an inverse association with respect to affiliation with a more fundamentalist religious denomination. However, no such association (inverse or otherwise) was found in relation to a correlated characteristic of "personal conservatism" (as expressed in a personal commitment to teaching and living according to creed). Chen and colleagues (Chen, 2003; Chen *et al.*, 2004a, b) found evidence that religion and religiosity may influence cannabis involvement by constraining or delaying first chances to try this drug. Generally supportive evidence about religion, religiosity, and spirituality has accumulated over the years (e.g., see Amey *et al.*, 1996; Johanson *et al.*, 1996; Tennant *et al.*, 1975; Wallace & Forman, 1998), with recent structural equations modeling to illuminate effects of theistic beliefs and religious/spiritual practices on drug-taking, as well as possible mediational pathways involving religious beliefs about the sinfulness of drug use and levels of peer religiousness. Twin studies suggest that the observed evidence of possible protective influences of religion are not simply due to some underlying common genetic susceptibility (e.g., see Heath *et al.*, 1999;

Kendler *et al.*, 1997), and potential gene–environment interactions merit close inspection (e.g., see Koopmans *et al.*, 1999).

## Parents and Parenting

Whereas parents can be positive sources of primary socialization, with suspected effects in the form of reduced risk of cannabis involvement (e.g., see Chilcoat & Anthony, 1996), they may also have other effects, as when parents are illegal drug users (e.g., see Lynskey *et al.*, 1998). Some of this early research on parents, parenting, and cannabis use had a focus on the influence parents might exert via supervision and monitoring of their children or via bonding or discipline processes. Neiderhiser *et al.* (1999) have marshaled evidence that adolescent children are not passive recipients of this parenting behavior – they are active shapers of the parenting behavior, and this reciprocity of child and parenting behaviors is important to study and to understand if we are to gain more definitive evidence on the suspected causal roles of parents and parenting in relation to cannabis involvement.

## Family History and Genetics

As described above, a growing body of evidence is consistent with the influences of genetic sources of variation in relation to the degree of cannabis involvement, including exposure to the first chances to try cannabis, the transition to first use, onset of cannabis dependence among users, and ultimate cessation of cannabis use. For example, epidemiological methods were used to obtain a nationally representative sample of twin pairs in the USA and to study MZ and DZ resemblance of recent (past year) cannabis use (Kendler *et al.*, 2002). In this study, a greater MZ concordance relative to DZ concordance led to an estimated heritability of 60%, a finding of some influence by family environment, and possibly by a special twin environment (i.e., unique to the twins within the family). Whereas the work of Kendler's program of research on female twins and male twins has led to similar estimates of heritability of cannabis involvement for males and females, this similarity has not always been true. A twin study by Lynskey *et al.* (1998) provides one exception, and it seems that in samples of American twins described by Maes *et al.* (1999) and by Miles *et al.* (2001), there is evidence of more influence of shared family environment than has been true for the samples assembled by Kendler and colleagues.

The work of Kendler's twin study program is of additional special interest because of its attention to some of the difficult methodological challenges faced in twin studies. For example, in their study of female twins and cannabis dependence, Kendler and Prescott (1998) consider the possibility that their estimates of cannabis dependence heritability might be inflated by social contact between the co-twins (e.g., via co-twin sharing of cannabis material). However, they also present evidence that, in their sample, the heritability estimate was no more than modestly inflated by such social contact.

The work of the HTS has been especially important for the epidemiology of cannabis dependence because of its decomposition of cannabis involvement into stages, with cannabis transitions being found to be subject to some degree of genetic influence, as also was true for amphetamine and cocaine, but not for three other drugs under study (Tsuang *et al.*, 1999). Lyons and colleagues (1997) have worked with the HTS twin data to illuminate subjective response to cannabis ingestion as a crucial element in the pathways leading from genetic influences to the transition from first use to increased levels of cannabis involvement.

In one of the most recent twin studies, with a focus specifically upon cannabis dependence, Lynskey *et al.* (2002) found an array of suspected causal factors in association with presence of cannabis dependence: educational attainment, exposure to parental conflict, sexual abuse, major depression, social anxiety, and childhood conduct disorder. After statistical control for these potentially influential covariates, there was evidence of substantial genetic influence on cannabis dependence, with some 15–72% of the variation explained by genetic factors, perhaps as much as 40% by shared environmental factors, and 26–45% by non-shared environmental factors. However, the wide confidence bounds associated with these estimates leads to tempered confidence. In addition, as contrasted with many other studies, no male–female difference in these estimates was found. However, Lynskey *et al.* (2002) were able to specify equally well-fitting models for males and females that did involve different relative emphases on these factors.

Interpretation of results from twin studies entails complexities that may not be apparent to all readers. For example, the observed variation in estimates of heritability of cannabis involvement may depend upon the relative availability of cannabis from place to place, the stage of cannabis involvement under study, whether the investigator has taken into account the environmental character of cannabis use, as well as other matters of a more general character. As an example of the latter, it is possible that active gene–environment correlations grow in importance during adolescence. This possibility has been examined by Elkins *et al.* (1997) and may be particularly pertinent when making comparisons of estimates and findings from studies of twin children as young as

8 years of age, who are at the beginning of the period of risk for starting cannabis use, versus studies of young adults as old as 25 years of age, who are at the end of that period of risk. Indeed, the challenges of gene–environment interaction often are swept under the rug in twin research, and generally deserve more attention than they are given by investigators and by readers.

### Directions for New Research

Under this third rubric of causal research on cannabis dependence, in the future we may see more hierarchical or multi-level research that will build upon the studies described above. For example, Diehr *et al.* (1993) offered a theoretically oriented overview of community contextual effects on individual health behaviors, which would encompass cannabis use and its consequences such as cannabis dependence. The work of Bobashev and Anthony (1998, 2000), described under the second rubric, depicts a pattern of clustering of cannabis involvement that might be induced by contextual effects. Wright and Zhang (1998) analyzed NHSDA data on perceptions and beliefs about cannabis use (e.g., the degree of risk or harm associated with regular cannabis smoking), using a multi-level model and found evidence of both neighborhood and family effects, in addition to individual-level sources of variation. Delva *et al.* (2001) used a hierarchical model and found positive associations between mothers using illegal drugs and their living in neighborhoods with higher occurrence of illegal drug use. These studies represent beginning steps in a line of causal research that will include the individual's "host" characteristics in the array of suspected causal determinants of cannabis involvement, and will nest these host characteristics within the context of family or larger neighborhood and community characteristics.

### Mechanisms: Pathogenesis, Natural History, and Consequences of Cannabis Dependence

Examples of epidemiological research on the pathogenesis, natural history, and consequences of cannabis use and dependence encompass studies of the "gateway" processes described by Kandel and Yamaguchi (1993), and the cessation of cannabis use (e.g., see Chen & Kandel, 1998), as well as investigations of cognitive, psychiatric, or other general medical complications of heavy cannabis use or cannabis dependence (e.g., see Chen *et al.*, 2002; Eisen *et al.*, 2002; Fried *et al.*, 2002; Wilcox *et al.*, 2002).

*Early Stages*

For cannabis dependence to occur, there must be a first chance to try cannabis, and for many populations in the world there is limited or no cannabis dependence because there is no chance to try cannabis. Investigations on the first chance to try cannabis have been reported by Chen *et al.* (2004a); Dormitzer *et al.* (2004); Grady *et al.* (1986); Stenbacka *et al.* (1993); Van Etten *et al.* (1997); Wagner and Anthony (2002b), among others. Wagner and Anthony (2002b) confirmed an initial finding by Van Etten and Anthony (1999) to the effect that in the USA, males are more likely than females to have had chance to try cannabis, but once females have the chance to try cannabis, they are just as likely as males to smoke cannabis. The "exposure opportunity" represented by this first chance to try cannabis appears to be central in the "gateway" phenomenon that links cannabis involvement to prior tobacco or alcohol use and onward to later use of illegal drugs like cocaine (e.g., see Wagner & Anthony, 2002b).

Research on early-onset drug use and later increased risk of drug problems has encompassed investigations into early-onset cannabis use as a suspected determinant of later increased risk of cannabis dependence. That is, initial observations about this association gave rise to optimism that it might be possible to prevent later, more serious drug involvement by delaying the onset of initial drug use (e.g., see Hanna & Grant, 1999; Lewinsohn *et al.*, 1999; Robins & Pryzbeck, 1985; Tennant *et al.*, 1975) or that it might be possible to prevent health or psychosocial complications in young adulthood if only we might delay or prevent early-onset cannabis use (e.g., see Brook *et al.*, 2002). Subsequently, some investigators have challenged this optimistic perspective. For example, Fergusson and Horwood (1997) presented Christchurch birth cohort study evidence that the observed associations linking early-onset cannabis use with later problems were largely explained by two facts: those with early cannabis use (a) were "a high risk population characterized by social disadvantage, childhood adversity, early onset behavioral difficulties and adverse peer affiliations," and (b) were more likely to have post-onset affiliation with delinquent and substance-using peers, to move away from home, and to drop out of school. If so, an intervention seeking a specific delay of early onset cannabis use without addressing these other contributory psychosocial liabilities may have much less impact on risk of later cannabis dependence than one might hope. On the other hand, the prognostic significance of early-onset cannabis use has withstood a series of methodologically-oriented challenges (e.g., see Anthony & Petronis, 1995; Chen & Anthony, 2003).

## Natural History In Relation to Clinical Features

Several research teams have tried to characterize the emergence of clinical features during the natural history of cannabis dependence, either in terms of frequency or in terms of order of appearance (Coffey *et al.*, 2002; Rosenberg & Anthony, 2001; Wagner & Anthony, 2002a). Wagner and Anthony (2002a) produced NCS-based estimates for risk of developing the DSM-IIIR cannabis dependence syndrome, for each year of use after first use, which are presented in Figure 4.3. First published in the journal *Neuropsychopharmacology*, these epidemiological estimates depict how the risk of DSM-IIIR cannabis dependence might climb from relatively low values during the 1st year of cannabis use to a value of almost 2% by the start of the 3rd year of use. Thereafter, the risk of developing cannabis dependence for someone in the 4th year of cannabis use is about 2%, and then in the 5th year the risk of becoming cannabis dependent drops toward zero values.

Figure 4.3 has special value because it provides comparative data to show how onset of cocaine dependence occurs explosively after first cocaine use, with a peak value of about 5% in the first 1–2 years after first cocaine use – that is, within 1–2 years of first cocaine use, about 5% of users have developed the DSM-IIIR cocaine dependence syndrome. Thereafter, the risk of developing cocaine dependence drops off, year by year, and by the 4th year after first

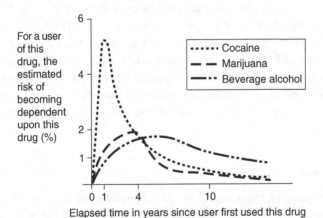

Figure 4.3 Estimated risk of developing DSM-IIIR dependence upon cocaine, marijuana, and beverage alcohol, plotted in relation to the number of elapsed years since the age at first use of the drug. From data reported by Wagner and Anthony (2002a), based upon estimates from the National Comorbidity Survey, USA, 1990–1992. Reproduction with permission of copyright holder or James C. Anthony (2002).

cocaine use, the risk has dropped to the 2% level. The risk curve for beverage alcohol is similar to that of marijuana until the 4th or 5th year after first use. Thereafter, during the 6–10th years after first use, risk of a drinker becoming alcohol dependent continues at a relatively stable level of about 1–2% per year, whereas risk of a cannabis user becoming cannabis dependent drops sharply toward values well under 1% in each successive year of use after the 5th year.

Analyzing the data from one of the large-sample longitudinal studies of young people in Australia (described in a prior section), Coffey *et al.* (2002) found that 91% of their cannabis dependent cases had experienced a persistent desire to stop or reduce use; 84% unintentional use; 74% withdrawal; 74% excessive time obtaining or using cannabis; 63% continued use despite health problems; 21% tolerance; 18% social consequences. As compared with alcohol-dependent users, the cannabis-dependent users were considerably more likely to report compulsive and out-of-control use, as well as withdrawal symptoms.

Rosenberg and Anthony (2001) conducted an epidemiologic study of the natural history of cannabis dependence by completing life-table analyses to show emergence of each clinical feature over the course of the condition and by providing statistical summaries in the form of mean and median age of onset of each clinical feature, and related indices. The data were from a follow-up of the Baltimore ECA sample, originally assessed in 1981 and re-assessed roughly 13–14 years later, and comparisons were made between the cannabis experiences of the 37 cannabis dependent cases in the sample versus 521 cannabis users with insufficient problems to qualify for the DSM-IIIR cannabis dependence diagnoses. These life table analyses showed that the most rapidly emerging clinical features among cannabis dependence cases were subjectively felt loss of control over cannabis and continued cannabis use despite knowledge of harm. In contrast, subjectively felt withdrawal symptoms tended to emerge later and for a much smaller proportion of both cannabis dependence cases and non-cases.

## Consequences

A very intriguing and provocative line of epidemiological research on the suspected consequences of cannabis use involves harnessing the monozygotic co-twin pair design to estimate long-term risk of subsequent harms as a function of the cannabis use of twin pairs ascertained epidemiologically. In this approach, there is a search within the epidemiological sample for MZ twins who are discordant for a suspected adverse consequence of cannabis use (e.g., divorce, hospitalization for a psychiatric problem), and then an application of appropriate matched pair statistical procedures to estimate an RR of the response as might be associated with the cannabis use of one twin but not the other. Eisen *et al.* (2002) have demonstrated an application of this method, studying a profile of medical and psychosocial adversities that might befall cannabis users, as well as health-related quality of life. The conclusion of their study was "Previous heavy marijuana use a mean of 20 years earlier by a group of men who reported no other significant illicit drug use does not appear to be associated with adverse sociodemographic, physical, or mental health adverse effects."

Against this evidence from a research design that holds constant underlying vulnerability traits (via MZ matching), it is of interest to note the results from a longitudinal study of school-attending youths, in which early adolescent cannabis use was found to be associated with a variety of psychosocial response variables in a profile that included personality traits such as rebelliousness as well as events such as being fired from a job and collecting welfare payments (D. W. Brook, J. S. Brook, *et al.*, 2002). This longitudinal study held constant many of the suspected alternative sources of variation in these responses, but did not have control over underlying vulnerability traits such as those discussed by Eisen *et al.* (2002) in the MZ co-twin study and by Fergusson and Horwood (1997) in their longitudinal study of the Christchurch (NZ) birth cohort. A similar critique may be offered in relation to the very interesting but incomplete study reported by Buchmueller and Zuvekas (1998). In this recent study of drug use and income in the USA, the investigators found that, for young adults, there was a positive relationship between drug use and income. This was not the case for young workers with daily drug use. In addition, for "prime-age" men (age 30–45 years), there was an indication of lower income in association with problematic drug use (e.g., as exemplified in the clinical features of cannabis dependence). However, in the study design, there was too little consideration of possible confounding via common vulnerability factors (i.e., vulnerabilities that lead toward co-occurrence of daily cannabis use and lower income).

Working within the domain of psychiatric disturbances, Hall and Degenhardt (2000) as well as Buhler *et al.* (2002) recently have summarized the available epidemiological evidence on cannabis use and psychosis, leaving room for doubt that cannabis use causes psychoses, with more substantial evidence that cannabis use may complicate the lives and clinical pictures of individuals who already have started to suffer the clinical features of schizophrenia or who fall within the spectrum of schizophrenia. It should be said, however, that there is some supportive epidemiological evidence to link cannabis use with psychosis or psychosis-like experiences. For example, Tien and Anthony's nested case-control study within the ECA sample, with prospectively gathered data and experimental control of suspected confounding covariates, disclosed an excess risk of delusion- and hallucination-like experiences among daily cannabis users as compared to non-users (Tien & Anthony, 1990). Furthermore, van Os *et al.* (2002) recently published results from a larger and more definitive study, including some additional evidence that cannabis use may be linked to an increased risk of newly incident psychoses. This domain of inquiry will remain a fruitful one for some time, given that it is not possible to conduct experiments that expose individuals to cannabis at random, and there are many possibilities for uncontrolled confounding – given lifestyle and other differences between cannabis users and non-users.

Differences between cannabis users and non-users also complicate other inquiries into the health and social consequences of cannabis involvement. For example, also within the psychiatric and neuropsychological domains, there are now mixed results from studies of the impact of cannabis on cognitive functioning and the affective disorders. For example, some studies indicate minimal or no long-term cognitive impairments associated with cannabis use (e.g., see Fried *et al.*, 2002; Lyketsos *et al.*, 1999); other studies suggest impairments of apparent clinical significance (e.g., see Solowij *et al.*, 2002).

Degenhardt *et al.* (2001a, b) found that statistical adjustments for neuroticism, sociodemographic variables, and other drug use were sufficient to yield a null association between cannabis use and rates of affective and anxiety disorders. Some studies have suggested otherwise (e.g., Rey *et al.*, 2002).

Focusing upon DSM-III MDE in a recent analysis of NCS data, Chen *et al.* (2003) found a modestly excess risk of MDE in association with prior use of cannabis, especially in relation to (a) levels of cannabis involvement as indexed by the cannabis dependence diagnosis, and (b) accumulated frequency of cannabis use. In this analysis, it was possible to include statistical controls for an array of suspected confounding covariates, including tobacco smoking, but measures of neuroticism were not available. For this reason, and because the strength of the observed association was relatively modest with an RR estimate of about 2.0, the authors concluded that cannabis use and cannabis dependence probably were not strong predictors or causes of major depression. Quite clearly, new prospective research on these associations is needed if this field is to make new progress. In order to secure definitive evidence about a causal role of cannabis use or cannabis dependence in the context of psychiatric comorbidities, it may be necessary to use randomized experiments in which cannabis use or dependence is experimentally ameliorated, with follow-up of the experimental subjects to see if risk of major depression is reduced with effective clinical intervention directed toward the cannabis involvement. This conclusion was also reached recently after completion of generally inconclusive and mixed prospective studies of the tobacco–depression relationship (Wu & Anthony, 1999).

### Fetal Exposure

The long-term consequences of fetal exposure to maternal cannabis use have also been the subject of some epidemiological inquiries. In a series of papers on a prospective study, a Canadian research group led by Peter Fried has described neuropsychological impairments associated with fetal exposures to cannabis (e.g., Fried & Smith, 2001; Fried *et al.*, 2002). Fergusson *et al.* (2002a) studied self-reports of cannabis use within a large epidemiological sample of mothers recruited during pregnancy and found that frequent and regular cannabis use during pregnancy might be a contributing cause to small but statistically detectable decrements in birthweight. However, the overall conclusion was that use of cannabis during pregnancy was not associated with increased risk of perinatal mortality or morbidity.

With respect to future research in this domain, we may anticipate an increasing use of multivariate statistical models that express transitions and progressions from the earlier to the later stages of cannabis dependence as a function of suspected causal determinants, with due consideration for buffering or moderating influence. Studies of recurrent events should also become increasingly frequent, in accompaniment with development of new statistical models for handling data on times to recurrent event. Of course, this increased reliance upon statistical modeling can lead to complications, not only in relation to complicated structural equations models, but also in relation to the less complex approach of multiple logistic regression (e.g., see Hays & Revetto, 1990; McKnight *et al.*, 1999).

### Prevention, Intervention, Amelioration, and Control

To date, epidemiology's contribution to research on prevention, intervention, amelioration, and control of cannabis dependence has been indirect. The past cannabis-oriented epidemiological studies on these topics have been concerned with use of cannabis and not with altering the probability of transitioning from first use to first appearance of a cannabis dependence syndrome. Regrettably, there is meager evidence of prevention impact on cannabis use, except in some relatively small but important and especially vulnerable subgroups of the population (e.g., see Palmgreen *et al.*, 2001). The work of Holder *et al.* (1999) and a report from an NAS/NRC task panel led by Professor Charles Manski (Manski *et al.*, 2001) offer some important directions for future research on this topic in specific and on the more general topic of drug policy research. In addition, it should be noted that crop substitution and youth employment programs are beginning to be discussed, if not already implemented within the total matrix of drug control instruments directed toward cannabis use and the hazards of cannabis use, such as the dependence syndromes.

**Future Directions**

Aside from the just-mentioned opportunities for prevention and intervention research, there are some potentially useful directions for the future research of investigators who seek to improve our current epidemiological evidence on cannabis dependence. Susser and Susser (1996a, b) have provided an important set of guiding principles for new epidemiological research on suspected causal mechanisms; these suggestions are consistent with a move to abandon what we disparagingly call "black box risk factor research." This form of research consists of studies that are based upon overly simplified impulse–response models, without due attention to multivariate relationships and a systems approach.

There is no question that the domain of genetic epidemiology will progress by leaps and bounds, but the most promising developments are likely to start with genome-wide scans and then more focused evaluations of candidate genes, gene products, and modifications through gene–environment interactions. The heyday of twin studies to estimate heritability of cannabis dependence via oversimplified approaches may be over or nearing its end. The discordant MZ co-twin design used by Eisen *et al.* (2002) represents an important advance, and we may expect to see more of this design in research on the causes and consequences of cannabis dependence, as well as innovative sibling, family, and case-control designs with a capacity to disclose gene–environment interactions more clearly (e.g., see Khoury *et al.*, 2000; Risch & Merikangas, 1996; Rowe *et al.*, 1992).

As represented within this chapter, epidemiological research pertinent to cannabis dependence already has progressed by leaps and bounds, with major advances since the cannabis dependence concept was formalized some 20–25 years ago. During the next decade, epidemiologists and epidemiologically oriented investigators will continue to make advances, drawing mainly upon conceptual models and approaches learned during the 20th century. Among the challenges for new investigators with an epidemiological orientation will be avoiding the mistakes of the past, developing enthusiasm for truly innovative 21st century investigations as opposed to the "me too" and "bandwagon" research that represents no more than an incremental improvement in light of 20th century accomplishments, and cultivating optimism regarding sustained federal funds for new and innovative research in this important domain of inquiry.

## References

American Psychiatric Association (1980). *Diagnostic and Statistical Manual of Mental Disorders* (3rd ed.). Washington DC: American Psychiatric Association.

American Psychiatric Association (1987). *Diagnostic and Statistical Manual of Mental Disorders* (3rd ed., revised). Washington DC: American Psychiatric Association.

Amey, C. H., Albrecht, S. L., & Miller, M. K. (1996). Racial differences in adolescent drug use: the impact of religion. *Substance Use and Misuse, 31*, 1311–1332.

Anthony, J. C. (1991). The epidemiology of drug addiction. In N. S. Miller (Ed.), *Comprehensive handbook of drug and alcohol addiction* (pp. 55–86). New York: Marcel Dekker, Inc.

Anthony, J. C. (2002). Death of the "stepping-stone" hypothesis and "gateway" model? Comments on Morral *et al. Addiction, 97*, 1505–1507.

Anthony, J. C., & Helzer, J. E. (1991). Syndromes of drug abuse and dependence. In L. N. Robins, & D. A. Regier (Eds.), *Psychiatric disorders in America: The Epidemiological Catchment Study* (pp. 116–154). New York: The Free Press.

Anthony, J. C., & Petronis, K. R. (1995). Early-onset drug use and risk of later drug problems. *Drug and Alcohol Dependence, 40*, 9–15.

Anthony, J. C., & Van Etten, M. L. (1998). Epidemiology and its rubics. In A. Bellack, & M. Hersen (Eds.), *Comprehensive clinical psychology* (pp. 355–390). Oxford, UK: Elsevier Science Publications.

Anthony, J. C., Warner, L. A., & Kessler, R. C. (1994). Comparative epidemiology of dependence on tobacco, alcohol, controlled substances, and inhalants: Basic findings from the National Comorbidity Survey. *Experimental and Clinical Psychopharmacology, 2*, 244–268.

Anthony, J. C., Neumark, Y., & Van Etten, M. L. (2000). Do I do what I say? A perspective of self report methods in drug dependence epidemiology. In A. A. Stone, J. S. Turkon, & C. A. Bachrach (Eds.), *The science of self report implications for research and practice* (pp. 175–198). Mahwah, NJ: Lawrence C. Erlbaum Associates, Inc.

Anthony, J. C., Reboussin, B. A., Storr, C. L., Wagner-Echeagaray, F., & Chen, C. Y. (2004). *New epidemiological evidence on cannabis dependence syndromes in the United States.* Unpublished manuscript.

Block, L. G., Morwitz, V. G., Putsis Jr., W. P., & Sen, S. K. (2002). Assessing the impact of antidrug advertising on adolescent drug consumption: results from a behavioral economic model. *Americal Journal of Public Health, 92*, 1346–1351.

Bobashev, G. V., & Anthony, J. C. (1998). Clusters of marijuana use in the United States. *American Journal of Epidemiology, 148*, 1168–1174.

96                                                        *James C. Anthony*

Bobashev, G. V., & Anthony, J. C. (2000). Use of alternating logistic regression in studies of drug-use clustering. *Substance Use and Misuse, 35,* 1051–1073.

Brook, J. S., Whiteman, M., Finch, S., Cohen, P. (1998). Mutual attachment, personality, and drug use: pathways from childhood to young adulthood. *Genetic Social General Psychology Monographs, 124*(4), 492–510.

Brook, J. S., Brook, D. W., De La Rosa, M., Whiteman, M., & Montoya, I. D. (1999a). The role of parents in protecting Colombian adolescents from delinquency and marijuana use. *Archives of Pediatric Adolescent Medicine, 153,* 457–464.

Brook, J. S., Kessler, R. C., & Cohen, P. (1999b). The onset of marijuana use from preadolescence and early adolescence to young adulthood. *Developmental Psychopathology, 11,* 901–914.

Brook, D. W., Brook, J. S., Rosen, Z., & Montoya, I. (2002). Correlates of marijuana use in Colombian adolescents: a focus on the impact of the ecological/cultural domain. *Journal of Adolescent Health, 31,* 286–298.

Brook, J. S., Adams, R. E., Balka, E. B., & Johnson, E. (2002). Early adolescent marijuana use: risks for the transition to young adulthood. *Psychological Medicine, 32,* 79–91.

Bruins, M. R., Okano, C. K., Lyons, T. P., & Lukey, B. J. (2002). Drug-positive rates for the Army from fiscal years 1991 to 2000 and for the National Guard from fiscal years 1997 to 2000. *Military Medicine, 167,* 379–383.

Buchmueller, T. C., & Zuvekas, S. H. (1998). Drug use, drug abuse, and labour market outcomes. *Health Economics, 7,* 229–245.

Buhler, B., Hambrecht, M., Loffler, W., an der Heiden, W., & Hafner, H. (2002). Precipitation and determination of the onset and course of schizophrenia by substance abuse – a retrospective and prospective study of 232 population-based first illness episodes. *Schizophrenia Research, 54,* 243–251.

Chen, C. Y. (2003). *Drugs in context: a cross national study of adolescents and their behavioral repertoire.* Baltimore, MD: Johns Hopkins University.

Chen, C. Y., & Anthony, J. C. (2003). Possible age-associated bias in reporting of clinical features of drug dependence: epidemiological evidence on adolescent-onset marijuana use. *Addiction, 98*(1), 71–82.

Chen, C. Y., Wagner, F. A., & Anthony, J. C. (2003). Marijuana use and the risk of major depressive episode. Epidemiological evidence from the United States National Comorbidity Survey. *Social Psychiatry and Psychiatric Epidemiology, 37,* 199–206.

Chen, C. Y., Dormitzer, C. M., Gutierrez, U., Vittetoe, K., Gonzalez, G. B., & Anthony, J. C. (2004a). The adolescent behavioral repertoire as a context for drug exposure: behavioral autarcesis at play. *Addiction, 99*(7), 897–906.

Chen, C. Y., Dormitzer, C. M., Bejarano, J., & Anthony, J. C. (2004b). Religiosity and the earliest stages of adolescent drug involvement in seven countries of Latin America. *American Journal of Epidemiology, 159*(12), 1180–1188.

Chen, C. Y., O'Brien, M. S., & Anthony, J. C. (2005). Who becomes cannabis dependent soon after onset of use? Epidemiological evidence from the United States: 2000–2001. *Drug and Alcohol Dependence, 79*(1), 11–22.

Chen, K., & Kandel, D. B. (1995). The natural history of drug use from adolescence to the mid-thirties in a general population sample. *Americal Journal of Public Health, 85,* 41–47.

Chen, K., & Kandel, D. B. (1998). Predictors of cessation of marijuana use: an event history analysis. *Drug and Alcohol Dependence, 50,* 109–121.

Chen, K., Kandel, D. B., & Davies, M. (1997). Relationships between frequency and quantity of marijuana use and last year proxy dependence among adolescents and adults in the United States. *Drug and Alcohol Dependence, 46,* 53–67.

Chen, V., & Anthony, J. C. (1991). Risk of becoming drug dependent. In J. C. Anthony (Ed.), *Comprehensive handbook of drug and alcohol addiction* (pp. 55–86). New York: Marcel Dekker, Inc.

Chilcoat, H. D., & Anthony, J. C. (1996). Impact on parent monitoring on initiation of drug use through late adulthood. *Journal of the American Academy of Child and Adolescent Pschiatry, 35,* 91–100.

Coffey, C., Carlin, J. B., Degenhardt, L., Lynskey, M., Sanci, L., & Patton, G. C. (2002). Cannabis dependence in young adults: an Australian population study. *Addiction, 97,* 187–194.

Compton, D. R., Dewey, W. L., & Martin, B. R. (1990). Cannabis dependence and tolerance production. *Advances in Alcohol and Substance Abuse, 9,* 129–147.

Compton, W. M., Grant, B. F., Colliver, J. D., Glantz, M. D., & Stinson, F. S. (2004). Prevalence of marijuana use disorders in the United States: 1991–1992 and 2001–2002. *Journal of the American Medical Association, 291*(17), 2114–2121.

Degenhardt, L., Hall, W., & Lynskey, M. (2001a). Alcohol, cannabis and tobacco use among Australians: a comparison of their associations with other drug use and use disorders, affective and anxiety disorders, and psychosis. *Addiction, 96,* 1603–1614.

Degenhardt, L., Hall, W., & Lynskey, M. (2001b). The relationship between cannabis use, depression and anxiety among Australian adults: findings from the National Survey of Mental Health and Well-Being. *Social Psychiatry and Psychiatric Epidemiology, 36,* 219–227.

Degenhardt, L., Lynskey, M., Coffey, C., & Patton, G. (2002). "Diagnostic orphans" among young adult cannabis users: persons who report dependence symptoms but do not meet diagnostic criteria. *Drug and Alcohol Dependence, 67,* 205–212.

Delva, J., Mathiesen, S. G., & Kamata, A. (2001). Use of illegal drugs among mothers across racial/ethnic groups in the United States: a multi-level analysis of individual and community level influences. *Ethnicity and Disease, 11,* 614–625.

Dennis, M., Babor, T. F., Roebuck, M. C., & Donaldson, J. (2002). Changing the focus: the case for recognizing and treating cannabis use disorders. *Addiction, 97* (Suppl. 1), 4–15.

DeWit, D. J. (1998). Frequent childhood geographic relocation: its impact on drug use initiation and the development of alcohol and other drug-related problems among adolescents and young adults. *Addictive Behaviors, 23,* 623–634.

DeWit, D. J., Offord, D. R., & Wong, M. (1997). Patterns of onset and cessation of drug use over the early part of the life course. *Health Education and Behavior, 24,* 746–758.

Diehr, P., Koepsell, T., Cheadle, A., Psaty, B. M., Wagner, E., & Curry, S. (1993). Do communities differ in health behaviors? *Journal of Clinical Epidemiology, 46,* 1141–1149.

Dormitzer, C. M., Gonzalez, G. B., Penna, M., Bejarano, J., Obando, P., Sanchez, M., *et al.* (2004). The PACARDO research project: youthful drug involvement in Central America and the Dominican Republic. *Rev Panam Salud Publica [Journal of the Pan American Health Organization], 15*(6), 400–416.

Eisen, S. A., Chantarujikapong, S., Xian, H., Lyons, M. J., Toomey, R., True, W. R., *et al.* (2002). Does marijuana use have residual adverse effects on self-reported health measures, socio-demographics and quality of life? A monozygotic co-twin control study in men. *Addiction, 97,* 1137–1144.

El-Guebaly, N. A. (2002). International aspects of epidemiology in substance use. Discussion of "The epidemiology of opiate dependence in Canada". Paper presented at the *XII World Congress of Psychiatry,* Yokohama, Japan.

Elkins, I. J., McGue, M., & Iacono, W. G. (1997). Genetic and environmental influences on parent–son relationships: evidence for increasing genetic influence during adolescence. *Developmental Psychology, 33,* 351–363.

Farrell, M. (1999). Cannabis dependence and withdrawal. *Addiction, 94,* 1277–1278.

Fergusson, D., & Horwood, L. (1997). Early onset cannabis use and psychosocial adjustment in young adults. *Scandinavian Journal of Social Medicine, 94,* 279–296.

Fergusson, D. M., & Horwood, L. J. (2000). Cannabis use and dependence in a New Zealand birth cohort. *The New Zealand Medical Journal, 113,* 156–158.

Fergusson, D. M., Lynskey, M. T., & Horword, L. J. (1993). Patterns of cannabis use among 13–14 year old New Zealanders. *The New Zealand Medical Journal, 106,* 247–250.

Fergusson, D. M., Horwood, L. J., & Northstone, K. (2002a). Maternal use of cannabis and pregnancy outcome. *BJOG: An International Journal of Obstetrics and Gynecology, 109,* 21–27.

Fergusson, D. M., Swain-Campbell, N. R., & Horwood, L. J. (2002b). Deviant peer affiliations, crime and substance use: a fixed effects regression analysis. *Journal of Abnormal Child Psychology, 30,* 419–430.

Fried, P., Watkinson, B., James, D., & Gray, R. (2002). Current and former marijuana use: preliminary findings of a longitudinal study of effects on IQ in young adults. *Canadian Medical Association Journal, 166,* 887–891.

Fried, P. A., & Smith, A. M. (2001). A literature review of the consequences of prenatal marihuana exposure. An emerging theme of a deficiency in aspects of executive function. *Neurotoxicology and Teratology, 23,* 1–11.

Furr-Holden, C. D. M., & Anthony, J. C. (2003). Epidemiologic difference in drug dependence: a US–UK cross-national comparison. *Social Psychiatry and Psychiatric Epidemiology, 38,* 165–172.

Gfroerer, J. C., Wu, L.-T., & Penne, M. A. (2002). *Initiation of marijuana use: trends, patterns, and implications.* Rockville, MD: Substance Abuse and Mental Health Services, Office of Applied Sciences.

Golub, A., & Johnson, B. D. (2001). Variation in youthful risks of progression from alcohol and tobacco to marijuana and to hard drugs across generations. *American Journal of Public Health, 91*, 225–232.

Grady, K., Gersick, K. E., Snod, D. L., & Kessen, M. (1986). The emergence of adolescent substance use. *Journal of Drug Education, 16*(3), 203–220.

Grant, B. F. (1996). Prevalence and correlates of drug use and DSM-IV drug dependence in the United States: results of the National Longitudinal Alcohol Epidemiologic Survey. *Journal of Substance Abuse, 8*, 195–210.

Hall, W., & Degenhardt, L. (2000). Cannabis use and psychosis: a review of clinical and epidemiological evidence. *Australia and New Zealand Journal of Psychiatry, 34*, 26–34.

Hall, W., & Swift, W. (2000). The THC content of cannabis in Australia: evidence and implications. *The Australian and New Zealand Journal of Public Health, 24*, 503–508.

Hanna, E. Z., & Grant, B. F. (1999). Parallels to early onset alcohol use in the relationship of early onset smoking with drug use and DSM-IV drug and depressive disorders: findings from the National Longitudinal Epidemiologic Survey. *Alcoholism, Clinical and Experimental Research, 23*, 513–522.

Hays, R. D., & Revetto, J. P. (1990). Peer cluster theory and adolescent drug use: a reanalysis. *Journal of Drug Education, 20*, 191–198.

Heath, A. C., Madden, P. A., Grant, J. D., McLaughlin, T. L., Todorov, A. A., & Bucholz, K. K. (1999). Resiliency factors protecting against teenage alcohol use and smoking: influences of religion, religious involvement and values, and ethnicity in the Missouri Adolescent Female Twin Study. *Twin Research, 2*, 145–155.

Hofler, M., Lieb, R., Perkonigg, A., Schuster, P., Sonntag, H., & Wittchen, H. U. (1999). Covariates of cannabis use progression in a representative population sample of adolescents: a prospective examination of vulnerability and risk factors. *Addiction, 94*, 1679–1694.

Holder, H., Flay, B., Howard, J., Boyd, G., Voas, R., & Grossman, M. (1999). Phases of alcohol problem prevention research. *Alcoholism, Clinical and Experimental Research, 23*, 183–194.

Johanson, C. E., Duffy, F. F., & Anthony, J. C. (1996). Associations between drug use and behavioral repertoire in urban youths. *Addiction, 91*, 523–534.

Johnston, L. D., O'Malley, P. M., & Bachman, J. G. (2001). *Monitoring the future national results on adolescent drug use: overview of key findings 2001.* Bethesda, MD: National Institute on Drug Abuse.

Kandel, D., & Yamaguchi, K. (1993). From beer to crack: developmental patterns of drug involvement. *American Journal of Public Health, 83*, 851–855.

Kandel, D. B., & Raveis, V. H. (1989). Cessation of illicit drug use in young adulthood. *Archives of General Psychiatry, 46*, 109–116.

Karkowski, L. M., Prescott, C. A., & Kendler, K. S. (2000). Multivariate assessment of factors influencing illicit substance use in twins from female–female pairs. *American Journal of Medical Genetics, 96,* 665–670.

Kendler, K. S., & Prescott, C. A. (1998). Cannabis use, abuse, and dependence in a population-based sample of female twins. *The American Journal of Psychiatry, 155,* 1016–1022.

Kendler, K. S., Gardner, C. O., & Prescott, C. A. (1997). Religion, psychopathology, and substance use and abuse: a multimeasure, genetic–epidemiologic study. *The American Journal of Psychiatry, 154,* 322–329.

Kendler, K. S., Neale, M. C., Thornton, L. M., Aggen, S. H., Gilman, S. E., & Kessler, R. C. (2002). Cannabis use in the last year in a US national sample of twin and sibling pairs. *Psychological Medicine, 32,* 551–554.

Khoury, M., Burke, W., & Thomson, E. (2000). *Genetics and public health in the 21st century: using genetic information to improve health and prevent disease.* New York: Oxford University Press.

Kokkevi, A., Terzidou, M., Politikou, K., & Stefanis, C. (2000). Substance use among high school students in Greece: outburst of illicit drug use in a society under change. *Drug and Alcohol Dependence, 58,* 181–188.

Koopmans, J. R., Slutske, W. S., van Baal, G. C., & Boomsma, D. I. (1999). The influence of religion on alcohol use initiation: evidence for genotype X environment interaction. *Behavior Genetics, 29,* 445–453.

Krausz, M., Haasen, C., Reimer, J., Basdekis, R., & Karow, A. (2002). International aspects of epidemiology in substance use. Discussion of "Epidemiological aspects of opiate dependence in Europe". Paper presented at the *XII World Congress of Psychiatry,* Yokohama, Japan.

Labouvie, E., Bates, M. E., & Pandina, R. J. (1997). Age of first use: its reliability and predictive utility. *Journal of Studies on Alcohol, 58,* 638–643.

Lanza, S. T., & Collins, L. M. (2002). Pubertal timing and the onset of substance use in females during early adolescence. *Prevention Science, 3,* 69–82.

Lewinsohn, P. M., Rohde, P., & Brown, R. A. (1999). Level of current and past adolescent cigarette smoking as predictors of future substance use disorders in young adulthood. *Addiction, 94,* 913–921.

Lynskey, M. T., Fergusson, D. M., & Horwood, L. J. (1998). The origins of the correlations between tobacco, alcohol, and cannabis use during adolescence. *Journal of Child Psychology and Psychiatry, and Allied Disciplines, 39,* 995–1005.

Lyketsos, C. G., Garret, E., Liang, K. Y., & Anthony, J. C. (1999). Cannabis use and cognitive decline in persons under 65 years of age. *American Journal of Epidemiology, 149,* 794–800.

Lynskey, M. T., Heath, A. C., Nelson, E. C., Bucholz, K. K., Madden, P. A., Slutske, W. S., et al. (2002). Genetic and environmental contributions to cannabis dependence in a national young adult twin sample. *Psychological Medicine, 32,* 195–207.

Lyons, M. J., Toomey, R., Meyer, J. M., Green, A., Eisen, S. A., Goldberg, J., et al. (1997). How do genes influence marijuana use? The role of subjective effects. *Addiction, 92,* 409–417.

Maes, H. H., Woodard, C. E., Murrelle, L., Meyer, J. M., Silberg, J. L., Hewitt, J. K., et al. (1999). Tobacco, alcohol and drug use in eight- to sixteen-year-old twins: the Virginia Twin Study of Adolescent Behavioral Development. *Journal of Studies on Alcohol, 60,* 293–305.

Manski, C. F., Pepper, J. V., & Petrie, C. V. (Eds.) (2001). *Informing America's policy on illegal drugs.* Washington, DC: National Academy Press.

Masse, L. C., & Tremblay, R. E. (1997). Behavior of boys in kindergarten and the onset of substance use during adolescence. *Archives of General Psychiatry, 54,* 62–68.

McKnight, B., Cook, L. S., & Weiss, N. S. (1999). Logistic regression analysis for more than one characteristic of exposure. *American Journal of Epidemiology, 149,* 984–992.

Miles, D. R., van den Bree, M. B., Gupman, A. E., Newlin, D. B., Glantz, M. D., & Pickens, R. W. (2001). A twin study on sensation seeking, risk taking behavior and marijuana use. *Drug and Alcohol Dependence, 62,* 57–68.

Miller, L., Davies, M., & Greenwald, S. (2000). Religiosity and substance use and abuse among adolescents in the National Comorbidity Survey. *Journal of the American Academy of Child and Adolescent Psychiatry, 39,* 1190–1197.

Morgenstern, J., Langenbucher, J., & Labouvie, E. W. (1994). The generalizability of the dependence syndrome across substances: an examination of some properties of the proposed DSM-IV dependence criteria. *Addiction, 89,* 1105–1113.

Morris, J. N. (1957). *Uses of epidemiology.* London, England: Livingstone.

Neiderhiser, J. M., Reiss, D., Hetherington, E. M., & Plomin, R. (1999). Relationships between parenting and adolescent adjustment over time: genetic and environmental contributions. *Developmental Psychology, 35,* 680–692.

Nelson, C. B., Rehm, J., Ustun, T. B., Grant, B., & Chatterji, S. (1999). Factor structures for DSM-IV substance disorder criteria endorsed by alcohol, cannabis, cocaine and opiate users: results from the WHO reliability and validity study. *Addiction, 94,* 843–855.

O'Malley, P. M., & Johnston, L. D. (2002). Epidemiology of alcohol and other drug use among American college students. *Journal of Studies on Alcohol, 14*(Suppl.), 23–39.

Oetting, E. R. (1999). Primary socialization theory. Developmental stages, spirituality, government institutions, sensation seeking, and theoretical implications. V. *Substance Use and Misuse, 34,* 947–982.

Palmgreen, P., Donohew, L., Lorch, E. P., Hoyle, R. H., & Stephenson, M. T. (2001). Television campaigns and adolescent marijuana use: tests of sensation seeking targeting. *American Journal of Public Health, 91,* 292–296.

Pandina, R. J., & Johnson, V. (1990). Serious alcohol and drug problems among adolescents with a family history of alcoholism. *Journal of Studies on Alcohol, 51,* 278–282.

Perkonigg, A., Lieb, R., & Wittchen, H. U. (1998). Prevalence of use, abuse and dependence of illicit drugs among adolescents and young adults in a community sample. *European Addiction Research, 4*, 58–66.

Perkonigg, A., Lieb, R., Hofler, M., Schuster, P., Sonntag, H., & Wittchen, H. U. (1999). Patterns of cannabis use, abuse and dependence over time: incidence, progression and stability in a sample of 1228 adolescents. *Addiction, 94*, 1663–1678.

Petraitis, J., Flay, B. R., Miller, T. Q., Torpy, E. J., & Greiner, B. (1998). Illicit substance use among adolescents: a matrix of prospective predictors. *Substance Use and Misuse, 33*, 2561–2604.

Pickens, R., & Meisch, R. A. (1973). Behavioral aspects of drug dependence. *Minnesota Medicine, 56*, 183–186.

Plant, M., & Miller, P. (2001). Young people and alcohol: an international insight. *Alcohol and Alcoholism, 36*, 513–515.

Poulton, R. G., Brooke, M., Moffitt, T. E., Stanton, W. R., & Silva, P. A. (1997). Prevalence and correlates of cannabis use and dependence in young New Zealanders. *The New Zealand Medical Journal, 110*, 68–70.

Rey, J. M., Sawyer, M. G., Raphael, B., Patton, G. C., & Lynskey, M. (2002). Mental health of teenagers who use cannabis. Results of an Australian survey. *The British Journal of Psychiatry, 180*, 216–221.

Rios-Bedoya, C., Samuels, J. F., Wood, N. P., & Anthony, J. C. (2004). Children taking risks: the association with cocaine and other drug use later in life. Manuscript submitted for publication.

Risch, N., & Merikangas, K. (1996). The future of genetic studies of complex human diseases. *Science, 273*, 1516–1517.

Robins, L. N. (1998). The intimate connection between antisocial personality and substance abuse. *Social Psychiatry and Psychiatric Epidemiology, 33*, 393–399.

Robins, L. N., & Przybeck, T. R. (1985). Age of onset of drug use as a factor in drug and other disorders. *National Institute on Drug Abuse Research Monograph, 56*, 178–192.

Rosenberg, M. F., & Anthony, J. C. (2001). Early clinical manifestations of cannabis dependence in a community sample. *Drug and Alcohol Dependence, 64*, 123–131.

Rowe, D. C., Rodgers, J. L., & Meseck-Bushey, S. (1992). Sibling delinquency and the family environment: shared and unshared influences. *Child Development, 63*, 59–67.

Russell, J. M., Newman, S. C., & Bland, R. C. (1994). Epidemiology of psychiatric disorders in Edmonton. Drug abuse and dependence. *Acta Psychiatrica Scandinavica, 376*(Suppl.), 54–62.

Solowij, N., Stephens, R. S., Roffman, R. A., Babor, T., Kadden, R., Miller, M., *et al.* (2002). Cognitive functioning of long-term heavy cannabis users seeking treatment. *The Journal of the American Medical Association, 287*, 1123–1131.

Stenbacka, M., Allebeck, P., & Romelsjo, A. (1993). Initiation into drug abuse: the pathway from being offered drugs to trying cannabis and progression to intravenous drug abuse. *Scandinavian Journal of Social Medicine, 21*, 31–39.

Substance Abuse and Mental Health Services Administration, Office of Applied Studies (2001). *Summary of findings from the 2000 National Household Survey on Drug Abuse* (NHSDA Series H-13, DHHS Publication No. (SMA) 01-3549). Rockville, MD: Substance Abuse and Mental Health Services Administration, Office of Applied Studies.

Substance Abuse and Mental Health Services Administration, Office of Applied Studies (2002a). *The DASIS report: marijuana treatment admissions increase 1993–1999.* Rockville, MD: Substance Abuse and Mental Health Services Administration, Office of Applied Studies.

Substance Abuse and Mental Health Services Administration, Office of Applied Studies (2002b). *National Household Survey on Drug Abuse: Main findings 1998.* Rockville, MD: Substance Abuse and Mental Health Services Administration, Office of Applied Studies.

Substance Abuse and Mental Health Services Administration, Office of Applied Studies (2002c). *National Survey on Drug Use and Health.* Retrieved June 1, 2004, from http://www.oas.samhsa.gov/NHSDA/2k2NSDUH.

Substance Abuse and Mental Health Services Administration, Office of Applied Studies (2002d). *Results from the 2001 National Household Survey on Drug Abuse: Volume I. Summary of National Findings* (NHSDA Series H-17, DHHS Publication No. (SMA) 02-3758). Rockville, MD: Substance Abuse and Mental Health Services Administration, Office of Applied Studies.

Susser, M., & Susser, E. (1996a). Choosing a future for epidemiology. I. Eras and paradigms. *American Journal of Public Health, 86,* 668–673.

Susser, M., & Susser, E. (1996b). Choosing a future for epidemiology. II. From black box to Chinese boxes and eco-epidemiology. *American Journal of Public Health, 86,* 674–677.

Swift, W., Hall, W., & Teesson, M. (2001a). Cannabis use and dependence among Australian adults: results from the National Survey of Mental Health and Well-Being. *Addiction, 96,* 737–748.

Swift, W., Hall, W., & Teesson, M. (2001b). Characteristics of DSM-IV and ICD-10 cannabis dependence among Australian adults: results from the National Survey of Mental Health and Well-Being. *Drug and Alcohol Dependence, 63,* 147–153.

Tennant Jr., F. S. Detels, R., & Clark, V. (1975). Some childhood antecedents of drug and alcohol abuse. *American Journal of Epidemiology, 102,* 377–385.

Tien, A. Y., & Anthony, J. C. (1990). Epidemiological analysis of alcohol and drug use as risk factors for psychotic experiences. *The Journal of Nervous and Mental Disease, 178,* 473–480.

True, W. R., Heath, A. C., Scherrer, J. F., Xian, H., Lin, N., Eisen, S. A., *et al.* (1999). Interrelationship of genetic and environmental influences on conduct disorder and alcohol and marijuana dependence symptoms. *American Journal of Medical Genetics, 88,* 391–397.

Tsuang, M. T., Lyons, M. J., Meyer, J. M., Doyle, T., Eisen, S. A., Goldberg, J., et al. (1998). Co-occurrence of abuse of different drugs in men: the role of drug-specific and shared vulnerabilities. *Archives of General Psychiatry, 55,* 967–972.

Tsuang, M. T., Lyons, M. J., Harley, R. M., Xian, H., Eisen, S., Goldberg, J., et al. (1999). Genetic and environmental influences on transitions in drug use. *Behavior Genetics, 29,* 473–479.

Tsuang, M. T., Bar, J. L., Harley, R. M., & Lyons, M. J. (2001). The Harvard Twin Study of Substance Abuse: what we have learned. *Harvard Review of Psychiatry, 9,* 267–279.

United Nations Office for Drug Control and Crime Prevention. (2002). *Global illicit drug trends 2002.* New York: United Nations Office on Drugs and Crime.

United States National Commission on Marihuana and Drug Abuse (1972). *Marihuana: a signal of misunderstanding.* Washington, DC: US Government Printing Office.

Van Etten, M. L., & Anthony, J. C. (1999). Comparative epidemiology of initial drug opportunities and transitions to first use: marijuana, cocaine, hallucinogens and heroin. *Drug and Alcohol Dependence, 54,* 117–125.

Van Etten, M. L., Neumark, Y. D., & Anthony, J. C. (1997). Initial opportunity to use marijuana and the transition to first use: United States 1979–1994. *Drug and Alcohol Dependence, 49,* 1–7.

van Os, J., Bak, M., Hanssen, M., Bijl, R. V., de Graaf, R., & Verdoux, H. (2002). Cannabis use and psychosis: a longitudinal population-based study. *American Journal of Epidemiology, 156,* 319–327.

Vega, W. A., Aguilar-Gaxiola, S., Andrade, L., Bijl, R., Borges, G., Caraveo-Anduaga, J. J., et al. (2002). Prevalence and age of onset for drug use in seven international sites: results from the international consortium of psychiatric epidemiology. *Drug and Alcohol Dependence, 68*(3), 285–297.

Vlahov, D., Galea, S., Resnick, H., Ahern, J., Boscarino, J. A., Bucuvalas, M., et al. (2002). Increased use of cigarettes, alcohol, and marijuana among Manhattan, New York, residents after the September 11th terrorist attacks. *American Journal of Epidemiology, 155,* 988–996.

von Sydow, K., Lieb, R., Pfister, H., Hofler, M., Sonntag, H., & Wittchen, H. U. (2001). The natural course of cannabis use, abuse and dependence over four years: a longitudinal community study of adolescents and young adults. *Drug and Alcohol Dependence, 64,* 347–361.

von Sydow, K., Lieb, R., Pfister, H., Hofler, M., & Wittchen, H. U. (2002). What predicts incident use of cannabis and progression to abuse and dependence? A 4-year prospective examination of risk factors in a community sample of adolescents and young adults. *Drug and Alcohol Dependence, 68,* 49–64.

Wagner, F. A., & Anthony, J. C. (2002a). From first drug use to drug dependence: developmental periods of risk for dependence upon marijuana, cocaine, and alcohol. *Neuropsychopharmacology, 26,* 479–488.

Wagner, F. A., & Anthony, J. C. (2002b). Into the world of illegal drug use: exposure opportunity and other mechanisms linking the use of alcohol, tobacco, marijuana, and cocaine. *American Journal of Epidemiology, 155,* 918–925.

Wallace Jr., J. M., & Forman, T. A. (1998). Religion's role in promoting health and reducing risk among American youth. *Health Education Behavior, 25*, 721–741.

Wallace Jr., J. M., Forman, T. A., Guthrie, B. J., Bachman, J. G., O'Malley, P. M., & Johnston, L. D. (1999). The epidemiology of alcohol, tobacco and other drug use among black youth. *Journal of Studies on Alcohol, 60*, 800–809.

Warner, L. A., Kessler, R. C., Hughes, M., Anthony, J. C., & Nelson, C. B. (1995). Prevalence and correlates of drug use and dependence in the United States. Results from the National Comorbidity Survey. *Archives of General Psychiatry, 52*, 219–229.

West, R. (2001). Theories of addiction. *Addiction, 96*, 3–13.

Wilcox, H. C., Wagner, F. A., & Anthony, J. C. (2002). Exposure opportunity as a mechanism linking youth marijuana use to hallucinogen use. *Drug and Alcohol Dependence, 66*, 127–135.

World Health Organization (1992). The ICD-10 classification of mental and behavioral disorders: clinical descriptions and diagnostic guidelines. Geneva: World Health Organization.

Wright, D., & Zhang, Z. (1998). *Hierarchical models applied to the National Household Survey on Drug Abuse*. www.amstat.org/sections/SRMS/proceedings/papers/1998_128.pdf

Wu, L. T., & Anthony, J. C. (1999). Tobacco smoking and depressed mood in late childhood and early adolescence. *American Journal of Public Health, 89*, 1837–1840.

Wu, L., Korper, S. P., Marsden, M. S., Lewis, C., & Bray, R. M. (2003). *Use of incidence and prevalence in the substance use literature: a review*. Rockville, MD: Substance Abuse and Mental Health Services Administration, Office of Applied Studies.

Zoccolillo, M., Vitaro, F., & Tremblay, R. F. (1999). Problem drug and alcohol use in community sample adolescents. *Journal of the American Academy of Child and Adolescent Psychiatry, 38*, 900–907.

# 5

# The Adverse Health and Psychological Consequences of Cannabis Dependence

WAYNE HALL AND NADIA SOLOWIJ

People who become dependent on cannabis are more likely than infrequent users to experience any of the adverse health effects that are caused by chronic cannabis use. Dependent cannabis use is rare in comparison with the more prevalent pattern of experimental and intermittent use (Bachman *et al.*, 1997), but it may nonetheless affect as many as 1% of adults in the USA and Australia in any 1 year (Anthony *et al.*, 1994; Hall *et al.*, 1999a). Dependent cannabis users typically smoke two or more cannabis cigarettes a day over periods of years or decades in a minority of cases (Copeland *et al.*, 2001; Solowij, 2002; Swift *et al.*, 1998b).

This chapter summarizes the most probable adverse health effects that cannabis-dependent persons are at increased risk of experiencing. With few exceptions (e.g., Solowij *et al.*, 2002; Taylor *et al.*, 2000), the literature does not directly assess the adverse health effects of cannabis dependence. The most probable effects can nonetheless be inferred from the more common studies of the effects of long-term daily cannabis use because many daily users are dependent on cannabis (Swift *et al.*, 1998a, 2001). The chapter reviews evidence on the adverse health effects of more or less daily use over periods of years during young adulthood, and among those who seek treatment in their mid-thirties who have used cannabis more or less daily for the past 15–20 years. These effects are organized in approximate order of prevalence and confidence that the relationship is causal (Hall & Babor, 2000a).

## Assessing Health Effects of Chronic Cannabis Use

A major difficulty in appraising the adverse health effects of chronic cannabis use is a dearth of good epidemiological evidence on the long-term health consequences of cannabis use, and problems in interpreting the evidence that is available (Hall & Pacula, 2003; Hall *et al.*, 1999b). Much of the evidence comes from North America, although more work is beginning to be reported from Australia (e.g., Swift *et al.*, 1998a), the Netherlands (e.g., van Os *et al.*, 2002), and New Zealand (e.g., Fergusson *et al.*, 2000), where there are relatively high rates of cannabis use among young adults.

The value of these epidemiological studies is often weakened by difficulties in excluding alternative explanations of associations observed between cannabis use and adverse health outcomes (Hall *et al.*, 1999b). Heavy cannabis use, for example, is correlated with alcohol and tobacco use, both of which adversely affect health in ways that may be difficult to distinguish from the effects of cannabis (e.g., respiratory disease and motor vehicle accidents). These interpretative issues are highlighted in the following review.

**The Respiratory Risks of Cannabis Smoking**

Over the past two decades, cross-sectional and longitudinal studies in the USA have shown that people who are regular smokers of cannabis but not tobacco have more symptoms of chronic bronchitis than non-smokers (see Tashkin, 1999, for a review). The immunological competence of the respiratory system in people who only smoke cannabis is also impaired, increasing their susceptibility to infectious diseases, such as pneumonia (Tashkin, 1999).

A prospective study was recently conducted by Taylor *et al.* (2000, 2002) who studied symptoms of respiratory disease and respiratory function in 1037 New Zealand youths who were followed from birth until age 21. They compared symptoms of respiratory disease and respiratory function in those who were cannabis dependent, cigarette smokers, and non-smokers of tobacco and cannabis. After adjusting for the effects of tobacco use, it was found that cannabis-dependent subjects had higher rates of wheezing, shortness of breath, chest tightness, and morning sputum production in comparison to non-smokers. The effects of cannabis dependence on respiratory symptoms were "generally similar to and occasionally greater than for tobacco smokers of 1–10 cigarettes/day" (Taylor *et al.*, 2000, p. 1673). A significantly higher proportion of cannabis-dependent subjects also had evidence of impaired respiratory function. The adverse effects of tobacco and cannabis smoking were additive.

Taylor *et al.* (2002) reported a follow-up of this cohort to age 26 years in which analyses were undertaken of the cumulative effects of cannabis on respiratory function (objectively assessed by forced expiratory volume and vital capacity). The study assessed cannabis use at ages 18, 21, and 26 years, and carefully controlled for the effects of cigarette smoking assessed at the same ages. The heaviest cannabis users (900 or more occasions of use by age 26 years) had

2.6–7% reductions in lung function. The authors argued that given the short time frame of the follow-up, "the trend suggests that continued cannabis smoking has the potential to result in clinically important impairment of lung function" (p. 1055).

In very long-term cannabis users who are also often regular tobacco smokers, cannabis smoking appears to exacerbate the adverse respiratory effects of tobacco smoking (Tashkin, 1999). For example, half of the participants who had smoked cannabis for 20 years studied in Australia reported symptoms of chronic bronchitis (Swift *et al.*, 1998b) and most of these were or had also been regular tobacco smokers. This was double the rate of symptoms reported by their age peers who did not smoke cannabis.

### Chronic Cannabis Use and Respiratory Cancers

Cannabis smoking could be a cause of cancer if tetrahydrocannabinol (THC) or the substances generated when cannabis is burnt produced genetic mutations in somatic cells exposed to cannabis smoke (such as those in the lung). There is only weak evidence that THC is "mutagenic" in this sense (MacPhee, 1999). THC can produce changes in cellular processes in animal cells in the test tube, altering cell metabolism, DNA synthesis, and cell division (MacPhee, 1999). These changes, however, probably delay or stop cell division rather than produce cellular changes that may lead to cancer (MacPhee, 1999). There is no evidence that THC and other cannabinoids produce mutations in microbial assays used to assess mutagenicity, such as the Ames test (MacPhee, 1999; Marselos & Karamanakos, 1999). Indeed, there is some evidence that THC and other cannabinoids may have anti-tumor activity in cell cultures and in animals (Guzman, 2003).

Cannabis *smoke* is mutagenic in the test tube, and hence is a potential carcinogen (Marselos & Karamanakos, 1999). Cannabis smoke produces chromosomal aberrations, is mutagenic in the Ames test, and causes cancers in the mouse skin test (MacPhee, 1999). The fact that cannabis smoke is carcinogenic suggests that any cancers caused by cannabis smoking are most likely to occur in organs that receive long-term exposure to carcinogens in cannabis smoke, such as the lungs, the aerodigestive tract (mouth, tongue, esophagus), and the bladder (Hall & MacPhee, 2002).

There are good reasons for suspecting that cannabis may cause cancers of the lung and the aerodigestive tract (Hall & MacPhee, 2002). First, tobacco is a cause of respiratory cancer and cannabis smoke contains many of the same carcinogens as tobacco smoke (Marselos & Karamanakos, 1999). Second, chronic cannabis smokers show many of the pathological changes in lung cells that precede the development of cancer in tobacco smokers (Tashkin, 1999).

Cancers have been reported in the aerodigestive tracts of young adults who have been chronic cannabis smokers (Donald, 1991; Taylor, 1988). In many cases, members of this group were also cigarette smokers and alcohol consumers, but Caplan and Brigham (1990) reported two cases of cancer of the tongue in men aged 37 and 52 years who neither smoked tobacco nor consumed alcohol. A history of long-term daily cannabis use was their only shared risk factor. These reports raise a suspicion but provide limited support for the hypothesis that cannabis use is a cause of upper respiratory tract cancers. They do not compare rates of cannabis use in cases and controls, and cannabis exposure has been assessed retrospectively, knowing that the user has cancer.

Sidney *et al.* (1997) studied cancer incidence during an 8.6-year follow-up of 64,855 members of the Kaiser Permanente Medical Care Program. Participants were asked about cannabis use during medical screening (average age 33 years) between 1979 and 1985 and followed up for a mean of 8.6 years. At study entry, 38% had never used cannabis, 20% had used it less than 6 times, 20% were former users, and 22% were current cannabis users. There were no more cases of cancer at follow-up when those who had ever used cannabis and current cannabis users were compared to those who had never used cannabis at study entry. There were more tobacco-related cancers among tobacco smokers (regardless of cannabis use) but no more among cannabis smokers. Males who had ever smoked cannabis had an increased risk of prostate cancer (relative risk, RR = 3.1), and so did males who were current cannabis smokers (RR = 4.7).

Zhang *et al.* (1999) compared rates of cannabis use among 173 persons with primary squamous cell carcinoma of the head and neck and 176 controls who were blood donors matched on age and sex from the same hospital. Cases were more likely to have used cannabis than controls (14% and 10%, respectively), with a 2.6 odds ratio (OR) for cannabis smoking after adjusting for cigarette smoking, alcohol use, and other risk factors. The cases with cancer smoked cannabis more often and for longer than the controls. The relationship between cannabis smoking and these cancers was stronger among adults under the age of 55 years (OR = 3.1).

Two recent studies of oral squamous cell carcinoma have failed to find any association between cannabis use and oral cancers. Llewellyn *et al.* (2004) reported a case–control study of 116 cases (identified from a cancer register) and 207 age and sex matched controls (sampled from the same general practices as the cases). They failed to find any association between self-reported cannabis use and oral cancers in young adults but they only compared people who had used cannabis heavily (10% of the sample) with the majority who reported no use and the prevalence of cannabis use was low.

Rosenblatt *et al.* (2004) reported a more convincing null finding in a larger community-based study of 407 cases and 615 controls aged 18–65 years in Washington state. They found no relationship between the risk of oral squamous cell carcinoma and various indices of cannabis use, including ever versus never used, frequency of use, and duration. They argued that the Zhang *et al.* (1999) study findings arose from bias introduced by the use of blood donors as controls. The prevalence of cannabis use was lower than it should have been among controls, thereby producing a spurious association. By contrast, the prevalence of cannabis use among the controls in Rosenblatt *et al.*'s study was exactly that predicted from population surveys of cannabis use in the USA adult population.

The conflicting findings mean that it is unclear what the risk of oral cancer is among cannabis smokers. The risk appears to be small when compared to those of tobacco and alcohol, especially given the modest increase in RR observed in the only positive study and the good statistical power in the study that failed to detect an association of this size (Rosenblatt *et al.*, 2004). There is also uncertainty about whether the risks of cannabis smoking interact with those of alcohol and tobacco, which many cannabis users also use. Larger cohort studies and larger, well-designed case–control studies of cancers are needed to clarify the relationship between cannabis smoking and cancer risk. These risks may become clearer as the baby boomer birth cohorts (who were the first to smoke cannabis in any numbers) enter the age groups in which cancer incidence begins to rise steeply (Hall & MacPhee, 2002; Rosenblatt *et al.*, 2004).

## Chronic Cannabis Use and Brain Function

Cannabis exerts its most prominent effects on the central nervous system where it acts on an endogenous cannabinoid system that is involved in regulating mood, emotion, memory, attention, and other cognitive functions (Solowij, 1998). Recent animal research has established that cannabinoid receptors play a role in memory storage and retrieval processes (see Iversen, 2003; Piomelli, 2003; Solowij, 2002). The findings from both human and animal research suggest that prolonged use of cannabis alters the functioning of the brain's cannabinoid system but that this does not translate to serious impairment (for recent reviews of the literature, see Ameri, 1999; Solowij, 1999, 2002).

Evidence for structural brain damage in humans following prolonged exposure to cannabis has generally not been sustained (see Solowij, 1998, 1999 for reviews). A recent study used sophisticated measurement techniques to show that frequent but relatively short-term use of cannabis produces neither structural brain abnormalities nor global or regional changes in brain tissue volume or composition that are assessable by magnetic resonance imaging (MRI) (Block *et al.*, 2000a). More recent research has found reduced cortical gray matter and increased white matter in those who commenced using cannabis before the age of 17 years compared to those who started using later (Wilson *et al.*, 2000). The possibility that there may be greater neurotoxic and adverse hormonal and developmental effects of cannabis use in adolescence deserves further attention in research.

A number of studies have demonstrated altered brain function and metabolism in humans following acute and chronic use of cannabis using cerebral blood flow (CBF), positron emission tomography (PET), and electroencephalographic (EEG) techniques. In the most recent carefully controlled study, Block and colleagues (2000b) found that after more than 26 h of supervised abstinence, frequent cannabis users (17 times per week for approximately 4 years) showed substantially lower resting levels of brain blood flow (up to 18%) than controls in a large region of posterior cerebellum and in prefrontal cortex. Similarly, Lundqvist *et al.* (2001) showed lower mean hemispheric and frontal blood flow shortly after cessation of cannabis use. These changes may have direct or indirect effects on cognitive function.

Loeber and Yurgelun-Todd (1999) have proposed that chronic cannabis use results in changes at the cannabinoid receptors that affect the dopamine system. This, in turn, produces a global reduction in brain metabolism, particularly in the frontal lobe and cerebellum. Recent research is increasingly using functional imaging techniques to examine brain activation during the performance of cognitive tasks (e.g., Porrino *et al.*, 2004; Smith *et al.*, 2004; Solowij *et al.*, 2004). Preliminary studies have shown diminished activity in the brains of chronic marijuana users relative to controls, even when the cannabis users abstained from cannabis for 28 days prior to testing (Block *et al.*, 2002; Loeber & Yurgelun-Todd, 1999).

## Chronic Cannabis Use and Cognitive Impairment

Cognitive impairments, particularly short-term memory deficits, are reported by many cannabis-dependent persons who seek help to cease using cannabis, and are often given as one of the main reasons for wanting to stop using cannabis (Solowij, 1998). The evidence from controlled studies, however, indicates that long-term heavy use of cannabis does not appear to produce severe or grossly debilitating impairment of cognitive function like that produced by chronic heavy alcohol use (Solowij, 1998). There is, nonetheless, evidence that long-term or heavy cannabis users show more subtle types of cognitive impairment that are detected in well-controlled studies using sensitive measures.

A major concern with earlier studies of the cognitive effects of chronic cannabis use was that cannabis users might have had poorer cognitive functioning than controls before they started to use cannabis (Solowij, 1998). Recent studies have addressed this problem by matching users and non-users on estimated premorbid intellectual functioning (Solowij, 1998) or on test performance prior to the onset of cannabis use (Block & Ghoneim, 1993; Block *et al.*, 2002; Pope & Yurgelun-Todd, 1996). These studies have found cognitive impairments associated with frequent and/or long-term cannabis use. Frequent users (using at least 7 times per week for 2 years) showed impairment in tests assessing verbal expression, mathematics, and memory (Block & Ghoneim, 1993; Block *et al.*, 2002). Heavy users (using at least 22 of the past 30 days) were more susceptible to interference, made more perseverative errors, had poorer recall, and showed deficient learning compared to light users (who had used no more than 9 times in the past month) (Pope & Yurgelun-Todd, 1996).

Solowij *et al.* (2002) found few impairments when comparing the neuropsychological performance of dependent, heavy cannabis users (near daily) with an average 10 years of regular use to a non-user control group. Heavy users with an average 24 years of regular use, however, showed impaired attention and a generalized memory deficit with impaired verbal learning, retention, and retrieval. Both groups of users showed impaired temporal judgment. In a series of earlier studies, Solowij (1998) used more sensitive measures of brain function (event-related potentials) to demonstrate attentional impairments in shorter-term users (5+ years). In every study, Solowij found that impairment increased with the number of years of cannabis use (Solowij, 1998; Solowij *et al.*, 2002).

While specific deficits in verbal learning, memory, and attention continue to be the most consistently replicated impairments in this population, the deficits are variously attributed to duration of cannabis use (Solowij *et al.*, 2002), frequency of cannabis use (Pope *et al.*, 2001), or cumulative dosage effects (Bolla *et al.*, 2002). The differential effects of the various parameters of cannabis use (frequency, duration, and dose) have not been investigated consistently, and debate continues about whether these deficits should be attributed to lingering acute effects, drug residues, abstinence effects, or gradual changes occurring in the brain as a result of cumulative exposure to cannabis (Pope *et al.*, 1995; Solowij, 1998, 2002; Solowij *et al.*, 2002).

Research continues to investigate the propensity for recovery of cognitive functioning following cessation of cannabis use. Solowij (1998) found partial recovery following a median 2 years abstinence (range 3 months–6 years) in a small group of ex-users performing a selective attention task. Sensitive brain event-related potential measures, however, continued to show impaired information processing that was correlated with the number of years of cannabis use. Bolla *et al.* (2002) found persistent dose-related decrements in neurocognitive performance after 28 days abstinence in heavy young users (mean age 20, 5 years use). Pope *et al.* (2001) reported that memory impairments may recover after 28 days abstinence from cannabis, while in another report based on the same sample (Pope *et al.*, 2002), they found that verbal and memory deficits persisted in those who had commenced cannabis use prior to the age of 17 years but not in those who started later in life. Subjects were between the ages of 30 and 55 years at the time of the study. This finding accords with other findings of adverse effects in those commencing regular cannabis use before versus after the age of 17 years (Ehrenreich *et al.*, 1999; Wilson *et al.*, 2000). Further research is needed to elucidate the impact of cannabis use on the developing brain.

The hippocampus, prefrontal cortex, and cerebellum are major sites of endogenous cannabinoid activity and strongly implicated in the cognitive impairments associated with chronic cannabis use. Functional brain imaging studies hold promise for further investigation of the parameters of cannabis use that are associated with specific short- or long-lasting cognitive deficits and the neurocognitive concomitants of dysfunction (e.g., Porrino *et al.*, 2004; Smith *et al.*, 2004; Solowij *et al.*, 2004).

Lyketsos *et al.* (1999) have reported the only large-scale prospective epidemiological study of the effect of cannabis use on cognitive functioning. They assessed cognitive decline on the Mini Mental State Examination (MMSE) in 1318 adults over 11.5 years. They found no relationship between cannabis use and decline in MMSE score, and this persisted when adjustments were made for age, sex, education, minority status, and use of alcohol and tobacco. The Lyketsos *et al.* study is consistent with other evidence that cannabis use does not produce *gross* cognitive impairment (Solowij, 1998), but for the following reasons it does not exclude the possibility that cannabis use causes more subtle cognitive impairment.

First, only 57% of those initially interviewed were followed up, and those who were not followed up had poorer MMSE scores at first assessment. Second, the MMSE is a screening test for gross cognitive impairment. It tests a restricted set of very simple cognitive functions and it is, therefore, not sensitive to smaller changes in specific cognitive functions. Third, any effect of cannabis use may have been diluted by the inclusion among "heavy users" of people who reported smoking daily or more often for over 2 weeks during any one of the study wave periods. Since cannabis use declines steeply with age (Bachman *et al.*, 1997), few in this sample were likely to be daily cannabis users for any length of time.

## Accidental Injury and Chronic Cannabis Use

Cannabis intoxication produces dose-related impairments in cognitive and behavioral performance, slowing reaction time and information processing, impairing perceptual-motor coordination and motor performance, short-term memory, attention, signal detection, tracking behavior, and time perception (Hall *et al.*, 1994; Solowij, 1998; Ramaekers *et al.*, 2004). These effects increase with the dose of THC, and are larger and more persistent in tasks that require sustained attention (Chait & Pierri, 1992; Hall *et al.*, 1994).

It has been unclear until recently whether these impairments increase the risk of motor vehicle accidents in most cannabis users (Hall *et al.*, 2001). Studies of the effects of cannabis upon on-road driving performance, for example, found modest impairments (Smiley, 1999) as cannabis-intoxicated persons drive more slowly and take fewer risks than alcohol-intoxicated drivers, probably because they are more aware of their psychomotor impairment than alcohol-affected drivers (Smiley, 1999). Epidemiological evidence on the role of cannabis use in fatal motor vehicle accidents had also been equivocal because blood levels of the cannabinoids often studied did not indicate whether a driver or pedestrian was intoxicated at the time of an accident (see Hall *et al.*, 2001 for a review). Moreover, many drivers with cannabinoids in their blood also have a high blood alcohol level at the time of the accident (Hall *et al.*, 2001). The fact that cannabis was rarely found on its own in motor vehicle fatalities was consistent with the epidemiological evidence that cannabis is often used with alcohol (e.g., Hall *et al.*, 2001). The separate effects of alcohol and cannabis on psychomotor impairment and driving performance were approximately additive (Chesher, 1995).

More recent evidence supports an increased risk of accidents among cannabis users who drive. Gerberich *et al.* (2003) analyzed the relationship between self-reported cannabis use and hospitalization for accidental injury in a cohort of 64,657 patients from a Health Maintenance Organization (HMO). Current cannabis users had higher rates of all-cause injury, self-inflicted injury, motor vehicle accidents, and assaults than former cannabis users or non-users, in both men and women. These relationships persisted for all-cause injury after controlling for other variables including alcohol and tobacco use among both men (RR = 1.28) and women (RR = 1.37). The relationships for motor vehicle accidents (RR = 1.96) and assault (RR = 1.90) persisted after statistical adjustment among men but not among women, reflecting much lower rates of both cannabis use and accidents in women than men in the cohort.

Mura *et al.* (2003) reported a case–control study of the relationship between THC and its metabolites in the serum of 900 persons hospitalized for injuries sustained in motor vehicle accidents and 900 controls of the same age and sex admitted to the same French hospitals for reasons other than trauma. The proportion with THC in their sera was higher in cases (10%) than controls (5%) (OR = 2.5). The highest proportion was found among those under the age of 27 years. They did not statistically adjust for blood alcohol level in these analyses but in 60% of their cases THC was found alone.

The convergence of recent evidence suggests that cannabis does increase the risk of motor vehicle crashes (Ramaekers *et al.*, 2004). Studies that have measured THC in blood (rather than inactive metabolites that reflect past use) have found a dose–response relationship between THC and risk of accident. The combination of THC and alcohol produces more marked impairment and increased accident risk (Ramaekers *et al.*, 2004).

**Cardiovascular Effects**

The most consistent physiological effect of cannabis in humans and animals is to increase heart rate (Chesher & Hall, 1999; Jones, 2002). This change parallels the experienced "high" and is related to amount of THC in the blood (Chesher & Hall, 1999). The hearts of healthy young adults are only mildly stressed by these effects (Institute of Medicine, 1999; Jones, 2002; Sidney, 2002). An increased heart rate is most obvious in occasional cannabis users because users become tolerant to these effects of THC within 24 h in laboratory studies and, in some cases, even large amounts of cannabis had little effect on heart rate (Chesher & Hall, 1999; Jones, 2002). The development of tolerance to these effects has also been observed in field studies of chronic heavy cannabis users in Costa Rica, Greece, and Jamaica. These studies failed to find any evidence of cardiac toxicity related to cannabis use (Chesher & Hall, 1999).

There are a number of concerns about the effects of cannabis use on patients with ischemic heart disease, hypertension, and cerebrovascular disease (Jones, 2002; Sidney, 2002). These include the possibilities of cardiac arrhythmias, chest pain, and myocardial infarction (heart attack). As THC has analgesic effects, it may mask chest pain, delaying treatment seeking. Cannabis smoking also increases the level of carboxyhaemoglobin in the blood, decreasing oxygen delivery to the heart, increasing the work of the heart and, perhaps, the risk of atheroma formation (Jones, 2002). Patients with cerebrovascular disease may

116                                          *Wayne Hall and Nadia Solowij*

also experience strokes caused by changes in blood pressure and patients with hypertension may experience exacerbations of their disease for the same reason (Chesher & Hall, 1999).

Mittleman *et al.* (2001) reported a case-crossover study to assess whether smoking cannabis may trigger an acute myocardial infarction. They asked 3882 patients who had had a myocardial infarction in the previous 4 days about their use of marijuana in the day on which it occurred. They compared this with the rate of cannabis use on another recent day when they had not had an infarct. Cannabis use was found to increase the risk of a myocardial infarction 4.8 times in the hour after use. The risk dropped rapidly after the first hour, as expected from the time course of the effects that THC and carbon monoxide have on heart function. Mittleman *et al.* estimated that a 44-year-old adult who used cannabis daily would increase their annual risk of an acute cardiovascular event by 1.5–3%.

The findings of this study are consistent with laboratory studies that have found that smoking cannabis cigarettes adversely affects patients with heart disease. Aronow and Cassidy (1974) compared the effect of smoking a cannabis and a high nicotine cigarette on heart rate and the time required to induce chest pain in an exercise tolerance test. Heart rate increased by 43%, and the time taken to produce chest pain halved after smoking a cannabis cigarette. Aronow and Cassidy (1975) compared the effects of smoking a single cannabis cigarette and a high nicotine cigarette in 10 men with heart disease, all of whom were cigarette smokers. Smoking cannabis produced a 42% increase in heart rate, compared with a 21% increase after smoking the tobacco cigarette. Exercise tolerance time was halved after smoking a cannabis cigarette by comparison with a tobacco cigarette. These findings have been confirmed by Gottschalk *et al.* (1977).

## Special Populations of Cannabis-Dependent Persons

### *The Educational Consequences of Adolescent Cannabis Dependence*

Adolescents who initiate cannabis use in their early teens are more likely to become regular cannabis users and are more likely to discontinue a high school education and to experience job instability in young adulthood (Hall & Pacula, 2003a; Lynskey & Hall, 2000). The strength of these relationships in cross-sectional studies is reduced in longitudinal studies when account is taken of the fact that adolescents who are heavy cannabis users have lower academic aspirations and poorer high school performance prior to using cannabis than do their peers who do not use at the same age (Hall & Pacula, 2003a; Lynskey & Hall, 2000).

A causal interpretation of the link between early cannabis use and subsequent educational performance has been supported by studies that have statistically controlled for a range of variables on which cannabis users and non-users differ prior to their cannabis use (e.g., Fergusson & Horwood, 1997, 2000; Macleod *et al.*, 2004). In these and other studies, early cannabis use predicts an increased risk of cannabis dependence, early school leaving, and precocious transitions to adult roles by engaging in early sexual activity, unplanned parenthood during adolescence, unemployment, and leaving the family home early (Hall & Pacula, 2003a; Hall *et al.*, 2001; Lynskey & Hall, 2000). Fergusson *et al.* (2003a) attribute the lower educational achievement in young people to the effects of the social context in which cannabis is used, rather than any specific effect of cannabis itself on intellectual ability or motivation. It is still possible that poorer cognitive functioning might contribute to poor school performance and hence to early school leaving.

### The Gateway Hypothesis

Research on drug use in adolescence and adulthood among American adolescents in the 1970s has consistently found a regular pattern of initiation into the use of illicit drugs in which cannabis use typically follows alcohol and tobacco use and precedes the use of stimulants and opioids (Hall & Lynskey, 2003; Hall *et al.*, 2001).

The interpretation of this sequence of drug initiation remains controversial (Hall & Lynskey, 2003b). Some argue that the pattern arises because the pharmacological effects of cannabis increase the likelihood of using more hazardous drugs later in the sequence, a hypothesis for which there is some supportive animal evidence (Hall & Lynskey, 2003b). There is also support for two other hypotheses that are not mutually exclusive:

1. that there is a selective recruitment into cannabis use of non-conforming adolescents who have a propensity to use a range of intoxicating substances, including other illicit drugs;
2. that once recruited to dependent cannabis use, the regular social interaction with drug using peers and the illicit drug market increases the likelihood of their using other illicit drugs (Hall *et al.*, 2001).

When compared to non-using peers, adolescents who start cannabis use early and become daily cannabis users are at a higher risk of using other illicit drugs (Fergusson & Horwood, 1997, 2000; Fergusson *et al.*, 2002). This increased risk is attributed to factors that are in place even before the cannabis use begins (i.e., family backgrounds and school performance), in addition to the finding that early users are more likely to keep company with other drug using peers (Fergusson & Horwood, 2000). Nonetheless, the better-controlled longitudinal studies show that heavy cannabis use in adolescence predicts an increased risk of using "harder" drugs that persists after controlling for pre-existing differences between adolescents who do and do not use cannabis (Fergusson & Horwood, 2000; Fergusson *et al.*, 2002; Hall & Lynskey, 2003b).

One possibility is that this unexplained association is due to uncontrolled factors, such as a genetic vulnerability to become dependent on a variety of different drugs. Studies of alcohol, tobacco, and other drug use in identical and non-identical twins indicate that there is a genetic vulnerability to developing dependence on alcohol (Heath, 1995), cannabis (Kendler & Prescott, 1998), and tobacco (Han *et al.*, 1999). More importantly, a component of the genetic vulnerability to dependence on these three drug classes is shared or common (True *et al.*, 1999), and so are the shared family and environmental factors that influence alcohol and cannabis dependence (Lynskey *et al.*, 1998; True *et al.*, 1999).

The hypothesis of common genes for regular use of cannabis and other illicit drugs has been directly tested using a discordant twin design by Lynskey *et al.* (2003). In this study, Lynskey *et al.* examined the relationship between cannabis and other illicit drug use in 311 monozygotic (136) and dizygotic (175) Australian twin pairs in which one twin had and the other twin had not used cannabis before the age of 17 years. If the association was attributable to a shared environment, then discordant twins raised together should not differ in the use of other illicit drugs. Similarly, if the association was attributable to a shared genetic vulnerability to drug dependence, then there should be no difference in the use of other illicit drugs between monozygotic twins who did and did not use cannabis before the age of 17 years. Lynskey *et al.* found that the twin who had used cannabis before the age of 17 years was more likely to have used sedatives, hallucinogens, stimulants, and opioids than their co-twin who had not used cannabis before the age of 17 years. Twins who had used cannabis were also more likely to report symptoms of abuse or dependence on cannabis and other illicit drugs than their twin who did not. These relationships persisted after controlling for other non-shared environmental factors that predicted an increased risk of developing drug abuse or dependence.

The findings of Lynksey *et al.* (2003), when taken together with those of Fergusson and Horwood (2000), suggest that shared genes and/or shared environment explain a substantial part of the association between cannabis use and other illicit drug use. The size of the association in the study of twins after statistical adjustment was substantially smaller (RR ~ 2–4) than that reported in the study of Fergusson and Horwood (2000) (RR ~ 59) but this may reflect in part the cruder measure of cannabis use in the Lynskey *et al.* study.

### Psychosis and Schizophrenia

Until recently, the most convincing evidence that cannabis use precipitates schizophrenia came from a 15-year prospective study of cannabis use and schizophrenia in 50,465 Swedish conscripts (Andreasson *et al.*, 1987). Andreasson *et al.* found that those who had tried cannabis by age 18 years were 2.4 times more likely to receive a diagnosis of schizophrenia than those who had not. The likelihood of receiving a diagnosis of schizophrenia increased with the number of times cannabis had been used. Compared to those who had not used cannabis, the risk of developing schizophrenia was 1.3 times higher for those who had used cannabis 1–10 times, 3 times higher for those who had used cannabis between 1 and 50 times, and 6 times higher for those who had used cannabis more than 50 times. These risks were substantially reduced after statistical adjustment for variables that were related to the risk of developing schizophrenia but they nevertheless remained statistically significant. Compared to those who had never used cannabis, those who had used cannabis 1–10 times were 1.5 times more likely, and those who had used 10 or more times were 2.3 times more likely to receive a diagnosis of schizophrenia.

Zammit *et al.* (2002) reported a 27-year follow-up of the Swedish cohort study. Zammit *et al.* found a dose–response relationship between frequency of cannabis use at baseline and risk of schizophrenia during the follow up and demonstrated that the relationship between cannabis use and schizophrenia persisted when they statistically controlled for the effects of other drug use and other potential confounding factors, including a history of psychiatric symptoms at baseline. They estimated that 13% of cases of schizophrenia could be averted if all cannabis use were prevented (i.e., the attributable risk of cannabis to schizophrenia was 13%). The relationship was a little stronger in cases observed in the first 5 years, probably reflecting the decline in cannabis use that occurs with age.

Zammit *et al.*'s (2002) findings have been supported by a study conducted by van Os and colleagues (2002). This was a 3-year longitudinal study of the relationship between self-reported cannabis use and psychosis in a community sample of 4848 people in the Netherlands. van Os *et al.* substantially replicated the Swedish cohort in a number of important ways. First, cannabis use at baseline predicted an increased risk of psychotic symptoms during the follow-up period in individuals who had not reported psychiatric symptoms at baseline. Second, there was a dose–response relationship between frequency of cannabis use at baseline and risk of psychotic symptoms during the follow up period. Third, the relationship between cannabis use and psychotic symptoms persisted when they statistically controlled for the effects of other drug use. Fourth, the relationship between cannabis use and psychotic symptoms was stronger for cases with more severe psychotic symptoms. van Os *et al.* estimated the attributable risk of cannabis to psychosis was 13% for psychotic symptoms and 50% for cases with psychotic disorders adjudged to need psychiatric treatment. Fifth, those who reported any psychotic symptoms at baseline were more likely to develop schizophrenia if they used cannabis than were individuals who were not so vulnerable.

These findings have been replicated in two smaller New Zealand cohort studies. Arseneault *et al.* (2002) reported a prospective study of the relationship between adolescent cannabis use and psychosis in young adults in a New Zealand birth cohort ($N = 759$) whose members had been assessed on risk factors for psychotic symptoms and disorders since birth. Arsenault *et al.* found a relationship between cannabis use by age 15 years and an increased risk of psychotic symptoms by age 26 years. So too did Fergusson *et al.* (2003b), who have reported a longitudinal study of the relationship between cannabis dependence at age 18 years and the number of psychotic symptoms reported at age 21 years in the Christchurch birth cohort in New Zealand. They found that cannabis dependence at age 18 years predicted an increased risk of psychotic symptoms at age 21 years (RR of 2.3). This association was smaller but still significant after adjustment for potential confounds (RR of 1.8).

In all of these studies, the relationship between cannabis use and the timing of the onset of psychotic symptoms was uncertain. Subjects were assessed once a year or less often and reported retrospectively on their cannabis use during the preceding year. Moreover, cannabis use was often only assessed by the number of times that cannabis had been used or the number of times used per week or month. A recent French study examined the relationship between cannabis use and psychotic symptoms in more detail using an experience sampling method (Verdoux *et al.*, 2002). These investigators asked 79 college students to report on their drug use and experience of psychotic symptoms at randomly selected time points, several times each day, over 7 consecutive days. The students gave their ratings after being randomly prompted to do so by a signal sent to a portable electronic device that they carried. The students were a stratified sample from a larger group in which high cannabis users ($N = 41$) and students identified as vulnerable to psychosis ($N = 16$) were over-represented. Verdoux *et al.* found that in time periods when cannabis was used, users reported more unusual perceptions. In vulnerable individuals, cannabis use was more strongly associated with strange impressions and unusual perceptions than in individuals who lacked this vulnerability. There was no relationship between reporting unusual experiences and using cannabis, as would be expected if self-medication were involved.

A major epidemiological puzzle, given this evidence, is that the treated incidence of schizophrenia, particularly early onset acute cases, has declined (or remained stable) during the 1970s and 1980s despite very substantial increases in cannabis use among young adults in Australia and North America (Hall & Degenhardt, 2000b). Although there are complications in interpreting such trends, a large reduction in treated incidence has been observed in a number of countries which have a high prevalence of cannabis use and in which the reduction is unlikely to be a diagnostic artifact (Hall, 1998; Degenhardt *et al.*, 2003).

A number of retrospective and prospective studies that have controlled for confounding variables give evidence that cannabis use exacerbates the symptoms of schizophrenia (e.g., Linszen *et al.*, 1994). In Australia, a third of persons with schizophrenia and other psychoses have been found to be daily users of cannabis (Jablensky *et al.*, 2000), a much higher rate than the 2% reported in the general population. It is biologically plausible that cannabis can exacerbate psychosis because psychotic disorders involve disturbances in the dopamine neurotransmitter systems, and THC increases dopamine release (Stahl, 2000).

**Conclusions**

The harms to health that could be caused by cannabis dependence are not as well understood as they could be. The adverse health effect that dependent users are most likely to experience is chronic bronchitis caused by regular smoking of cannabis preparations. These adverse effects will be amplified in cannabis smokers who also smoke tobacco. A birth cohort in New Zealand has found respiratory function changes in cannabis-dependent young adults that are comparable to respiratory changes attributed to low levels of daily tobacco cigarettes. There is suggestive evidence that regular cannabis smoking over a period of decades increases the risk of cancers of the upper respiratory system.

Frequent cannabis use alters brain blood flow and metabolism, but the functional significance of these findings remains obscure. Cannabis dependence is not associated with severe cognitive impairment of the type found in some alcohol-dependent persons, but there is evidence for more subtle impairments of memory, attention, and executive functions associated with long-term or heavy cannabis use. These may persist for weeks following cessation of cannabis use, and may be greater among those who commenced cannabis use during adolescence.

Some populations of cannabis-dependent persons seem at increased risk of experiencing adverse effects of their cannabis use. Foremost among these are adults with cardiovascular disease who may precipitate myocardial infarctions by smoking cannabis; adolescents whose school performance and psychosocial development may be adversely affected and who may be at increased risk of using other illicit drugs; persons with schizophrenia and other psychoses whose illnesses may be exacerbated by continued use of cannabis; and probably persons with a family history of psychoses in whom regular cannabis use may precipitate the onset of a psychosis.

## References

Ameri, A. (1999). The effects of cannabinoids on the brain. *Progress in Neurobiology, 58*(4), 315–348.

Andreasson, S., Engstrom, A., Allebeck, P., & Rydberg, U. (1987). Cannabis and schizophrenia: a longitudinal study of Swedish conscripts. *Lancet, 2*(8574), 1483–1486.

Anthony, J. C., Warner, L., & Kessler, R. (1994). Comparative epidemiology of dependence on tobacco, alcohol, controlled substances and inhalants: basic findings from the National Comorbidity Survey. *Experimental and Clinical Psychopharmacology, 2*(3), 244–268.

Aronow, W., & Cassidy, J. (1974). Effect of marihuana and placebo marihuana smoking on angina pectoris. *New England Journal of Medicine, 291*, 65–67.

Aronow, W., & Cassidy, J. (1975). Effect of smoking marijuana and of a high nicotine cigarette on angina pectoris. *Clinical Pharmacology and Therapeutics, 17*, 549–554.

Arseneault, L., Cannon, M., Poulton, R., Murray, R., Caspi, A., Moffitt, T. E., *et al.* (2002). Cannabis use in adolescence and risk for adult psychosis: longitudinal prospective study. *British Medical Journal, 325*(7374), 1212–1213.

Bachman, J. G., Wadsworth, K. N., O'Malley, P. M., Johnston, L. D., & Schulenberg, J. (1997). *Smoking, drinking, and drug use in young adulthood: the impacts of new freedoms and new responsibilities.* Mahwah, NJ: Lawrence Erlbaum.

Block, R. I., & Ghoneim, M. M. (1993). Effects of chronic marijuana use on human cognition. *Psychopharmacology (Berlin), 110*(1–2), 219–228.

Block, R. I., O'Leary, D. S., Ehrhardt, J. C., Augustinack, J. C., Ghoneim, M. M., Arndt, S., *et al.* (2000a). Effects of frequent marijuana use on brain tissue volume and composition. *Neuroreport, 11*(3), 491–496.

Block, R. I., O'Leary, D. S., Hichwa, R. D., Augustinack, J. C., Boles Ponto, L. L., Ghoneim, M. M., *et al.* (2000b). Cerebellar hypoactivity in frequent marijuana users. *Neuroreport, 11*(4), 749–753.

Block, R. I., O'Leary, D. S., Hichwa, R. D., Augustinack, J. C., Boles Ponto, L. L., Ghoneim, M. M., *et al.* (2002). Effects of frequent marijuana use on memory-related regional cerebral blood flow. *Pharmacology, Biochemistry and Behavior, 72*(1–2), 237–250.

Bolla, K. I., Brown, K., Eldreth, D., Tate, K., & Cadet, J. L. (2002). Dose-related neuro-cognitive effects of marijuana use. *Neurology, 59*(9), 1337–1343.

Caplan, G. A., & Brigham, B. A. (1990). Marijuana smoking and carcinoma of the tongue: Is there an association? *Cancer, 66*(5), 1005–1006.

Chait, L. D., & Pierri, J. (1992). Effects of smoked marijuana on human performance: a critical review. In L. Murphy, & A. Bartke (Eds.), *Marijuana/cannabinoids: neurobiology and neurophysiology* (pp. 387–423). Boca Raton, FL: CRC Press.

Chesher, G. (1995). Cannabis and road safety: an outline of research studies to examine the effects of cannabis on driving skills and actual driving performance. In Parliament of Victoria Road Safety Committee (Ed.), *The effects of drugs (other than alcohol) on road safety* (pp. 67–96). Melbourne: Road Safety Committee.

Chesher, G., & Hall, W. D. (1999). Effects of cannabis on the cardiovascular and gastro-intestinal systems. In H. Kalant, W. Corrigall, W. D. Hall, & R. Smart (Eds.), *The health effects of cannabis* (pp. 435–458). Toronto: Centre for Addiction and Mental Health.

Copeland, J., Swift, W., & Rees, V. (2001). Clinical profile of participants in a brief intervention program for cannabis use disorder. *Journal of Substance Abuse Treatment, 20*(1), 45–52.

Degenhardt, L., Hall, W. D., & Lynskey, M. (2003). Testing hypotheses about the relationship between cannabis use and psychosis. *Drug and Alcohol Dependence, 71*(1), 37–48.

Donald, P. (1991). Marijuana and upper aerodigestive tract malignancy in young patients. In G. Nahas, & C. Latour (Eds.), *Physiopathology of illicit drugs: cannabis, cocaine, opiates* (pp. 39–54). Oxford: Pergamon.

Ehrenreich, H., Rinn, T., Kunert, H. J., Moeller, M. R., Poser, W., Schilling, L., et al. (1999). Specific attentional dysfunction in adults following early start of cannabis use. *Psychopharmacology (Berlin), 142*(3), 295–301.

Fergusson, D. M., Horwood, L. J., & Health, C. (2000). Cannabis use and dependence in a New Zealand birth cohort. *New Zealand Medical Journal, 113*(1109), 156–158.

Fergusson, D. M., & Horwood, L. J. (1997). Early onset cannabis use and psychosocial adjustment in young adults. *Addiction, 92*(3), 279–296.

Fergusson, D. M., & Horwood, L. J. (2000). Does cannabis use encourage other forms of illicit drug use? *Addiction, 95*(4), 505–520.

Fergusson, D. M., Horwood, L. J., & Swain-Campbell, N. R. (2002). Cannabis use and psychosocial adjustment in adolescence and young adulthood. *Addiction, 97*, 1123–1135.

Fergusson, D. M., Horwood, L. J., & Beautrais, A. L. (2003a). Cannabis and educational achievement. *Addiction, 98*(12), 1681–1692.

Fergusson, D. M., Horwood, L. J., & Swain-Campbell, N. R. (2003b). Cannabis dependence and psychotic symptoms in young people. *Psychological Medicine, 33*, 15–21.

Gerberich, S. G., Sidney, S., Braun, B. L., Tekawa, I. S., Tolan, K. K., & Queensberry, C. P. (2003). Marijuana use and injury events resulting in hospitalization. *Annals of Epidemiology, 13*(4), 230–237.

Gottschalk, L., Aronow, W., & Prakash, R. (1977). Effect of marijuana and placebo-marijuana smoking on psychological state and on psychophysiological and cardiovascular functioning in angina patients. *Biological Psychiatry, 12*(2), 255–266.

Guzman, M. (2003). Cannabinoids: potential anticancer agents. *Nature Reviews Cancer, 3,* 745–755.

Hall, W. D. (1998). Cannabis use and psychosis. *Drug and Alcohol Review, 17*(4), 433–444.

Hall, W. D., & Babor, T. F. (2000a). Cannabis use and public health: assessing the burden. *Addiction, 95*(4), 485–490.

Hall, W. D., & Degenhardt, L. (2000b). Cannabis use and psychosis: a review of clinical and epidemiological evidence. *Australian and New Zealand Journal of Psychiatry, 34*(1), 26–34.

Hall, W. D., & MacPhee, D. (2002). Cannabis use and cancer. *Addiction, 97*(3), 243–247.

Hall, W. D., & Pacula, R. L. (2003a). *Cannabis use and dependence: public health and public policy.* Cambridge: Cambridge University Press.

Hall, W. D., & Lynskey, M. (2003b). Testing hypotheses about the relationship between the use of cannabis and the use of other illicit drugs. *Drug and Alcohol Review, 22*(2), 125–133.

Hall, W. D., Solowij, N., & Lemon, J. (1994). *The health and psychological consequences of cannabis use,* National Drug Strategy Monograph, Vol. 25. Canberra: Australian Government Publishing Service.

Hall, W. D., Teesson, M., Lynskey, M. T., & Degenhardt, L. (1999a). The 12-month prevalence of substance use and ICD-10 substance use disorders in Australian adults: findings from the National Survey of Mental Health and Well-Being. *Addiction, 94*(10), 1541–1550.

Hall, W. D., Johnston, L. D., & Donnelly, N. (1999b). Assessing the health and psychological effects of cannabis use. In H. Kalant, W. Corrigall, W. D. Hall, & R. Smart (Eds.), *The health effects of cannabis* (pp. 1–17). Toronto: Centre for Addiction and Mental Health.

Hall, W. D., Degenhardt, L., & Lynskey, M. T. (2001). *The health and psychological effects of cannabis use,* National Drug Strategy Monograph, Vol. 44. Canberra: Commonwealth Department of Health and Aged Care.

Han, C., McGue, M. K., & Iacono, W. G. (1999). Lifetime tobacco, alcohol and other substance use in adolescent Minnesota twins: univariate and multivariate behavioral genetic analyses. *Addiction, 94*(7), 981–993.

Heath, A. C. (1995). Genetic influences on alcoholism risk: a review of adoption and twin studies. *Alcohol Health and Research World, 19*(3), 166–171.

Institute of Medicine (1999). *Marijuana and medicine: assessing the science base.* Washington, DC: National Academy Press.

Iversen, L. (2003). Cannabis and the brain. *Brain, 126,* 1252–1270.

Jablensky, A., McGrath, J., Herrman, H., Castle, D., Gureje, O., & Evans, M. (2000). Psychotic disorders in urban areas: an overview of the Study on Low Prevalence Disorders. *Australian and New Zealand Journal of Psychiatry, 34*(2), 221–236.

Jones, R. T. (2002). Cardiovascular system effects of marijuana. *Journal of Clinical Pharmacology, 42*(11 Suppl.), 58S–63S.

Kendler, K. S., & Prescott, C. A. (1998). Cannabis use, abuse, and dependence in a population-based sample of female twins. *American Journal of Psychiatry, 155*(8), 1016–1022.

Linszen, D. H., Dingemans, P. M., & Lenior, M. E. (1994). Cannabis abuse and the course of recent-onset schizophrenic disorders. *Archives of General Psychiatry, 51*(4), 273–279.

Llewellyn, C. D., Linklater, K., Bell, J., Johnson, N. W., & Warnakulasuriya, S. (2004). An analysis of risk factors for oral cancer in young people: a case–control study. *Oral Oncology, 40*(3), 304–313.

Loeber, R. T., & Yurgelun-Todd, D. A. (1999). Human neuroimaging of acute and chronic marijuana use: implications for frontocerebellar dysfunction. *Human Psychopharmacology – Clinical and Experimental, 14*(5), 291–304.

Lundqvist, T., Jonsson, S., & Warkentin, S. (2001). Frontal lobe dysfunction in long-term cannabis users. *Neurotoxicology and Teratology, 23*(5), 437–443.

Lyketsos, C. G., Garrett, E., Liang, K. Y., & Anthony, J. C. (1999). Cannabis use and cognitive decline in persons under 65 years of age. *American Journal of Epidemiology, 149*(9), 794–800.

Lynskey, M. T., & Hall, W. D. (2000). The effects of adolescent cannabis use on educational attainment: a review. *Addiction, 96*(3), 433–443.

Lynskey, M. T., Fergusson, D. M., & Horwood, L. J. (1998). The origins of the correlations between tobacco, alcohol, and cannabis use during adolescence. *Journal of Child Psychology and Psychiatry, 39*(7), 995–1005.

Lynskey, M. T., Heath, A. C., Bucholz, K. K., & Slutske, W. S. (2003). Escalation of drug use in early-onset cannabis users vs co-twin controls. *Journal of the American Medical Association, 289*(4), 427–433.

Macleod, J., Oakes, R., Copello, A., Crome, I., Egger, M., Hickman, M., *et al.* (2004). Psychological and social sequelae of cannabis and other illicit drug use by young people: a systematic review of longitudinal, general population studies. *Lancet, 363*(9421), 1579–1588.

MacPhee, D. (1999). Effects of marijuana on cell nuclei: a review of the literature relating to the genotoxicity of cannabis. In H. Kalant, W. Corrigall, W. D. Hall, & R. Smart (Eds.), *The health effects of cannabis* (pp. 435–458). Toronto: Centre for Addiction and Mental Health.

Marselos, M., & Karamanakos, P. (1999). Mutagenicity, developmental toxicity and carcinogeneity of cannabis. *Addiction Biology, 4*(1), 5–12.

Mittleman, M. A., Lewis, R. A., Maclure, M., Sherwood, J. B., & Muller, J. E. (2001). Triggering myocardial infarction by marijuana. *Circulation, 103*, 2805–2809.

Mura, P., Kintz, P., Ludes, B., Gaulier, J. M., Marquet, P., Martin-Dupont, S., *et al.* (2003). Comparison of the prevalence of alcohol, cannabis and other drugs between 900 injured drivers and 900 control subjects: results of a French collaborative study. *Forensic Science International, 133*(1–2), 79–85.

van Os, J., Bak, M., Hanssen, M., Bijl, R.V., de Graaf, R., *et al.* (2002). Cannabis use and psychosis: a longitudinal population-based study. *American Journal of Epidemiology, 156*(4), 319–327.

Piomelli, D. (2003). The molecular logic of endocannabinoid signalling. *Nature Reviews Neuroscience, 4*(11), 873–884.

Pope, H. G., & Yurgelun-Todd, D. (1996). The residual cognitive effects of heavy marijuana use in college students. *Journal of the American Medical Association, 275*(7), 521–527.

Pope, H. G., Gruber, A. J., & Yurgelun-Todd, D. (1995). The residual neuropsychological effects of cannabis: the current status of research. *Drug and Alcohol Dependence, 38*(1), 25–34.

Pope, H. G., Gruber, A. J., Hudson, J. I., Huestis, M. A., & Yurgelun-Todd, D. (2001). Neuropsychological performance in long-term cannabis users. *Archives of General Psychiatry, 58*(10), 909–915.

Pope, H. G., Gruber, A. J., Hudson, J. I., Huestis, M. A., & Yurgelun-Todd, D. (2002). Cognitive measures in long-term cannabis users. *Journal of Clinical Pharmacology, 42*(11 Suppl.), 41S–47S.

Porrino, L. J., Whitlow, C. T., Lamborn, C., Laurienti, P. J., Livengood, L. B., & Liguori, A. (2004). Impaired performance on a decision-making task by heavy marijuana users: an fMRI study. In *2004 Symposium on the Cannabinoids* (p. 239). Burlington, VT: International Cannabinoid Research Society.

Ramaekers, J. G., Berghaus, G., van Laar, M., & Drummer, O. H. (2004). Dose related risk of motor vehicle crashes after cannabis use. *Drug and Alcohol Dependence, 73*(2), 109–119.

Rosenblatt, K. A., Daling, J. R., Chen, C., Sherman, K. J., & Schwartz, S. M. (2004). Marijuana use and risk of oral squamous cell carcinoma. *Cancer Research, 64*(11), 4049–4054.

Sidney, S. (2002). Cardiovascular consequences of marijuana use. *Journal of Clinical Pharmacology, 42*(11 Suppl.), 64S–70S.

Sidney, S., Quesenberry Jr., C. P., Friedman, G. D., & Tekawa, I. S. (1997). Marijuana use and cancer incidence (California, United States). *Cancer Causes and Control, 8*(5), 722–728.

Smiley, A. (1999). Marijuana: on road and driving simulator studies. In H. Kalant, W. Corrigall, W. D. Hall, & R. Smart (Eds.), *The health effects of cannabis* (pp. 171–191). Toronto: Centre for Addiction and Mental Health.

Smith, A. M., Fried, P. A., Hogan, M. J., & Cameron, I. (2004). Effects of prenatal marijuana on response inhibition: an fMRI study of young adults. *Neurotoxicology and Teratology*, 26(4), 533–542.

Solowij, N. (1998). *Cannabis and cognitive functioning*. Cambridge, UK: Cambridge University Press.

Solowij, N. (1999). Long-term effects of cannabis on the central nervous system. I. Brain function and neurotoxicity. II. Cognitive functioning. In H. Kalant, W. Corrigall, W. D. Hall, & R. Smart (Eds.), *The health effects of cannabis* (pp. 195–265). Toronto: Centre for Addiction and Mental Health.

Solowij, N. (2002). Marijuana and cognitive function. In E. S. Onaivi (Ed.), *Biology of marijuana: from gene to behaviour* (pp. 308–332). London: Taylor and Francis.

Solowij, N., Stephens, R. S., Roffman, R. A., Babor, T., Kadden, R., Miller, M., et al. (2002). Cognitive functioning of long-term heavy cannabis users seeking treatment. *Journal of the American Medical Association*, 287(9), 1123–1131.

Solowij, N., Respondek, C., & Ward, P. (2004). Functional magnetic resonance imaging indices of memory function in long-term cannabis users. In *2004 Symposium on the Cannabinoids* (p. 89). Burlington, VT: International Cannabinoid Research Society.

Stahl, S. M. (2000). *Essential psychopharmacology: neuroscientific basis and practical applications* (2nd ed.). Cambridge, UK: Cambridge University Press.

Swift, W., Hall, W. D., & Copeland, J. (1998a). Characteristics of long-term cannabis users in Sydney, Australia. *European Addiction Research*, 4(4), 190–197.

Swift, W., Hall, W. D., Didcott, P., & Reilly, D. (1998b). Patterns and correlates of cannabis dependence among long-term users in an Australian rural area. *Addiction*, 93(8), 1149–1160.

Swift, W., Hall, W. D., & Teesson, C. (2001). Characteristics of DSM-IV and ICD-10 cannabis dependence among Australian adults: results from the National Survey of Mental Health and Well-being. *Drug and Alcohol Dependence*, 63(2), 147–153.

Tashkin, D. P. (1999). Effects of cannabis on the respiratory system. In H. Kalant, W. Corrigall, W. D. Hall, & R. Smart (Eds.), *The health effects of cannabis* (pp. 311–345). Toronto: Centre for Addiction and Mental Health.

Taylor, I. F. (1988). Marijuana as a potential respiratory tract carcinogen: a retrospective analysis of a community hospital population. *Southern Medical Journal*, 81(10), 1213–1216.

Taylor, D. R., Poulton, R., Moffitt, T. E., Ramankutty, P., & Sears, M. R. (2000). The respiratory effects of cannabis dependence in young adults. *Addiction*, 95(11), 1669–1677.

Taylor, D. R., Fergusson, D. M., Milne, B. J., Horwood, L. J., Moffitt, T. E., Sears, M. R., et al. (2002). A longitudinal study of the effects of tobacco and cannabis exposure on lung function in young adults. *Addiction*, 97(8), 1055–1061.

True, W. R., Heath, A. C., Scherrer, J. F., Xian, H., Lin, N., Eisen, S. A., et al. (1999). Interrelationship of genetic and environmental influences on conduct disorder and alcohol and marijuana dependence symptoms. *American Journal of Medical Genetics, 88*(4), 391–397.

Verdoux, H., Gindre, C., Sorbara, F., Tournier, M., & Swendsen, J. (2002). Cannabis use and the expression of psychosis vulnerability in daily life. *European Psychiatry, 17*(Suppl.), 180S–190S.

Wilson, W., Mathew, R., Turkington, T., Hawk, T., Coleman, R. E., & Provenzale, J. (2000). Brain morphological changes and early marijuana use: a magnetic resonance and positron emission tomography study. *Journal of Addictive Diseases, 19*(1), 1–22.

Zammit, S., Allebeck, P., Andreasson, S., Lundberg, I., & Lewis, G. (2002). Self-reported cannabis use as a risk factor for schizophrenia in Swedish conscripts of 1969: historical cohort study. *British Medical Journal, 325*(7374), 1199–1201.

Zhang, Z. F., Morgenstern, H., Spitz, M. R., Tashkin, D. P., Yu, G. P., Marshall, J. R., *et al.* (1999). Marijuana use and increased risk of squamous cell carcinoma of the head and neck. *Cancer Epidemiology Biomarkers and Prevention, 8*(12), 1071–1078.

# Part II

Interventions with Cannabis-Dependent Adults

# 6

# Cognitive-Behavioral and Motivational Enhancement Treatments for Cannabis Dependence

ROBERT S. STEPHENS, ROGER A. ROFFMAN, JAN COPELAND, AND WENDY SWIFT

Cognitive-behavioral (CBT) and motivational enhancement treatments (MET) are two of the most researched and most empirically supported approaches to the treatment of alcohol and drug use disorders (e.g., Carroll *et al.*, 1998; Miller *et al.*, 1995; Project MATCH Research Group, 1997). They were the first to be adapted for the treatment of cannabis dependence in controlled research trials and, consequently, have generated the most research. Although theoretically distinct, CBT and MET may be complementary (e.g., Baer *et al.*, 1999) and have often been combined into a single intervention in the treatment of cannabis dependence. In this chapter we provide an overview of these therapeutic strategies, discuss their application to cannabis dependence treatment, and review the empirical literature on their efficacy.

The core of CBT is the development of coping skills to deal with high-risk situations for drug use (Marlatt & Gordon, 1985; Monti *et al.*, 2002). As an action-oriented set of strategies, CBT is perhaps best suited to individuals who already have a commitment to changing their substance using behavior. MET, on the other hand, uses principles of motivational interviewing (MI) and was developed specifically to deal with ambivalence regarding change (Miller & Rollnick, 1991, 2002). As such, MET may be most appropriate for those contemplating change or those who would profit from solidifying their commitment to change before engaging in additional treatment. However, studies have shown that brief motivational interventions alone were sufficient to engender reductions in drug use. Subsequently, MET was codified as a bona fide, stand alone treatment approach in Project MATCH (Miller *et al.*, 1992).

At the time of the first controlled treatment study with cannabis users (Stephens *et al.*, 1994) there was little information on the prevalence or nature of cannabis dependence to guide treatment development. Several early clinical perspectives recognized the need for assessment and intervention with this population of drug users (Miller & Gold, 1989; Tennant, 1986; Zweben & O'Connell,

1988), but there were few empirical studies upon which to base clinical strategies. Adaptations of 12-step approaches had been suggested (Miller *et al.*,
1989; Zweben & O'Connell, 1988) but there were no data to support their
efficacy. CBT seemed particularly appropriate for cannabis users for both
philosophical and clinical reasons (see Stephens & Roffman, 1993). At the
philosophical level CBT is a non-judgmental, compensatory model based on
principles of learning that does not blame the individual for the development
of the problem (Brickman *et al.*, 1982). This view of the nature of cannabis
dependence is likely to be consistent with the experience of many dependent
users who used marijuana recreationally and without apparent problems for
many years. In contrast, the relatively mild withdrawal symptoms associated
with cannabis dependence and the historical belief that cannabis is not physically addictive diminished the plausibility of biological explanations for many
users.

Similarly, it seemed likely that MET approaches would be appealing and
useful with cannabis-dependent adults. Early trials of this approach were effective in reaching and helping alcohol users who were reluctant to label themselves as having a problem or ambivalent about making changes (Miller &
Sovereign, 1989; Miller *et al.*, 1988). Ambivalence about quitting or substantially reducing drug use is common in those seeking treatment but may be particularly strong in cannabis users (e.g., Budney *et al.*, 1998). The relative
absence of severe and immediate negative effects on health and social functioning may fuel ambivalence about change. The most frequently reported
problems across several treatment studies have been self-deprecation, lowered
energy, and procrastination (Copeland *et al.*, 2001; Stephens *et al.*, 1993, 2000,
2002). Perceived memory problems and lower productivity are also frequently
reported, but negative familial or financial consequences were only noted by
approximately one-half of the participants. Legal and other health problems
were even less frequently endorsed (see Copeland *et al.*, 1999 for an exception). Smoking cannabis is related to impairments in respiratory functioning
and a variety of laboratory studies suggest it is a risk factor for lung cancer
and other life-threatening pulmonary diseases (Tashkin, 1999), but the lack of
clear epidemiological findings showing these associations leaves many users
unconvinced of the threat. Rather, it seems to be a more gradual awareness of
signs of dependence that brings the chronic, daily user to the point of considering change. Therapists need skills to help users identify and focus on these
subtle intrinsic feelings of dissatisfaction with oneself and one's accomplishments in order to sustain motivation for quitting or reduced use. MET is ideally
suited for this task and, when coupled with CBT techniques, may provide

an optimal treatment combination for addressing both motivational and coping skill issues.

## MET Principles and Techniques

MET is based on MI, an empathic, reflective therapeutic style designed to resolve ambivalence and develop self-motivation for change (Miller & Rollnick, 1991, 2002; Miller *et al.*, 1992). Ambivalence can be thought of as a balance between opposing forces. On one side are the perceived benefits of drug use and the costs of quitting or reducing use. On the other side are the negative effects of current drug use and the benefits of change. In order to tip the scale in favor of change, the therapist follows a set of four general principles: express empathy, develop discrepancy, roll with resistance, and support self-efficacy. Accurate empathy regarding the client's feelings about drug use shows respect, understanding, and acceptance. In addition to establishing rapport and building a collaborative relationship, it normalizes feelings of ambivalence and reduces defensiveness. Acceptance is fundamental to facilitating change because it creates a context in which the client does not have to defend or rationalize continued drug use. In this context, the therapist develops discrepancy by eliciting the client's "not-so-positive" feelings about drug use. Motivation for change is achieved as the client becomes more aware of the way in which drug use is inconsistent with personal goals and values. Rolling with resistance refers to the avoidance of confrontation. The client, not the therapist, should be arguing for change. Confronting or arguing with the client regarding the need for change promotes resistance and when resistance is encountered it is a sign to change strategies. The therapist supports the client's self-efficacy for change whenever possible because belief in one's ability to change is an important motivator. As the therapist expresses confidence in the client's ability to make changes, the client's confidence grows.

A wide variety of therapeutic techniques and strategies that embody the principles of MI are described elsewhere and detailed presentation is beyond the scope of this chapter (see Miller & Rollnick, 1991, 2002; Miller *et al.*, 1992). However, five techniques are central and are used throughout the course of treatment. They include the use of open-ended questions, reflective listening, affirmation of the client, periodic summaries of client's thoughts and feelings regarding drug use, and the elicitation of self-motivational statements. Open-ended questions encourage the client to do the talking and to explore feelings about drug use and change. Therapists avoid closed-ended questions that typically lead to brief answers and the need for another question. Reflective listening

expresses accurate empathy, encourages further disclosure, and conveys acceptance. Reflections facilitate exploration of the client's thoughts and feelings
regarding drug use. Affirmation of the client is another way to build rapport
and facilitate exploration. Therapists note accomplishments, directly compli-
ment the client, and express appreciation and understanding of the client's perspectives. Periodically summarizing what the client has said about drug use
and interest in change allows the client to hear again what she or he has been
saying. Summaries can be used to link what the person is saying with feedback
based on assessment data and they can provide a transition to another focus. In
general, the therapist chooses what to summarize so as to reinforce material
relevant to resolving ambivalence.

Eliciting self-motivational statements or change talk is the fifth strategy.
Self-motivational statements include recognition of the disadvantages of continued drug use or the advantages of change. They also include statements that
express optimism about the likelihood of successful change and intentions to
initiate change. For some clients, these statements may emerge from open-
ended questions and reflective listening. However, for more ambivalent clients,
additional strategies may be needed. Miller and Rollnick (1991, 2002) provide
examples of open-ended questions and other strategies intended to evoke self-
motivational statements. In each case, the goal is to get the person to talk more
about what they do not like about drug use or the way in which the drug use is
inconsistent with values or future goals.

As the client expresses increasing interest in modifying his or her substance
use, the therapist assesses and builds efficacy for making a change. It is important to avoid prescribing the change too early because it may elicit resistance.
Instead, when the client seems to be committed, the therapist enquires about
the steps or methods that will be used in accomplishing the change and the degree
of confidence the client has in being successful. The therapist then attempts
to bolster confidence and may offer a menu of self-change and assisted-
change options depending upon the client's inclinations and past experience
in making changes. At this stage, giving advice is appropriate as long as the
client clearly wants it. Ideally, the therapist and client work together to negotiate
a plan for change.

In order to facilitate the exploration of feelings about drug use, the first MET
session often involves reviewing a personalized feedback report (PFR) generated from an initial assessment (e.g., Miller *et al.*, 1992). A wide range of
assessment instruments have been created or adapted for cannabis users that
can be used to construct the PFR (see Stephens & Roffman, 2005). PFRs typically organize assessment results in sections such as: Your Cannabis Use (i.e.,

frequency and pattern of use); Risk Factors (presence of dependence symptoms or other severity indicators); Consequences of Use (self-reported problems); Anticipated Consequences of Reducing Use (costs and benefits of changing); and Confidence in Avoiding Cannabis Use (perceived ability to avoid use in specific types of situations). Each section presents information from the initial assessment, often in graphic form with specific responses listed to promote discussion. It is useful to provide normative data in the PFR so that the client's responses or scores can be seen in relation to those of others. Epidemiological data from community samples can often be used for this purpose, but another variation is to present scores in relation to diagnostic cutoffs, other risk indicators, or to data from those in treatment for cannabis dependence. After each piece of information on the PFR is presented and briefly explained, the therapist pauses and uses the techniques of MI to elicit the client's reaction. The intent is to encourage the participant to explore the meaning of the information. Any self-motivational statements are reinforced via reflective listening and resistance is avoided by acknowledging any expressions of ambivalence about change. It is useful to assess the client's perceptions of the positive aspects of cannabis use and to include them on the PFR in order to acknowledge them explicitly. An accompanying document that explains the meaning of the scores in each section of the PFR (e.g., "Understanding Your Personal Feedback Report") may be given to participants to take home after the initial sessions.

MET interventions are typically brief and involve 1–4 sessions of 60–90 min duration, unless they are combined with CBT in multi-component programs. MET interventions grew out of findings that brief treatments with substance users are often as effective as longer ones and from observations that much of the change in substance use occurs relatively early in the course of longer interventions (Miller & Rollnick, 1991, 2002). MET is presumed to work by identifying, crystallizing, and harnessing the client's own motivation. The typical length of the MET in the research studies that have been conducted thus far suggests that this process is expected to happen relatively quickly or not at all. The brevity of the intervention also conveys that the client is responsible for making changes. The timing of multiple MET sessions may vary and often has been driven by the demands of research designs. However, there seems to be some wisdom in having initial assessment and feedback sessions spaced close together (e.g., weekly) in order to capitalize on whatever motivation initially brings the client to treatment. A space of a month or more may occur between later MET sessions in order to allow the client time to experiment with change on their own. Subsequent sessions then act as "boosters" that reinforce progress and efficacy for change or revisit ambivalence depending upon the client's experiences. Significant others (SO) have been included in some versions of MET interventions (e.g., MTPRG, 2004; Miller *et al.*, 1992; Stephens *et al.*, 2000). The therapist attempts to elicit the SO's perspective on the client's drug use and uses it to explore ambivalence, motivation for change, and goals. Principles and techniques for engaging SOs within the motivational framework of MI have been described (Miller *et al.*, 1992) but research has not yet systematically examined the contribution of SO participation to the effects of MET treatments.

## CBT Principles and Techniques

CBT for cannabis dependence typically lasts 6–12 sessions and may be conducted in either individual or group formats, both of which have been shown to be efficacious (Copeland *et al.*, 2001; MTPRG, 2004; Stephens *et al.*, 1994, 2000). CBT treatments are based on social learning theory and assume that drug dependence is at least in part an acquired behavior pattern, learned in the same way as other non-drug-related behaviors (e.g., Maisto *et al.*, 1999; Marlatt & Gordon, 1985). Parental and peer attitudes, and other vicarious sources of positive information about drug use combine to foster initial experimentation. If the acute effects of the drug are experienced positively, drug use may continue. As drug use continues various coping functions may be served that further reinforce the behavior pattern. For instance, cannabis use may become the means for releasing creativity, socializing with friends, reducing stress, avoiding unpleasant tasks, or perhaps dealing with more general psychological distress. This model predicts that individuals who are deficient in the skills needed to cope with a variety of life situations and who live in an environment supportive of drug use will be more likely to rely on drug use for coping. Reliance on drugs to cope results in the atrophy or failed development of alternative coping behaviors and increases the value of drug use to the individual. This pattern of increasing reliance on drug use is consistent with the notion of a dependence syndrome continuum (see Chapter 2).

CBT therefore targets the functional role that drug use plays in the individual's life. Clients learn to identify the antecedent feelings, thoughts, and situations that precipitate use, and then are helped to generate and master alternate responses (e.g., Marlatt & Gordon, 1985; Monti *et al.*, 2002). The theme of anticipating and avoiding relapse clearly conveys that the client must take personal responsibility for changing behavior. Self-monitoring assignments between treatment sessions and debriefing encounters with recent high-risk situations during therapy sessions help identify antecedents to drug use. The client and therapist then work together to master coping strategies for each high-risk situation. Coping strategies may include avoiding the situation entirely, relaxation techniques, positive imagery, delay, distraction, assertiveness, physical exercise, positive self-statements, and other forms of cognitive restructuring or self-talk. Although this list includes the most common coping strategies taught in protocol driven treatments, the particular coping skills that are needed will be idiosyncratic to the client and his or her particular situation. The therapist uses role-playing, modeling, and instruction to assist the client in practicing and ultimately mastering techniques for avoiding or coping with high-risk situations for drug use. The intent is to increase self-efficacy for dealing with high-risk situations without using drugs.

Two strategies systematically target the problem of relapse once clients have successfully eliminated, or substantially reduced, their drug use. First, clients may be asked to predict or anticipate future situations or circumstances that will lead them to use drugs again or they may be asked to identify a series of "apparently irrelevant decisions" that will place them in high-risk situations (Marlatt & Gordon, 1985). This process emphasizes vigilance and self-examination in order to identify rationalizations that may be used to justify a return to drug use. These cognitions and decision points can then be targeted preemptively with additional planning and coping skill training. Second, clients are educated about how cognitive and emotional reactions to an initial "slip" back into drug use may precipitate a full-blown relapse. Rather than blame themselves for inherent weaknesses, clients are helped to view slips as learning experiences. Cognitive restructuring is used to objectify the experience and consequences of the lapse and to minimize the negative self-evaluations that may foster further use. The therapist helps the client focus on how waning motivation or inadequate coping skills may have precipitated the slip and then helps the client to prepare for similar situations in the future.

CBT treatments sometimes incorporate more molar level interventions by encouraging lifestyle changes that will decrease encounters with high-risk situations. Most daily cannabis users seeking treatment use multiple times daily such that use is interwoven throughout their social, occupational, and familial roles. Becoming abstinent entails more than simply avoiding or coping with isolated high-risk situations. Monitoring of daily "shoulds" and "wants" (i.e., stresses and rewards) can be used to identify lifestyle imbalances that may foster stress, boredom, or other negative affective states that precipitate cannabis use (Marlatt & Gordon, 1985). Clients are encouraged to build frequent rewards into their daily or weekly schedules in order to offset the loss of a potent reinforcer. More comprehensive changes in lifestyle are fostered by helping the client to set both proximal and distal lifestyle goals, and by identifying manageable steps to take in reaching them.

## Combining MET and CBT Approaches

Although MET is conceptually best suited for those in the contemplation stage of change and CBT is more appropriate for those in preparation or action phases of the change process (Connors *et al.*, 2001; DiClemente *et al.*, 2004), research to date has failed to show that stage of change moderates response to either treatment (Burke *et al.*, 2003). Still, it seems clinically defensible to use MET at the beginning of treatment to enhance and solidify readiness for change and then shift to CBT techniques to aid the active process of making changes. Key issues that emerge when combining the approaches are how much time to devote to each, when to shift into CBT, and perhaps when to return to MET if a client is struggling with making changes. As noted above, MET therapists ideally make the decision to move into CBT or other action-oriented approaches when the client shows clear readiness and commitment to making changes. Whereas the signs that the client is ready may be clear in many cases, there are others where it is not. The therapist is left with a decision to continue with the MI approach or forge ahead with a change plan despite signs that the client is less than committed. Research is just beginning to systematically address these issues and for now we can only offer general guidelines based on clinical experience and the few relevant studies.

Treatment outcome studies combining MET and CBT have been protocol driven and generally have not given therapists much discretion in these matters. Rather, therapists are trained to follow manuals and to move from the MET approach to more action-oriented techniques during a specific session, which often has been toward the end of the first session (i.e., Budney *et al.*, 2000; Copeland *et al.*, 2001; Stephens *et al.*, 2000). The implication seems to be that 1 session is sufficient for MET. A more recent study provided 2 sessions of MET before shifting to CBT and explicitly gave therapists latitude to return to more of an MET approach if the client continued to appear ambivalent about change (MTPRG, 2004; Steinberg *et al.*, 2002). While this approach appears to be more clinically sensitive to issues in motivation for change, there are few hard and fast rules for when to shift techniques. Miller and colleagues (Miller & Rollnick, 1991, 2002; Miller *et al.*, 1992) list signs that the client may be more or less ready to start discussing a plan for change. More recently they provide detailed discussion of traps to avoid once the person is ready for change but is low in efficacy for doing so (Miller & Rollnick, 2002). In our on-going studies with less-motivated cannabis users, we are experimenting with asking clients directly at the beginning of sessions where they stand in their readiness to make changes and using the response to help focus the content and process of the session. Future reports from these projects may suggest additional techniques or guidelines.

**Group versus Individual Treatment**

Both group and individual CBT interventions have been found to be efficacious with cannabis-dependent adults, as well as with other drug-dependent populations. As we discuss below, research with cannabis dependence has not yet been designed to determine if one modality is superior to the other or whether there are identifiable characteristics of users that make them better suited for one or the other. In reality the decision to offer group or individual therapy is more often driven by the resources of the treatment provider, but it is worth considering the potential advantages of each. In an initial study (Stephens *et al.*, 1994), group CBT therapy was compared to a more support-oriented group intervention and both were equally successful in reducing cannabis use among participants. Group interventions in general may be particularly powerful because they provide multiple opportunities to "learn" from the experiences of others and, thus, may provide some of the benefits of CBT approaches. In that study, participants' post-treatment ratings of various treatment components indicated that "having time available to discuss issues related to cannabis use" and "being encouraged to discuss concerns with other group members" were judged to be as helpful as learning new coping techniques (Stephens & Roffman, 1993). During initial sessions, the sharing of common concerns about cannabis use is a powerful form of consciousness raising that may help dismantle myths regarding the lack of negative consequences and strengthen resolve to change. Group discussions may reveal potential coping techniques for accomplishing change and may guard against backsliding as group members challenge each others' rationalizations for drug use. Therefore, group versions of CBT can effectively harness the cumulative experience of the group in identifying high-risk situations, brainstorming and role-playing coping strategies, and providing support and reinforcement for change. The potential cost savings in terms of therapist time is another benefit of group therapy.

On the other hand, some potential clients may dislike the notion of sharing information regarding an illegal behavior in a group forum or more generally may not relate well in this environment. The use of delayed treatment control

(DTC) groups in two studies of cannabis dependence treatment may shed some light on the preferences of clients regarding group versus individual treatment. Participants who were randomly assigned to DTC conditions in these studies had the choice of receiving either of two active treatments following the pre-scribed waiting period. When the choice was between either a 14-session group treatment or a 2-session individual treatment, 64% chose the briefer individual treatment (Stephens *et al.*, 2000). However, in a similarly designed study where the choice was between a 9-sesssion individual treatment or a 2-session individual treatment, 64% chose the longer individual intervention (MTPRG, 2004). Thus, it may be that the group format of the longer intervention in the first study was less appealing. Individual CBT offers greater privacy and has the advantage of being able to tailor coping skills training to the specific needs of the client. It is therefore possible that fewer sessions would be needed to achieve the same level of coping skills and this savings may at least partially offset the apparent cost-effectiveness of group approaches. However, as we discuss below, it is not clear that coping skills training is essential to success-ful outcomes. Ultimately, relative efficacy and cost-effectiveness of individual and group approaches await future research.

The advantages and disadvantages of group versus individual MET inter-ventions are even less clear. No study of the treatment of cannabis dependence has used a group MET intervention and a review of group MET interventions with other addiction problems finds little support for the approach (Walters *et al.*, 2002). However, Walters and colleagues (2002) are careful to point out that most attempts have tried to directly translate the techniques of individual MET into a group format rather than develop an approach for groups that retains fidelity with the intent of MET. Their chapter discusses both the obstacles and possibilities in this approach.

### Issues in the Treatment of Cannabis Dependence

For the most part, MET and CBT treatments have been adapted and applied to cannabis-dependent adults in the same way they have been used with alcohol and other drug problems. The many similarities in the development of drug dependence across substances and the similar outcomes of treatment seem to justify this approach. Indeed, we have found both MET and CBT to be appeal-ing to cannabis-dependent adults and comparably effective (see below). Two related issues that are relatively unique to the treatment of cannabis depend-ence are the political turmoil surrounding the legal status of cannabis and the longstanding notion that cannabis is not "addictive." Clinicians working with cannabis users will frequently encounter clients who have strong feelings that cannabis should be legal because it is no more, and perhaps less, harmful than alcohol. Similarly, many users will question whether cannabis is really addictive like other drugs. Although clinicians should be able to provide information on recent research into cannabis dependence and its effects on health (see Chapter 5), they must be careful not to be the ones arguing for the need for change. In fact, many experts rate the addictive potential of cannabis low and the negative health effects of using the drug may not be as severe. As noted above, the primary reasons that cannabis users seek treatment seem to be related to more personal dissatisfactions with its effects on their motivation, productivity, and self-image. In keeping with the spirit of MI, therapists should use reflective listening regarding the clients' concerns about legal status or beliefs about addiction and should attempt to understand how these concerns relate to the clients' personal experiences with the drug. When clients bring up these issues it is likely an expression of their ambivalence about quitting or reducing use, and the therapist must acknowledge this ambivalence while identifying both the reasons for continued use and the reasons for change. Doing so avoids the trap of taking sides in a debate that cannot be won.

Another client-generated issue that is common across the treatment of most drugs of abuse concerns whether the treatment goal should be complete abstinence or should allow for some degree of moderate or recreational use. Again, beliefs that cannabis is not addictive and should be legal may make a moderate use goal seem attainable and justifiable. We know that, like alcohol users, the vast majority of cannabis users do not become dependent (see Chapter 4), yet there is no systematic research on the wisdom of either goal choice when treating those who are dependent on cannabis. All of the treatment outcome studies reviewed in the next section have promoted complete abstinence as the goal of treatment. When clients ask about the possibility of moderation we advise an abstinence goal based on the logic that it is actually easier to attain complete cessation than it is to try to limit the use of a drug over which they have already shown poor control. From the CBT perspective, abstinence is an easier goal to attain because cues and opportunities for use can be more drastically reduced by getting rid of all cannabis and associated paraphernalia. With the abstinence goal a single use or lapse becomes an immediate signal to the client to examine their behavior and motivations in order to regain abstinence. In contrast, moderating use would require setting a specific use goal, and then carefully and vigilantly monitoring the frequency and amount of use. Having cannabis available would provide a constant cue to use and leave the person open to rationalizing reasons to smoke. For those clients who have difficulty in accepting abstinence as the goal we leave open the possibility that they may be able to achieve a moderate use pattern in the future after they have demonstrated their ability to be completely abstinent for a significant length of time.

## Review of Treatment-Outcome Studies

In the first controlled treatment-outcome trial of CBT treatments for cannabis use, 212 adult users who wanted treatment were recruited from the community and randomly assigned either to a relapse prevention (RP) or discussion-oriented social support (SS) group treatment (Stephens *et al.*, 1994). The RP intervention closely followed Marlatt's CBT model (Marlatt & Gordon, 1985). The SS intervention emphasized the use of group support for change through discussion of topics related to cannabis cessation, but therapists did not provide skill-training or other CBT techniques. Both treatments consisted of ten 2-h group sessions with booster sessions at 3 and 6 months post-treatment. Participants were largely male (76%), in their early 30s, and had been using cannabis on average for 15 years. At pretreatment they had used on 81 of the 90 days preceding treatment and most used multiple times on a typical day of use. At the end of treatment, 63% of participants reported abstinence for at least the past 2 weeks. Continuous post-treatment abstinence rates at the 1-, 3-, 6-, 9-, and 12-month post-treatment follow-ups were 49%, 37%, 22%, 19%, and 14%, respectively. Significant reductions in the frequency of cannabis use and associated problems were observed at each follow-up and about 20% of non-abstinent participants in each condition were classified as "improved" at each follow-up based on at least a 50% reduction in the frequency of use and the absence of self-reported problems related to cannabis use. However, there were no differences between the RP and SS treatments on measures of cannabis use or negative consequences at any follow-up and findings did not support the hypothesis that the RP treatment based on CBT would yield superior outcomes. The lack of significant differences between treatments tempered conclusions regarding the success of treatment. High levels of motivation in the self-referred sample, rather than treatment, may have accounted for most of the change in cannabis use. Nevertheless, this study demonstrated that there was a subpopulation of adult cannabis users interested in treatment aimed at abstinence. Further, the overall success rates and the relapse rates during the post-treatment follow-up period were similar to those found in the treatment of other drugs of abuse.

In a second study, the same research group employed a DTC condition to examine change in cannabis use that might occur in the absence of intervention

(Stephens *et al.*, 2000). The final sample of 291 adults recruited from the community was assigned randomly to one of three conditions: a 14-session RP group intervention, a 2-session individualized assessment and intervention (IAI), or the DTC condition. Participants assigned to the DTC condition were reassessed after 4 months and then offered their choice of either of the other two treatments. Participant characteristics were similar to those in the first study with most participants being daily users in their mid-30s. Inclusion of a DSM-IIIR checklist of dependence symptoms suggested that most participants (98%) met criteria for cannabis dependence. The RP intervention was lengthened by 1 month and 4 additional sessions in order to provide more time for coping skill development. In addition, an optional 4-session group for spouses or SOs was included and focused on teaching them how they could help the participants in quitting cannabis use. A novel component of this group-based treatment was an attempt to train group members to keep meeting on their own to support abstinence after the end of the formal treatment period. The 2-session individual treatment was based on the success of brief interventions with problem drinkers and used a format modeled after the Drinkers' Check-Up (Bien *et al.*, 1993; Miller & Sovereign, 1989). Participants attended 2 individual sessions with a therapist, 1-month apart. During these sessions, MET was used to build motivation, a plan for change was negotiated, and CBT coping strategies for high-risk situations were discussed. At a 4-month follow-up, participants in both active treatment conditions reported significantly higher abstinence rates for the past month (42%) than those in the DTC condition (17%), as well as fewer days of cannabis use, number of times used per day, dependence symptoms, and problems related to use. However, there were no significant differences between the 14-session group RP and 2-session IAI conditions on any outcome measure. During the 16-month follow-up period, reductions in cannabis use and related consequences remained evident for participants in both the extended group and brief individual treatments, but no significant differences between the active treatments emerged. Analyses of DTC participants' reactions to being wait-listed suggested that neither feelings of disappointment nor relief over the assignment to this condition suppressed change in cannabis use that otherwise would have occurred. Overall, these results confirmed that reductions in cannabis use were not simply a function of client motivation at the outset and they suggested that a 2-session MET treatment may produce changes in cannabis use comparable to a much longer CBT-based intervention. However, differences in the mode of delivery (group versus individual) and experience of the therapists (the MET therapists were more experienced than the CBT therapists) made strong conclusions difficult.

In order to clarify the confounding of length and type of treatment, an Australian study compared the efficacy of 6-session and 1-session CBT-oriented treatments to a DTC condition. The study recruited 229 treatment-seeking adults from the general community in Sydney, Australia. The majority (69%) of participants were male with an average age of 32 years. Participants had been using cannabis at least weekly for around 14 years and the majority were daily or near daily users, consuming a median of eight waterpipes a day. Almost all (96%) received a current DSM-IV cannabis dependence diagnosis, while all met criteria for dependence according to the Severity of Dependence Scale (Swift *et al.*, 1998). Less than one-third (28.8%) had previously sought specialist assistance to moderate their cannabis use (Copeland *et al.*, 1999). In this study follow-up information was obtained on average 237 days from the completion of treatment for both treatment groups. Participants in the treatment groups reported better treatment outcomes than the DTC group. They were more likely to report abstinence with 15% of those in the 6-session group reporting continuous abstinence across the follow-up period compared with 5% in the 1-session group and 0% of the DTC. Similarly, when examining abstinence in the month prior to follow-up, verified with urinalysis for cannabinoids, 21% of the 6-session group; 17% of the 1-session group; and 4% of the DTC groups reported abstinence from cannabis use. The treatment groups were significantly less concerned about their control over cannabis use and reported significantly fewer cannabis-related problems than those in the DTC group. Those in the 6 sessions of CBT group also reported significantly reduced levels of cannabis consumption than the DTC group. While the therapist variable had no effect on any measure of outcome, a secondary analysis of the 6-versus 1-session groups showed that treatment compliance was significantly associated with decreased dependence and cannabis-related problems. This study supports the attractiveness of individual CBT and the potential for the application of even very brief versions in a variety of settings for individuals for cannabis dependence.

Another study randomly assigned 60 men and women to one of three conditions to compare the efficacy of CBT and MET treatments and the added effect of a contingency management approach that provided monetary incentives based on the absence of cannabis metabolites in weekly urine samples (Budney *et al.*, 2000). Participants were recruited from the community and had to meet diagnostic criteria for cannabis dependence in order to be eligible to participate. The average age was 32 years and most participants were men (83%). In this study the MET condition consisted of 4 individual sessions modeled after those in Project MATCH (Miller *et al.*, 1992) conducted over a 14-week period. The CBT condition consisted of 14 weekly individual sessions. The first session employed a motivational interview with feedback as in the MET condition, but subsequent sessions were designed to teach coping skills that were either directly (e.g., refusal skills, planning for high-risk situations, etc.) or indirectly (e.g., managing negative moods, enhancing social networks) related to achieving and maintaining abstinence. The third condition received the same 14 sessions of CBT with the addition of vouchers for negative urines during the 14 weeks of treatment. Vouchers had monetary values that escalated with consecutive weeks of abstinence such that someone who was continuously abstinent throughout treatment could earn $570. However, a positive urine result would reset the value of the vouchers to the initial level, providing a strong incentive to maintain continuous abstinence in order to maximize monetary reward. Indeed, the findings indicated that adding voucher-based monetary incentives to CBT significantly increased the number of weeks of continuous abstinence in comparison with MET- and CBT-based approaches. End-of-treatment abstinence rates for the preceding 30 days were also significantly greater in the voucher condition (35%) compared to the pure CBT (10%) and MET (5%) treatments. However, there were no significant differences between the three conditions on end-of-treatment frequency of cannabis use, which declined significantly in all conditions, nor on measures of negative consequences associated with use. These findings are consistent with previous data suggesting that complete abstinence is not necessary to achieve clinically meaningful improvement (MTPRG, 2004; Stephens *et al.*, 1994). The CBT condition outcomes tended to be somewhat better than those of the MET group but there were no significant differences perhaps because of small sample sizes and limited power. Although the absence of longer-term follow-ups precluded statements regarding the durability of the differences in abstinence, adding contingent reinforcement for verified abstinence to MET/CBT treatments appears promising and is discussed in more detail in Chapter 7.

The most recent published trial of CBT and MET treatments for cannabis dependence was a multi-site study (MTPRG, 2004; Stephens *et al.*, 2002). The study was developed to follow-up on the results from earlier trials that suggested very brief treatments (1–2 sessions) may be as effective as those of more moderate length (6–14) with this population. Since most of the prior trials had recruited fairly homogenous samples of white males in research settings an additional purpose of the study was to examine the efficacy of treatments for a more diverse group of cannabis-dependent adults. The study was conducted in parallel at drug treatment agencies in Farmington, CT, Miami, FL, and Seattle, WA. At each site participants were randomly assigned to a 9-session MET/CBT condition, a 2-session MET condition, or a 4-month DTC condition. The 9-session MET/CBT condition also included a case management component designed to help participants identify and address non-substance problems that could pose obstacles to reducing cannabis use (see Steinberg *et al.*, 2002). A total of 450 participants who met diagnostic criteria for cannabis dependence participated. The final sample was somewhat more diverse than in previous studies (32% female; 30% non-white), yet there were few meaningful differences in the cannabis use patterns and consequences across these geographically and ethnically diverse sites (Stephens *et al.*, 2002). Frequency of cannabis use decreased significantly in all three conditions at the 4-month follow-up, with participants in the 9-session MET/CBT treatment reducing their use of cannabis more than participants in the 2-session MET intervention, who in turn reduced use significantly more than those in the DTC condition. Abstinence rates for the preceding 90 days at the 4-month follow-up were significantly higher in the 9-session MET/CBT condition (23%) compared to the 2-session MET (9%) and DTC (4%) conditions. Although abstinence rates did not differ significantly between the 9-session (16%) and 2-session (10%) interventions at the 9-month follow-up, more 9-session participants (23%) reported 90 days of abstinence at a 15-month follow-up than those in the 2-session condition (13%). Further, significant differences in frequency of cannabis use continued to be present at both the 9-month and 15-month follow-ups with greater reductions for the 9-session treatment participants relative to those in the 2-session condition. Measures of the average amount of smoking per day and negative consequences associated with use generally showed parallel outcomes favoring the 9-session condition at the early follow-ups, but were no longer significantly different at 15 months. Importantly, the pattern of outcomes across treatments did not appear to be moderated by treatment site, sex, ethnicity, or employment status.

**Mechanisms of Change**

The presumed mechanisms of action of CBT and MET interventions have received relatively little attention in cannabis dependence treatment studies. CBT is proposed to work by increasing coping skills and self-efficacy for avoiding drug use. Self-efficacy for avoiding cannabis use and the use of situational coping strategies covaried as expected and both were predictive of cannabis use during follow-up periods (Stephens *et al.*, 1993, 1995). Self-efficacy was slightly higher following CBT compared to a group support condition, but a self-report measure of coping skill utilization did not differ between treatments and actually decreased significantly from baseline values (Stephens *et al.*, 1995). Thus, it was not clear that increases in the use of coping skills accounted for reductions in cannabis use. Budney and colleagues (2000) also found greater increases in situational self-efficacy for their MET/CBT treatment relative to the MET only condition, but did not relate these changes to the acquisition or use of coping skills. Self-efficacy and coping skill utilization may be affected similarly by a variety of effective interventions (Finney *et al.*, 1998) and other research fails to support strong relationships between coping skills and drug use outcomes (e.g., Finney *et al.*, 1999; Morgenstern & Longabaugh, 2000). Thus, it may be that CBT works through some unidentified process rather than by remediating coping skills deficits.

Some evidence was found for the importance of specific cognitions surrounding a relapse episode (Stephens *et al.*, 1994). The abstinence violation effect (AVE), more generally referred to as the rule violation effect, is proposed to occur when individuals make internal, stable, and global attributions for the cause of an initial use of a substance following a period of abstinence (Marlatt & Gordon, 1985). This particular constellation of attributions may lead the user to give up on remaining abstinent in the face of a single lapse and may increase the probability of a complete relapse. CBT treatments typically include education and cognitive restructuring regarding attributions for slips or lapses in order to prevent full-blown relapse. Indeed, analysis of data from one treatment-outcome study showed that those who made AVE attributions for a lapse were more likely to report increased use of cannabis both concurrently and at future follow-ups (Stephens *et al.*, 1994). However, the tendency to experience the AVE was not differentially affected by CBT relative to a group support treatment despite the inclusion of cognitive-restructuring techniques targeting this attributional style. Although there appears to be some predictive validity to the AVE, modification of AVE reactions may take more intensive cognitive therapy than has been provided in CBT studies to date.

Proposed mediators of the effects of MET interventions have been studied even less often in cannabis studies. MET presumably works by making reasons for change more salient, thereby increasing motivation. Only one study reported changes in motivation or readiness to change following treatment with results showing that motivation to change actually decreased (Budney *et al.*, 2000). A review of the larger literature on MET-type interventions concludes that there is little evidence that MET works by increasing motivation. Although studies have shown increases in motivation following MET interventions they generally have not been greater than increases in comparison treatments nor have they been shown to mediate the effects of treatment (see Burke *et al.*, 2002 for a review). Changes in self-efficacy may also account for MET treatment effects because a basic principle in these therapies is to support efficacy for change. Unpublished data from two studies shows that self-efficacy for avoiding cannabis use increases significantly following brief MET treatments (MTPRG, 2004; Stephens *et al.*, 2000), but the timing of efficacy measurements in these studies do not allow for an unequivocal assessment of whether efficacy is increased directly by the therapy or whether the change simply reflects the success in reducing cannabis use associated with the treatments. Another study failed to find a significant increase in self-efficacy with MET (Budney *et al.*, 2000). A recent analysis of treatment session tapes of drug users showed that clients who made stronger statements of commitment to change during MI treatment made greater reductions in drug use (Amrhein *et al.*, 2003). However, these types of analyses have not yet been conducted in studies focused on the treatment of cannabis dependence and questions also remain regarding how such statements function to engender change in drug use if it is not through increases in motivation.

## Summary and Future Directions

Taken together, the results from these studies indicate that some cannabis-dependent adults are interested in treatment and respond well to both CBT and MET interventions. The poorer outcomes of DTC groups in three studies demonstrate that these effects are not simply due to pre-existing motivation for change in the participants. Sustained abstinence was a relatively uncommon outcome and relapse rates following treatments were similar to those for other drugs of abuse. However, the substantial reductions in cannabis use, coupled with decreases in associated negative consequence supports the efficacy of MET and CBT treatments tailored specifically for cannabis users.

On the other hand, a clear superiority of CBT or MET has not been demonstrated and, in fact, no study has been designed specifically to examine this difference. Treatment type has frequently been confounded with treatment intensity or duration such that even when differences in outcomes emerge it is not clear whether they are related to the nature of the treatment or the number of sessions (Budney *et al.*, 2000; MTPRG, 2004; Stephens *et al.*, 2000). This confounding makes it difficult to understand several differences in the outcomes across trials. Unlike initial findings that a very brief MET intervention produced outcomes similar to longer CBT treatment (Stephens *et al.*, 2000), subsequent studies tended to show somewhat better outcomes for longer treatments. However, in only one study were the greater benefits of the longer intervention clear (MTPRG, 2004).

There are several possible reasons for the comparable outcomes in these studies that suggest avenues for future research. Stephens and colleagues (2000) delivered the CBT treatment in a group format whereas the MET treatment was delivered individually and by a different set of therapists with more experience. All subsequent studies used the same therapists to deliver both types of interventions individually. Thus, it is possible that either the group format diluted the impact of CBT or that the greater experience and professional credentials of the MET therapists augmented the impact of the brief intervention in that initial study. Stephens and colleagues (2000) was the only study to use doctoral level therapists to deliver the brief MET intervention. Others have discussed the complexity of training MET techniques and it is possible that greater treatment experience may facilitate learning and applying these subtle techniques in a way that maximizes change in a brief intervention. Research is needed that directly addresses the level of competency of therapists in relation to client outcomes.

It is also possible that the group therapy format diluted the effect of CBT in this study but the fact that post-treatment abstinence rates and reductions in frequency of use in the CBT treatment were equivalent or greater than those in any of the subsequent treatment trials argues against this interpretation (Stephens *et al.*, 2000). Of course, differences in the populations sampled across studies in terms of severity of dependence or motivation for change may also account for differences in outcomes, but the overall similarities in users across these studies suggest that the group CBT intervention was as potent in producing change as subsequent individual CBT treatments. No other studies have used the group modality for treatment of cannabis dependence and more research is needed with this potentially cost-effective approach.

The studies of MET and CBT to date have not generally tested pure versions of either approach. The CBT interventions usually have used some MET style techniques in the early sessions (Budney *et al.*, 2000; Copeland *et al.*, 2001; MTPRG, 2004) and some relatively pure MET interventions may have crossed the line into CBT by providing handouts related to coping skills and allowing therapists latitude of addressing specific high-risk situations during booster sessions (e.g., Stephens *et al.*, 2000). As we have noted, the two approaches are compatible and focus on different issues and stages in the change process, so there is no mandate to pair them in a horse race. Yet, the continual blending of these treatments may impede our understanding of why they work. Designs that systematically separate the techniques of each approach are needed to answer such questions (e.g., Sellman *et al.*, 2001).

## References

Amrhein, P. C., Miller, W. R., Yahne, C. E., Palmer, M., & Fulcher, L. (2003). Client commitment language during motivational interviewing predicts drug use outcomes. *Journal of Consulting and Clinical Psychology, 71,* 862–878.

Baer, J. S., Kivlahan, D. R., & Donovan, D. N. (1999). Integrating skills training and motivational therapies. *Journal of Substance Abuse Treatment, 17,* 15–23.

Bien, T. H., Miller, W. R., & Tonigan, S. (1993). Brief interventions for alcohol problems: a review. *Addiction, 88,* 315–336.

Brickman, P., Rabinowitz, V. V., Karuza, J., Coates, D., Cohn, E., & Kidder, L. (1982). Models of helping and coping. *American Psychologist, 37,* 368–384.

Budney, A. J., Higgins, S. T., Radonovich, K. J., & Novy, P. L. (2000). Adding voucher-based incentives to coping skills and motivational enhancement improves outcomes during treatment for marijuana dependence. *Journal of Consulting and Clinical Psychology, 8,* 1051–1061.

Budney, A. J., Radonovich, K. J., Higgins, S. T., & Wong, C. J. (1998). Adults seeking treatment for marijuana dependence: a comparison to cocaine-dependent treatment seekers. *Experimental and Clinical Psychopharmacology, 6,* 1–8.

Burke, B., Arkowitz, H., & Dunn, C. (2002). The efficacy of motivational interviewing. In W. R. Miller, & S. Rollnick (Eds.), *Motivational interviewing: preparing people for change* (2nd ed., pp. 217–250). New York: Guilford Press.

Burke, B. L., Arkowitz, H., & Menchola, M. (2003). The efficacy of motivational interviewing: a meta-analysis of controlled clinical trials. *Journal of Consulting and Clinical Psychology, 71,* 843–861.

Carroll, K. M., Nich, C. Ball, S. A., McCance, E., & Rounsaville, B. J. (1998). Treatment of cocaine and alcohol dependence with psychotherapy and disulfarim. *Addiction, 93,* 713–728.

Connors, G. J., Donovan, D. M., & DiClemente, C. C. (2001). *Substance abuse treatment and the stages of change: selecting and planning interventions.* New York: Guilford Press.

Copeland, J., Rees, V., & Swift, W. (1999). Health concerns and help-seeking among a sample entering treatment for cannabis dependence. Correspondence. *Australian Family Physician, 28,* 540–541.

Copeland, J., Swift, W., & Rees, V. (2001). Clinical profile of participants in a brief intervention for cannabis use disorder. *Journal of Substance Abuse Treatment, 20*(1), 45–52.

Copeland, J., Swift, W., Roffman, R., & Stephens, R. (2001). A randomised controlled trial of brief cognitive-behavioral interventions for cannabis use disorders. *Journal of Substance Abuse Treatment, 21,* 55–64.

DiClemente, C. C., Schlundt, D., & Gemmell, L. (2004). Readiness and stages of change in addiction treatment. *American Journal on Addictions, 13,* 103–119.

Finney, J. W., Moos, R. H., & Humphreys, K. (1999). A comparative evaluation of substance abuse treatment: II. Linking proximal outcomes of 12-step and cognitive-behavioral treatment to substance use outcomes. *Alcoholism: Clinical and Experimental Research, 23,* 537–544.

Finney, J. W., Noyes, C. A., Coutts, A. I., & Moos, R. H. (1998). Evaluating substance abuse treatment process models: I. Changes on proximal outcome variables during 12-step and cognitive-behavioral treatment. *Journal of Studies on Alcohol, 59,* 371–380.

Maisto, S. A., Carey, K., & Bradizza, C. M. (1999). Social learning theory. In K. E. Leonard, & H. T. Blane (Eds.), *Psychological theories of drinking and alcoholism* (2nd ed., pp. 106–163). New York: Guilford Press.

Marijuana Treatment Project Research Group (MTPRG). (2004). Brief treatments for cannabis dependence: findings from a randomized multisite trial. *Journal of Consulting and Clinical Psychology, 72,* 455–466.

Marlatt, G. A., & Gordon, J. R. (1985). *Relapse prevention: maintenance strategies in the treatment of addictive behaviors.* New York: Guilford.

Miller, W. R., Brown, J. M., Simpson, T. L., Handmaker, N. S., Bien, T. H., Luckie, L. F., Montgomery, H. A., Hester, R. K., & Tonigan, J. S. (1995). What works? A methodological analysis of the alcohol treatment outcome literature. In R. K. Hester, & W. R. Miller (Eds.), *Handbook of alcoholism and treatment approaches: effective alternatives* (2nd ed., pp. 12–44). Boston: Allyn and Bacon.

Miller, N. S., & Gold, M. S. (1989). The diagnosis of marijuana (cannabis) dependence. *Journal of Substance Abuse Treatment, 6,* 183–192.

Miller, N. S., Gold, M. S., & Pottash, A. C. (1989). A 12-step treatment approach to marijuana (*cannabis*) dependence. *Journal of Substance Abuse Treatment, 6,* 241–250.

Miller, W. R., & Rollnick, S. (1991). *Motivational interviewing: preparing people to change addictive behavior.* New York: Guilford Press.

Miller, W. R., & Rollnick, S. (2002). *Motivational interviewing: preparing people for change* (2nd ed.). New York: Guilford Press.

Miller, W. R., & Sovereign, R. G. (1989). The check-up: a model for early intervention in addictive behaviors. In T. Loberg, W. R. Miller, P. E. Nathan, & G. A. Marlatt (Eds.), *Addictive behaviors: prevention and early intervention* (pp. 219–231). Amsterdam: Swets and Zeitlinger.

Miller, W. R., Sovereign, R. G., & Krege, B. (1988). Motivational interviewing with problem drinkers: II. The drinker's check-up as a preventive intervention. *Behavioral Psychotherapy, 16,* 251–268.

Miller, W. R., Zweben, A., DiClemente, C. C., & Rychtarik, R. G. (1992). *Motivational enhancement therapy manual: a clinical research guide for therapists treating individuals with alcohol abuse and dependence* (DHHS Publication No. ADM 92–1894). Washington, DC: US Government Printing Office.

Monti, P. M., Kadden, R. M., Rohsenow, D. J., Cooney, N. L., & Abrams, D. B. (2002). *Treating alcohol dependence: a coping skills training guide.* New York: Guilford Press.

Morgenstern, J., & Longabaugh, R. (2000). Cognitive-behavioral treatment for alcohol dependence: a review of evidence for its hypothesized mechanisms of action. *Addiction, 95*, 1474–1490.

Project MATCH Research Group. (1997). Matching alcoholism treatments to client heterogeneity: Project MATCH posttreatment drinking outcomes. *Journal of Studies on Alcohol, 58*, 7–29.

Sellman, J. D., Sullivan, P. F., Dore, G. M., Adamson, S. J., & MacEwan, I. (2001). A randomized controlled trial of motivational enhancement therapy (MET) for mile to moderate alcohol dependence. *Journal of Studies on Alcohol, 62*, 389–396.

Steinberg, K. L., Roffman, R. A., Carroll, K. M., Kabela, E., Kadden, R., Miller, M., Duresky, D., & The Marijuana Treatment Project Research Group (MTPRG). (2002). Tailoring cannabis dependence treatment for a diverse population. *Addiction, 97* (Suppl. 1), 135–142.

Stephens, R. S., Babor, T. F., Kadden, R., Miller, M., & The Marijuana Treatment Project Research Group (MTPRG). (2002). The Marijuana Treatment Project: Rationale, design, and participant characteristics. *Addiction, 97*, 109–124.

Stephens, R. S., Curtin, L., Simpson, E. E., & Roffman, R. A. (1994). Testing the abstinence violation effect construct with marijuana cessation. *Addictive Behaviors, 19*, 23–32.

Stephens, R. S., & Roffman, R. A. (1993). Adult marijuana dependence. In J. S. Baer, G. A. Marlatt, & J. McMahon (Eds.), *Addictive behaviors across the lifespan: Prevention, treatment, and policy issues* (pp. 202–218). Newbury Park, CA: Sage.

Stephens, R. S., & Roffman, R. A. (2005). Assessment of cannabis use disorders. In D. Donovan, & G. A. Marlatt (Eds.), *Assessment of addictive behaviors* (2nd ed., pp. 248–273). New York: Guilford.

Stephens, R. S., Roffman, R. A., & Curtin, L. (2000). Comparison of extended versus brief treatments for marijuana use. *Journal of Consulting and Clinical Psychology, 68*, 898–908.

Stephens, R. S., Roffman, R. A., & Simpson, E. E. (1993). Adult marijuana users seeking treatment. *Journal of Consulting and Clinical Psychology, 61*, 1100–1104.

Stephens, R. S., Roffman, R. A., & Simpson, E. E. (1994). Treating adult marijuana dependence: a test of the relapse prevention model. *Journal of Consulting and Clinical Psychology, 62*, 92–99.

Stephens, R. S., Wertz, J. S., & Roffman, R. A. (1993). Predictors of marijuana treatment outcomes: the role of self-efficacy. *Journal of Substance Abuse, 5*, 341–353.

Stephens, R. S., Wertz, J. S., & Roffman, R. A. (1995). Self-efficacy and marijuana cessation: a construct validity analysis. *Journal of Consulting and Clinical Psychology, 63*, 1022–1031.

Swift, W., Copeland, J., & Hall, W. (1998). Choosing a diagnostic cut-off for cannabis dependence. *Addiction, 93*(11), 1681–1692.

Tashkin, D. P. (1999). Cannabis effects on the respiratory system. In H. Kalant, W. Corrigall, W. Hall, & R. Smart (Eds.), *The health effects of cannabis* (pp. 313–345). Toronto: Addiction Research Foundation.

Tennant, F. S. (1986). The clinical syndrome of marijuana dependence. *Psychiatric Annals, 16*, 225–242.

Walters, S. T., Ogle, R., & Martin, J. E. (2002). Perils and possibilities of group-based motivational interviewing. In W. R. Miller, & S. Rollnick (Eds.), *Motivational interviewing: preparing people for change* (2nd ed., pp. 377–419). New York: Guilford Press.

Zweben, J. C., & O'Connell, K. (1988). Strategies for breaking marijuana dependence. *Journal of Psychoactive Drugs, 20*, 121–127.

# 7

# Contingency-Management Interventions for Cannabis Dependence

ALAN J. BUDNEY, BRENT A. MOORE, STACEY C. SIGMON AND
STEPHEN T. HIGGINS

Individuals who seek treatment for substance abuse problems are notoriously difficult to retain in treatment and motivate to change. Even when clients make initial progress, frequently motivation wanes and relapse occurs. Contingency-management (CM) interventions represent one treatment approach that has great potential to effectively motivate and facilitate change in this challenging clinical population. CM may be particularly useful for treating individuals seeking treatment for cannabis abuse or dependence, as their motivation to change their cannabis use may not be as great as those seeking treatment for other types of drug abuse (Budney et al., 1997, 1998b). Cannabis-dependent clients report psychosocial problems similar to other drug abuse clients, but in general they do not experience the type of acute crises or severity of consequences that often drive alcohol-, cocaine-, or heroin-dependent individuals into treatment. Typically, they exhibit frequent and stable patterns of cannabis use with less financial burden and without as great a disruption to daily routines as individuals with other types of drug dependence. Perhaps, for reasons related to this issue, cannabis abusers appear to exhibit at least as much difficulty as other drug abusers in initiating and maintaining abstinence. Results from the few controlled clinical trials examining treatments for cannabis dependence indicate that even the most effective treatments do not engender abstinence among the majority of those who enroll, and the rates of relapse, like with other substance dependence treatments is relatively high (Budney et al., 2000; Copeland et al., 2001; Moore & Budney, 2003; Stephens et al., 1994, 2000). Thus, there exists significant room for enhancement of outcomes.

A recent resurgence of clinical trials examining CM interventions across various types of substance dependence provides compelling support for their efficacy for improving treatment outcome (Higgins & Silverman, 1999). CM interventions are based on extensive basic-science and clinical-research evidence demonstrating that drug use and abuse are heavily influenced by learning

154

and conditioning and are quite sensitive to systematically applied environmental consequences (Goldberg & Stollerman, 1986; Griffiths *et al.*, 1980; Higgins, 1997). These interventions arrange the environment such that reinforcing or punishing events occur contingent on drug abstinence, drug use, or other therapeutic targets. In treatment settings, CM has typically been integrated with other psychosocial or pharmacological therapies.

### Conceptual Framework

Behavior-analytic theory posits that drug use is a case of operant behavior that is maintained, in part, by the pharmacological actions of the drug in conjunction with social and other non-pharmacological reinforcement derived from the drug-abusing lifestyle (Goldberg & Stollerman, 1986; Higgins & Katz, 1998). Within the field of behavioral pharmacology, empirical research across species and drugs provides strong support for the position that reinforcement is a fundamental determinant of drug use and abuse. Hence, drug use is considered a normal, learned behavior that falls along a continuum ranging from patterns of little use and few problems to excessive use and dependence. All healthy humans are assumed to possess the necessary neurobiological systems to experience drug-produced reinforcement, and thus to have the potential to develop patterns of use or abuse. Genetic or acquired characteristics are accepted as contributors to the probability of developing drug abuse, but this model assumes that such special characteristics are not necessary for drug abuse to develop.

An important feature of this model of drug abuse is that it facilitates a direct connection between clinical practice and the scientific disciplines of behavior analysis and behavioral pharmacology. Those disciplines include an extensive research literature demonstrating principles and procedures that can be applied to modify behavior of all kinds, including drug abuse. Indeed, controlled studies with humans and laboratory animals have shown that drug use is an orderly form of behavior that is affected by environmental context and the reinforcement contingencies under which it occurs (Griffiths *et al.*, 1980; Higgins, 1997). Alterations in drug availability, drug dose, response requirement needed to obtain drug, and the availability of other non-drug reinforcers each have orderly and generalizable effects on drug use.

The CM treatment approach capitalizes on knowledge that drug seeking and drug use can be directly modified by manipulating relevant environmental contingencies. Treatment focuses on reorganizing the physical and social environments of the user. The goal is to systematically weaken the influence of reinforcement derived from drug use and the related lifestyle, and to increase the frequency and magnitude of reinforcement derived from healthier alternative activities. For example, the particular CM program for cannabis dependence that we describe below is structured such that abstinence from cannabis (documented by urinalysis testing) is reinforced by providing monetary-based vouchers that can be used to increase participation in non-drug related, prosocial activities.

## Basic Principles

CM interventions involve the use of positive reinforcement, negative reinforcement, positive punishment, or negative punishment contingencies to increase and decrease the frequency of a target behavior. In substance abuse settings, the most common target behavior has been drug use, although other therapeutic behaviors have been targeted, such as counseling attendance, completion of homework tasks, or medication compliance (Higgins & Silverman, 1999).

Positive reinforcement involves delivery of a desired consequence contingent on meeting a therapeutic goal. Examples of positive reinforcers used in CM programs for substance dependence are vouchers exchangeable for retail items, methadone take-home privileges, access to housing or employment, and increased opportunities to win prizes. Negative reinforcement involves removing an aversive or confining circumstance contingent on meeting a therapeutic goal, which might involve a reduction in the intensity of criminal justice supervision or schedule of counseling. Positive punishment involves delivery of a non-desirable consequence contingent on evidence of undesirable behavior (e.g., drug use). This might include increases in treatment participation requirements, termination of treatment, suspension of employment, or a specified period of incarceration. Negative punishment involves removal of a positive circumstance or condition contingent on evidence of undesirable behavior, such as a reduction in the monetary value of vouchers earned for drug abstinence, or removal of preferred schedules of medication dosing or counseling sessions. Reinforcement and punishment contingencies can both be effective tools in substance abuse treatment programs, but the former are generally preferred over the latter by clients and clinicians.

## Efficacy of CM

The scientific literature includes many examples of how creative and careful programming of a combination of contingencies can enhance therapeutic outcomes across a wide range of substance abuse treatment populations (Higgins & Silverman, 1999). Perhaps the most well researched CM intervention is an abstinence-based voucher program for cocaine dependence (Budney & Higgins, 1998). In this program, clients provide urine specimens on a thrice-weekly schedule, and monetary-based incentives (vouchers) are earned for each cocaine-negative urine specimen. Vouchers are exchangeable for retail goods or services that support healthy lifestyle changes. This outpatient program has demonstrated efficacy across five controlled clinical trials and its positive effects extend at least 15 months post-treatment (Higgins *et al.*, 1991, 1993, 1994, 2000, 2003).

Similar abstinence-based incentive programs effectively increase cocaine abstinence in methadone-maintained, opiate-dependent clients (Silverman *et al.*, 1996), inner-city crack abusers (Kirby *et al.*, 1998), pregnant cocaine abusers (Elk, 1999), and homeless, dually diagnosed cocaine abusers (Milby *et al.*, 2000). These type of CM programs can also improve retention and abstinence rates during treatment for opiate dependence (Bickel *et al.*, 1997) and alcohol dependence (Petry *et al.*, 2000). Of most importance here, we recently demonstrated (and describe in detail below) that an abstinence-based voucher program can increase cannabis abstinence during treatment for cannabis dependence when added to cognitive-behavioral and motivational enhancement therapies (Budney *et al.*, 2000).

**Principles of Application**

Behavioral-analytic theory and the empirical literature on behavior change in general suggests that the efficacy of CM interventions will be influenced by the schedule used to deliver consequences, the magnitude of the consequence, the choice of the target behavior, the selection of the type of consequence, and the monitoring of the target behavior (Sulzer-Azaroff & Meyer, 1991). In this section, we use examples from our cannabis CM program to describe these basic principles and illustrate their application.

The schedule of reinforcement or punishment refers to the temporal relation between the target behavior and the delivery of the consequence. Generally, efficacy is likely to improve as the temporal delay between the occurrence of the target behavior and delivery of the consequence decreases. For example, all else being equal, providing positive reinforcement for cannabis abstinence 5 min after a client submits a cannabis-negative urine specimen would likely generate greater rates of abstinence than waiting a week before reinforcement is delivered. In our CM program for cannabis dependence, on-site drug testing allows staff to provide reinforcement within 5 min or so following specimen collection.

Similarly, more frequent schedules of reinforcement are usually preferable to less frequent schedules in establishing an initial target behavior like cannabis abstinence or regular attendance at counseling sessions (Ferster & Skinner, 1957). In our cannabis program, we conduct urinalysis tests twice per week. Frequent schedules allow multiple opportunities to reinforce and thereby strengthen the target behavior. Once a target behavior is established, less frequent schedules are typically considered for maintenance of behavior change. One must also consider how often drug testing is needed to ensure that drug use does not go undetected between tests so that the probability of providing reinforcement when drug use has occurred is minimized.

The magnitude of reinforcement or punishment is also an important factor that will likely affect the efficacy of most CM interventions. For example, if the goal is cannabis abstinence, a voucher worth $10.00 for each cannabis-negative specimen is likely to be more effective in increasing cannabis abstinence than one worth $2.00. Given the resilience of substance-use patterns that typically develop over many years, strong reinforcers are likely necessary to compete with the reinforcement derived from such well-established behavior. In our cannabis and cocaine programs, the value of the vouchers earned escalates with each consecutive drug-negative specimen, and when an unexcused absence from a scheduled urinalysis or a drug-positive test occurs, the value of the voucher resets to the initial lower level. This schedule is designed to promote continuous periods of abstinence by increasing the amount of reinforcement earned in direct relation to the number of consecutive drug-negative specimens submitted, and by resetting the value of the vouchers back to low amounts of reinforcement if drug use occurs (Roll *et al.*, 1996). Of note, although one would generally expect higher magnitude reinforcement to generate greater amounts of abstinence than lower magnitude reinforcement, creative use of relatively low magnitude reinforcers and variable or intermittent schedules can successfully modify target behaviors among drug abusers (Petry & Martin, 2002; Petry *et al.*, 2000).

The choice of reinforcers or punishers used in a CM program can be critical to its success. Individuals vary greatly in terms of the types of goods and services that will serve as reinforcers. For example, a specific reinforcer (e.g., pizza or movie theater passes) that functions as an effective reinforcer for one client may not be reinforcing for another. In our voucher programs, clients can choose any appropriate item or service available in the community, and clinic staff make the purchase. This procedure allows for access to a wide range of reinforcers, while providing some control and guidance over reinforcer purchases. Reinforcers used in other CM programs include cash, on-site retail items, specific prizes, desirable clinic privileges, employment or housing opportunities, or refunds on treatment service fees (Higgins & Silverman, 1999). Each of these has its strengths and drawbacks. For example, providing cash would be highly reinforcing for most clients, but cash also may function as a trigger for drug use.

Most successful CM programs for drug dependence have selected drug abstinence as the target behavior. CM programs have also targeted medication compliance, counseling attendance, and completion of lifestyle change activities. When choosing such targets, one must be aware that successful change in such behavior may not result in drug abstinence. For example, treatment attendance may improve by providing vouchers contingent for coming to sessions, but drug use might not change (Iguchi *et al.*, 1996). The extant CM literature suggests that the first choice of a target behavior should be drug use. If other targets are selected, these should be specific, individualized behavioral goals that have a high probability for successful completion (Sulzer-Azaroff & Meyer, 1991).

Effective monitoring of the targeted behavior is essential to a CM program, because consequences must be applied systematically. With substance abusers, this typically involves some form of biochemical verification of drug abstinence, usually via urinalysis testing. With cannabis, urinalysis testing poses some unique issues that deserve comment. Regular, heavy cannabis users continue to test positive for cannabis use for 2–3 weeks at detection levels of 50 or 100 ng/ml, which are the accepted cutoff levels for documenting recent abstinence. Thus, in our voucher program, we provide a 2-week notice prior to initiating the voucher program that informs clients that it will take 2 weeks of abstinence from cannabis for them to achieve a cannabinoid-negative urinalysis result. Reinforcement must therefore be delayed because of the limitations of our technology. As technological advances are made in the field of urine toxicology perhaps this situation will be rectified. The importance of having a method for objectively and reliably verifying whether a target behavior occurred pertains as well to other target behaviors. Reliance on self-reports of drug use or completion of other therapeutic tasks is not adequate for these purposes.

**Effective Implementation**

CM approaches are novel to most substance abuse therapists and clients. Thus, here we offer some brief comment on clinical issues that are critical to successful implementation using our voucher program as an example. A more in-depth discussion of CM implementation issues can be found elsewhere (Budney & Higgins, 1998; Budney *et al.*, 2001; Petry, 2000). Therapists and clients must clearly understand the rationale for the program and how it works in order to maximize its acceptability and efficacy. Most clients who enroll in treatment for cannabis dependence expect to receive counseling that involves talking about their problems. They do not expect that they will be required to follow rules and complete specific tasks. CM programs use behavioral contracts to specify rationales for the program, and define client and staff roles and expectations. In addition, therapists are responsible for fostering understanding, interest, and compliance, and for ensuring that clients fully understand the monitoring and voucher programs.

Urinalysis testing is a hallmark of most CM substance abuse interventions, hence everyone involved must embrace it as a crucial element of the treatment process. Even therapists may be hesitant about the need for urine testing and how it may affect the client's willingness to participate. In our cannabis program, clients are required to provide two urine specimens per week, and the observation process is sometimes awkward at first. Hence, an explanation of the need for this procedure should include the following points:

- Testing permits careful and immediate evaluation of progress.
- Observation serves to maintain the integrity and credibility of the testing.
- Testing keeps the focus of treatment on the primary problem, cannabis use.
- Testing reduces the tendency to conceal use because of embarrassment, pride, etc.
- Results assist the therapist to detect and work on relapse triggers.
- Testing provides opportunities to document abstinence and gain credibility with family or friends.

Therapists and clients may also find the concept of directly "rewarding " abstinence with vouchers novel and perhaps perplexing. Thus, explanation and discussion of our cannabis program includes the following points:

- Research clearly demonstrates that incentive programs can increase drug abstinence.
- Voucher programs provide a clear positive reward for achieving the goal of not using cannabis, which contrasts with what typically happens, that is punishment for using.
- Voucher programs can enhance and maintain motivation to work hard on an abstinence goal.
- Earnings increase with each cannabis-negative urine specimen as a way to enhance investment in the goal of abstinence. Research indicates that continuous abstinence during treatment is a good predictor of longer-term abstinence.
- Voucher earnings can help provide non-drug alternative sources of fun and pleasure.

Last, the anticipation of problems unique to CM programs, such as the denial of use when positive testing occurs and disagreements over appropriate voucher spending, can enhance the overall efficacy of the program. Clinical responses to these types of issues that are in concert with the philosophy of CM programs can promote retention and treatment progress.

## Initial Treatment Study for a CM Voucher Program for Cannabis Dependence

As reviewed in Chapters 6 and 9, behavioral treatment approaches have demonstrated efficacy with cannabis-dependent adults. Thus, effective treatments for cannabis dependence are available, but as with treatments for other types of substance dependence, there remains room for improved success rates. The primary purpose of our initial trial examining a CM intervention for cannabis dependence was to determine if we could improve treatment outcome by adding an abstinence-based voucher program to treatments that had demonstrated efficacy in prior controlled studies (Budney *et al.*, 2000).

### *Study Design*

Three behaviorally based outpatient treatments were compared: a brief motivational therapy (M), brief motivational therapy combined with cognitive-behavioral coping-skills therapy (MBT), and a combination of the brief motivational therapy, the coping-skills therapy and an abstinence-based voucher program (MBTV). The comparison of the M and MBT treatments was a replication and extension of Stephens and colleagues' study in which no differences were observed between a brief two-session intervention and a 14-session cognitive-behavioral intervention, but both were more effective than a delayed treatment control group (Stephens *et al.*, 2000). Most important to the aims of this chapter were the comparisons of MBTV with MBT and with M. These comparisons provided a clear test of whether adding the voucher-based CM program to previously demonstrated effective treatments could enhance treatment efficacy.

### *Participants*

Sixty adults (43 men and 17 women) seeking treatment for cannabis dependence enrolled in this study. All participants met DSM-III-R diagnostic criteria for current cannabis dependence. Individuals were excluded if they were currently dependent on alcohol or any other drug except nicotine. The resulting sample appears representative of those seeking treatment for cannabis dependence as only 10 individuals seeking treatment were excluded. Most participants used cannabis on an almost daily basis ($M$ = 22.5, SD = 8.6 days/month), smoked multiple times per day ($M$ = 3.7, SD = 2.6 episodes/day), and had used cannabis regularly for many years ($M$ = 15.2, SD = 8.3 years). Most participants were Caucasian (83%) with an average age of 32 (SD = 8.5) years. Sixty-five percent were employed full time, and 92% had at least a high school education or its equivalent. Substantial psychiatric symptomatology was noted, as 65% of the sample scored in the clinically significant range of the Global Symptom Index of the Brief Symptom Inventory (Derogatis, 1993).

*Treatments*

Participants were randomly assigned to one of the three treatment conditions and stratified on two variables: involvement with the legal system and gender. Each treatment lasted 14 weeks and was manual-driven. All participants provided urine specimens on a twice-weekly schedule throughout treatment. The M treatment was adapted from the motivational enhancement therapy used in the Project Match alcohol treatment study (NIAAA, 1992b). Participants received four, 60–90-min individual therapy sessions scheduled during Weeks 1, 2, 6, and 12. A written assessment feedback report was provided, and therapists used a motivational interviewing style to encourage changes in marijuana use. The MBT treatment combined the motivational enhancement therapy with an adapted version of the Behavioral Coping Skills Therapy used in Project Match (NIAAA, 1992a). The coping-skills therapy involved once weekly 60-min, individual therapy sessions throughout the 14-week treatment. These sessions focused on increasing motivation, developing skills to help achieve and maintain cannabis abstinence, and setting lifestyle change goals. Examples of the coping skills included in MBT were: craving management, planning for high-risk situations, drug refusal, managing mood, and enhancing social networks.

The therapy for the MBTV condition was almost identical to that provided in MBT. The only difference was that, in MBTV, therapists regularly reviewed and discussed voucher earnings and purchases with the goal of using the vouchers to promote abstinence and to facilitate healthy lifestyle change goals. The voucher program did not begin until the third week of treatment because, as discussed above, cannabis remains detectable via standard urinalysis testing for approximately 2 weeks following the initiation of abstinence in regular cannabis users. Hence, MBTV participants were informed about this "washout" period during the first session when the therapist explained and provided the rationale for the program. Participants also receive a "priming" reinforcer (choice of YMCA or movie theater pass) to demonstrate what can be gained from voucher earnings. During the program, participants received vouchers (i.e., a slip of paper indicating current and cumulative earnings) each time they provided a urine specimen negative for cannabis. Voucher earnings could then be redeemed at any time for retail goods or services chosen by the participant and agreed upon by their therapist. Staff would purchase selected items typically within 48 h.

The schedule of voucher earning is illustrated in Table 7.1. In general, earnings escalated with each consecutive cannabis-negative specimen provided. Cannabis-positive specimens or missed specimens resulted in no voucher earnings, and the value of the next cannabis-negative specimen was reset to the amount that was provided for the first negative specimen. If following a cannabis-positive specimen, three consecutive negative specimens were provided, the value of the vouchers returned to the level achieved prior to the submission of the positive specimen.

Table 7.1. *Voucher schedule used in Cannabis Dependence Treatment Program*

|  | Specimen 1 | Specimen 2 | Bonus | Total |
|---|---|---|---|---|
| Week 1 | $5.00 | $5.00 | – | $10.00 |
| (washout period) | (non-contingent) | (non-contingent) | | |
| Week 2 | $5.00 | $5.00 | – | $10.00 |
| (washout period) | (non-contingent) | (non-contingent) | | |
| Week 3* | $1.50 | $3.00 | $10.00 | $14.50 |
| Week 4 | $4.50 | $6.00 | $10.00 | $20.50 |
| Week 5 | $7.50 | $9.00 | $10.00 | $26.50 |
| Week 6 | $10.50 | $12.00 | $10.00 | $32.50 |
| Week 7 | $13.50 | $15.00 | $10.00 | $38.50 |
| Week 8 | $16.50 | $18.00 | $10.00 | $44.50 |
| Week 9 | $19.50 | $21.00 | $10.00 | $50.50 |
| Week 10 | $22.50 | $24.00 | $10.00 | $56.50 |
| Week 11 | $25.50 | $27.00 | $10.00 | $62.50 |
| Week 12 | $28.50 | $30.00 | $10.00 | $68.50 |
| Week 13 | $31.50 | $33.00 | $10.00 | $74.50 |
| Week 14* | $34.50 | $36.00 | $10.00 | $80.50 |
| Total | | | | $590.00 |

* Sample voucher earnings for patients who provide negative urine specimen during Weeks 3–14.

## Results

Rates of treatment acceptability (attended more than one session) and treatment completion were comparable and did not significantly differ across the three treatments. All but four participants returned for a second session and an approximately 55% of all participants completed treatment.

The primary treatment outcome variable of interest was the longest period of documented continuous cannabis abstinence based on the twice-weekly urinalysis testing. All missing urinalysis specimens were considered positive for cannabis. A significantly greater percentage of participants in the MBTV group were able to achieve specific periods of cannabis abstinence than in the MBT or M groups, and a greater percentage were abstinent at each treatment week (see Figure 7.1). The MBTV group achieved significantly longer periods of continuous

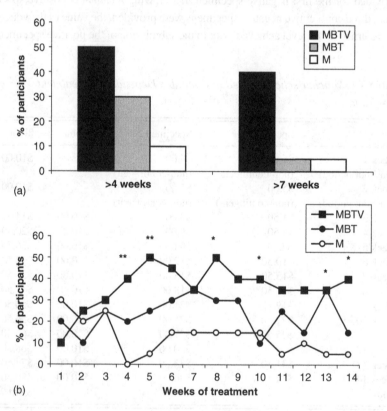

Figure 7.1 (a) Achieved periods of marijuana abstinence and (b) marijuana abstinence during consecutive treatment weeks.

cannabis abstinence ($M = 4.8 \pm 4.9$ weeks) than the MBT ($M = 2.3 \pm 3.0$ weeks) or M group ($1.6 \pm 2.4$ weeks). A greater percentage of MBTV participants were abstinent at the end of treatment (defined by cannabis-negative urinalysis in the last week of treatment and 30 days of self-reported abstinence) than MBT and M participants (35% versus 10% versus 5%; $p < 0.05$). MBTV participants also had significantly lower Addiction Severity Index drug composite scores (McLellan *et al.*, 1985) at the end of treatment than both MBT and M participants.

No treatment group differences were detected on other outcome measures of drug use or psychosocial functioning. However, significant improvement from intake to treatment completion was noted within all groups on the self-reported days of cannabis use, Addiction Severity Index, psychiatric, family, employment, and legal composite scores, the Marijuana Consequences Questionnaire (Stephens *et al.*, 1994), and the Global Symptom Index of the Brief Symptom Inventory (Derogatis, 1993).

Of note, no significant differences were observed between the MBT and M groups; however, outcome measures for MBT tended to indicate a more positive treatment response than for M. Due to the relatively low power to detect differences in this study, we hesitate to conclude that the non-significant outcome differences between these groups are not important. The two studies comparing similar treatments using larger samples sizes reviewed in Chapter 6 of this book provide additional information regarding the comparative efficacy of these interventions.

This study demonstrated that the addition of an abstinence-based voucher program to previously documented effective therapies enhanced abstinence during treatment for cannabis dependence. Of note, the specific effect of the voucher program was to increase continuous periods of abstinence, which was the hypothesized outcome based on the design of the reinforcement schedule (i.e., escalating value of vouchers for consecutive cannabis-negative specimens, and a substantial reduction in value for cannabis use). Overall, this study represents an initial step towards extending the treatment efficacy literature on CM approaches for drug dependence to the treatment of cannabis-dependent adults.

Many unanswered questions emanate from this initial study. As the voucher component was integrated with MBT, we could not determine how this therapy contributed to the effects of the voucher program. Likewise we have no information on whether the voucher program is effective if delivered without MBT. Last, we do not know whether the positive effects of the voucher program observed during treatment maintain post-treatment. We have conducted a second study with cannabis-dependent adults designed to answer these questions. Preliminary findings indicate that (a) the voucher effect is maintained post-treatment, (b) vouchers delivered alone is an effective treatment option, and (c) behavior therapy appears to enhance the maintenance of the voucher effect post-treatment (Budney *et al.*, in press).

## Using CM to Engage Probation-Referred Marijuana Abusers in Treatment

Almost half of those seeking treatment for marijuana abuse have criminal justice involvement and are referred to treatment by the legal system, and the majority are less than 25-year old (SAMHSA, 2001; Sinha *et al.*, 2003a, b). Such client characteristics are associated with poor engagement in the treatment process, and many of those who fit this profile are characterized as being in the *pre-contemplation* stage of change regarding their marijuana use. Hence, using CM to enhance motivation and effort to change in this population of marijuana abusers might prove particularly beneficial.

Sinha and colleagues (2003b) evaluated the efficacy of a modified voucher program for increasing treatment attendance among probation-referred young adults referred to outpatient treatment for marijuana abuse. Sixty-five 18–25-year olds were randomly assigned to receive a three-session motivational enhancement treatment (MET) or MET plus a contingent voucher program (MET/V) designed to reinforce attendance at counseling sessions. An escalating voucher program provided a $25 voucher for attendance at the first session, $35 for the second and $45 for the third, and missing a session reset the voucher value back to $25. A $5 bonus voucher was a provided for arriving at the session within 5 min of the scheduled appointment time. Vouchers could be redeemed for prosocial items or services. Significantly more MET/V clients completed treatment (64% versus 39%), and MET/V clients attended more sessions (2.3 versus 1.8). Additionally, more MET/V clients continued with treatment after completing the three scheduled MET sessions (14 versus 8), but this difference was not statistically significant. No between-groups differences were observed for marijuana use or other psychosocial outcome measures. This study demonstrated the efficacy of a CM intervention designed to enhance attendance at counseling session in a sample of young, unmotivated, marijuana abusers. It also showed that successful use of reinforcement to enhance treatment attendance does not necessarily produce concomitant changes in drug use outcome.

**Cannabis as a Secondary Drug of Abuse**

Many individuals seeking treatment for other drug dependence also use cannabis regularly (Budney *et al.*, 1996, 1998a; Hubbard, 1990). Such secondary cannabis use is commonly viewed as a significant risk factor for relapse or treatment failure. However, there are data suggesting that cannabis use during treatment for cocaine and opiate dependence is not clearly associated with poor treatment outcome (Budney *et al.*, 1996, 1998a; Nirenberg *et al.*, 1996; Saxon *et al.*, 1993). Regardless of its relation to treatment outcome in these polydrug-using populations, treatment providers must have a plan to deal with such cannabis use. This issue presents a significant challenge because the majority of these individuals do not consider their cannabis use problematic, and their readiness to change is significantly lower for cannabis use than their primary substance of abuse (Budney *et al.*, 1997, 1998b). CM models, particularly those that use positive reinforcement contingencies, may offer a promising treatment avenue for these difficult treatment populations.

*Cannabis Abuse among Cocaine Abusers*

In a small-*N* study (Budney *et al.*, 1991), we examined a sequential strategy of initially reinforcing abstinence from the primary drug of abuse (cocaine) with vouchers, and then moving on to address abstinence from the secondary drug (cannabis). The rationale for this approach was that cocaine-dependent individuals who achieved abstinence with the voucher program might have increased desire to access non-drug, prosocial reinforcers, and find that cannabis use interfered with this goal. These circumstances might prompt them to participate in a program in which they could earn additional vouchers for abstaining from cannabis.

Using a multiple-baseline design, a 12-week voucher program first engendered cocaine abstinence in the two participants, but both continued to use cannabis regularly despite counseling that encouraged marijuana abstinence. These individuals were then offered a second 12-week treatment at staggered time intervals that involved a modified contingency requiring abstinence from both cocaine and cannabis in order to earn vouchers. Both participants achieved abstinence from both drugs with the initiation of a cannabis abstinence coinciding with the initiation of the modified voucher program. Following discontinuation of the vouchers, both participants resumed their cannabis use, but remained abstinent from cocaine. This small study illustrated that voucher programs can engender abstinence from cannabis in multiple-drug users who are ambivalent about their cannabis use, but also suggested that the effects may not endure if such use is not deemed highly problematic.

## Cannabis Abuse in the Methadone Clinic

Cannabis use among methadone-maintained, opiate-dependent individuals is common (Calsyn & Saxon, 1999). The significance of such use is typically minimized because the problems associated with cannabis use are considered negligible compared with those associated with heroin dependence. Accordingly, many methadone clinics do not conduct regular urinalysis testing for cannabis, or if they do, there are usually no negative consequences delivered for positive test results. In contrast, consequences are typically provided for use of most other drugs of abuse. Hence, the lack of consequences for cannabis use may give the impression that such use is condoned. Here we describe a quasi-experimental study evaluating an innovative CM intervention designed to address this issue (Calsyn & Saxon, 1999).

The intervention was an add-on to an existing CM program that required 6 months of drug-negative urinalysis tests (except for cannabis) in order to earn twice-a-week methadone dose take-home privileges. Take-home privileges are highly valued by this clinical population because methadone must be taken daily to avoid substantial opiate withdrawal symptoms. If take-home doses are not available, clients are burdened by the need to attend the clinic daily to obtain their methadone. The experimental CM program increased the requirement for obtaining twice-weekly take-home status to include cannabis-negative urinalysis test results.

Prior to initiating the study, eight clients who had earned the twice-per-week take-home were using cannabis regularly. A 6-month notice was provided informing all clients about the new cannabis requirement. Three of the eight cannabis users achieved abstinence during this 6-month period. The other five lost their privilege when the program began due to cannabis-positive urine tests. One of these earned back that privilege by providing a cannabis-negative urine specimen. The other four clients remained at a lower privilege status (thrice-weekly take-home) for the remainder of the 1-year study.

This study demonstrates the feasibility of implementing a CM program that can engender cannabis abstinence in a subset of methadone clients without having deleterious effects on other aspects of their treatment. In general, issues such as the relative harm of cannabis compared to other substances, the client's interest in abstaining from cannabis use, and the difficulty of abstaining from all substances versus just the primary one, must be given careful consideration when designing interventions to address secondary cannabis use.

## Cannabis Use in Individuals with Severe Psychiatric Illness

As with the general population, cannabis is the most common illicit drug used among individuals with schizophrenia (Kandel *et al.*, 1997; Zisook *et al.*, 1992). Cannabis use has been associated with problems related to schizophrenic illness such as: (a) earlier or more abrupt onset of symptomatology, (b) interfering with identification and diagnosis, (c) exacerbating symptomatology, (d) poor medication compliance, (e) antagonizing the efficacy of neuroleptic drugs, and (f) increasing risk for recurrent symptomatology or relapse (Dixon *et al.*, 1991; Negrete & Gill, 1999; Negrete *et al.*, 1986).

We conducted a study to examine the feasibility of using a CM intervention to reduce cannabis use in this population (Sigmon *et al.*, 2000). Participants were 18 adults with schizophrenia or other serious mental illness who were not seeking treatment, but rather were regular cannabis users willing to participate in a study in which they were offered monetary incentives to abstain from cannabis use. The study consisted of five conditions, each 5 weeks in duration. Urinalysis testing was performed twice weekly. During the first and fifth conditions, participants received payment ($25) each time they submitted a urine specimen independent of urinalysis results (baseline condition). During the three incentive conditions, participants received varying amounts of money ($25, $50, and $100) each time the urine specimen was cannabinoid negative.

The mean number of cannabis-negative specimens obtained was significantly greater during the three incentive conditions (mean number of positive specimens: $25 = 4.2 \pm 1.4$, $50 = 4.1 \pm 1.4$, $100 = 5.1 \pm 1.4$) than during the baseline conditions (B1 $= 1.3 \pm 0.6$, B2 $= 1.8 \pm 1.1$), but no differences were observed among incentive conditions. These results provided evidence that cannabis use among severely mentally ill individuals, like drug use among non-psychiatric populations, is sensitive to reinforcement contingencies. We have observed similar findings supporting this notion with cigarette smoking in individuals with schizophrenia (Roll *et al.*, 1998; Tidey *et al.*, 1999).

Others have begun to examine the efficacy of CM-based interventions to reduce substance use among the severely mentally ill by dispensing disability benefits contingent on drug abstinence (Ries *et al.*, 2004; Shaner *et al.*, 1999). The rationale for such an intervention originated from data indicating that individuals with comorbid substance abuse and schizophrenia tend to misuse disability benefits to purchase illicit substances (Shaner *et al.*, 1995). Although this research to date has focused on cocaine abuse, the high prevalence of cannabis use in this population suggests that spending disability monies on cannabis is most likely common. Arranging conditions such that disability income is used to positively reinforce drug abstinence rather than facilitate continued drug abuse would seem to warrant study.

## CM in the Treatment of Adolescent Marijuana Abusers

In Chapter 11, a number of treatment approaches for adolescent marijuana dependence are described. With the exception of one feasibility study demonstrating that a contingent positive reinforcement procedure can effectively reduce adolescent tobacco cigarette smoking (Corby *et al.*, 2000), CM has not yet been studied with adolescent drug abusers. We recently began work on a project with the aim of creating a developmentally appropriate CM intervention for adolescent cannabis abusers (Kamon *et al.*, 2005). The intervention combines individual cognitive-behavioral counseling with two CM-based treatment components. An abstinence-based voucher program similar to that used in our adult studies is used to enhance engagement in the treatment process and the initiation of cannabis and other drug abstinence. Second, a behavioral parent training program is used to assist parents develop CM skills that can increase drug abstinence and other prosocial behavior (Dishion & Andrews, 1995). This intervention teaches parents to (a) increase monitoring of their teen's behavior, (b) provide consistent consequences following drug use or abstinence and other related negative or positive behaviors, and (c) increase opportunities for their teens to engage in prosocial activities and to increase reinforcement for doing so. Preliminary data for a pilot group of 16 families receiving this intervention indicate that the program is acceptable to the majority of treatment seekers. Adolescents and parents attended the majority of scheduled sessions, and 75% completed treatment. Substance use, externalizing behaviors, and negative parenting behaviors all significantly decreased from treatment initiation to treatment end. Sixty-three percent of adolescents provided marijuana-negative urine specimens at the end of treatment, and mean number of days of self-reported marijuana use during the prior 30 days decreased from 12.9 to 3.1 ($p < 0.01$) from the intake to the end of treatment assessment. An ongoing randomized-controlled trial will determine whether this CM-based treatment enhances outcome when added to a standard individual and family treatment intervention.

## Concluding Comments

CM programs can effectively increase abstinence and facilitate other healthy lifestyle changes, yet dissemination of CM interventions to community clinics is likely to be challenging. CM interventions, like many other drug abuse treatments shown to be effective in research settings, are not the models of intervention commonly used in community clinics (Miller *et al.*, 1995). Hence, one primary obstacle to dissemination originates with treatment providers. Most therapists and administrators in the substance abuse treatment field have had no training in CM procedures or principles, and their existing models for treating substance abuse emanate from a very different conceptual understanding of substance dependence. Second, the logistics and cost of initiating CM programs can appear overwhelming, and thus even consideration of adopting such unfamiliar practices is likely to meet with dismissal.

The practical and clinical obstacles such as funding programs, educating and training treatment providers, and convincing program developers and policymakers of the value of this approach to substance abuse treatment have been discussed in depth elsewhere (Crowley, 1999; Kirby *et al.*, 1999). Creative ways to fund CM programs already appear in the literature. For example, a number of projects, including our adolescent pilot program have solicited donations from community businesses to use as reinforcers (Kirby *et al.*, 1999; Petry *et al.*, 2000). Of note, the National Institute on Drug Abuse has recently launched a multi-center study of a CM treatment for cocaine and heroin dependence that locates the research directly in community-based clinics with the hopes of indoctrinating community providers to the potential value of this treatment model (Petry, 2005). The education and training of treatment providers in both the theory and practice of CM and other effective-behavioral treatment discussed in this text must become a priority if we expect these professionals to accept and adopt a model that is not congruent with their current belief system and practices. Most substance abuse treatment providers, regardless of their theoretical background, would agree that more effective interventions are needed to better help clients with serious drug abuse problems including cannabis dependence. CM interventions clearly offer one avenue for enhancing outcomes, but much more must be done in the area of technology transfer before current treatment systems adopt these models.

An additional CM dissemination issue that is perhaps unique to the treatment for cannabis is the question of whether or not cannabis abuse is deemed a substantial problem in need of effective, more powerful, and perhaps more costly treatments. Historically, cannabis dependence has not been viewed as a significant problem and many still question whether cannabis dependence exists at all (Budney & Wiley, 2001; Stephens & Roffman, 1994). The task of building a consensus that cannabis dependence is a real disorder and that many youth and adults are in need of professional help for this problem may need to be addressed either prior to or simultaneous with dissemination efforts. Hopefully, efforts such as the publication of this book, continued clinical-research efforts, and national education campaigns will serve to educate the treatment community, policymakers, and the general public on cannabis' potential for abuse and dependence.

## References

Bickel, W. K., Amass, L., Higgins, S. T., Badger, G. J., & Esch, R. A. (1997). Effects of adding a behavioral treatment to opioid detoxification with buprenorphine. *Journal of Consulting and Clinical Psychology, 65*, 803–810.

Budney, A. J., & Higgins, S. T. (1998). *A community reinforcement plus vouchers approach: treating cocaine addiction.* Rockville, MD: United States Department of Health and Human Services.

Budney, A. J., & Wiley, J. (2001). Can marijuana use lead to dependence. In J. B. Overmeir, & M. E. Carroll (Eds.), *Animal research and human health: advancing human welfare through behavioral science* (pp. 115–126). Washington, DC: American Psychological Association.

Budney, A. J., Higgins, S. T., Delaney, D. D., Kent, L., & Bickel, W. K. (1991). Contingent reinforcement of abstinence with individuals abusing cocaine and marijuana. *Journal of Applied Behavior Analysis, 24*, 657–665.

Budney, A. J., Higgins, S. T., & Wong, C. J. (1996). Marijuana use and treatment outcome in cocaine-dependent patients. *Experimental and Clinical Psychopharmacology, 4*, 396–403.

Budney, A. J., Kandel, D., Cherek, D. R., Martin, B. R., Stephens, R. S., & Roffman, R. (1997). Marijuana use and dependence: college on problems of drug dependence annual meeting, Puerto Rico (June, 1996). *Drug and Alcohol Dependence, 45*(1–2), 1–11.

Budney, A. J., Bickel, W. K., & Amass, L. (1998a). Marijuana use and treatment outcome among opioid-dependent patients. *Addiction, 93*(4), 493–503.

Budney, A. J., Radonovich, K. J., Higgins, S. T., & Wong, C. J. (1998b). Adults seeking treatment for marijuana dependence: a comparison to cocaine-dependent treatment seekers. *Experimental and Clinical Psychopharmacology, 6*(4), 419–426.

Budney, A. J., Higgins, S. T., Radonovich, K. J., & Novy, P. L. (2000). Adding voucher-based incentives to coping-skills and motivational enhancement improves outcomes during treatment for marijuana dependence. *Journal of Consulting and Clinical Psychology, 68*, 1051–1061.

Budney, A. J., Sigmon, S. C., & Higgins, S. T. (2001). Implementing contingency management programs: using science to motivate change. In R. Coombs (Ed.), *Addiction recovery tools* (pp. 147–172). Thousand Oaks, CA: Sage Publications.

Budney, A. J., Moore, B. A., Higgins. S.T., & Rocha, H. L. (in press). Clinical trial of abstinence-based vouchers and cognitive-behavioral therapy for marijuana dependence. *Journal of Consulting and Clinical Psychology.*

Calsyn, D. A., & Saxon, A. J. (1999). An innovative approach to reducing cannabis use in a subset of methadone clients. *Drug and Alcohol Dependence, 53,* 167–169.

Copeland, J., Swift, W., Roffman, R., & Stephens, R. (2001). A randomized controlled trial of brief cognitive-behavioral interventions for cannabis disorder. *Journal of Substance Abuse Treatment, 21,* 55–64.

Corby, E. A., Roll, J. M., & Schuster, C. R. (2000). Contingency management interventions for treating substance abuse of adolescents: a feasibility study. *Experimental and Clinical Psychopharmacology, 8,* 371–376.

Crowley, T. J. (1999). Research on contingency management treatment of drug dependence: clinical implications and future directions. In S. T. Higgins, & K. Silverman (Eds.), *Motivating behavior change among illicit-drug abusers* (pp. 345–370). Washington, DC: American Psychological Association.

Derogatis, L. R. (1993). *Brief symptom inventory: administration, scoring and procedures manual.* Minneapolis, MN: National Computer Systems Inc.

Dishion, T. J., & Andrews, D. W. (1995). Preventing escalation in problem behaviors with high-risk young adolescents: immediate and 1-year outcomes. *Journal of Consulting and Clinical Psychology, 63*(4), 538.

Dixon, L., Haas, G., Weiden, P. J., Sweeney, J., & Frances, A. J. (1991). Drug abuse in schizophrenic patients: clinical correlates and reasons for use. *American Journal of Psychiatry, 148,* 224–230.

Elk, R. (1999). Pregnant women and tuberculosis-exposed drug abusers: reducing drug use and increasing treatment compliance. In S. T. Higgins, & K. Silverman (Eds.), *Motivating behavior change among illicit-drug abusers* (pp. 123–144). Washington, DC: American Psychological Association.

Ferster, C. B., & Skinner, B. F. (1957). *Schedules of reinforcement.* Englewood Cliffs, NJ: Prentice Hall.

Goldberg, S. R., & Stollerman, I. P. (1986). *Behavioral analysis of drug dependence.* Orlando: Academic Press.

Griffiths, R. R., Bigelow, G. E., & Henningfield, J. E. (1980). Similarities in animal and human drug-taking behavior. In N. K. Mello (Ed.), *Advances in substance abuse: behavioral and biological research* (pp. 1–90). Greenwich, CT: JAI Press.

Higgins, S. T. (1997). The influence of alternative reinforcers on cocaine use and abuse: a brief review. *Pharmacology, Biochemistry, and Behavior, 57,* 419–427.

Higgins, S. T., & Katz, J. L. (1998). *Cocaine abuse: behavior, pharmacology, and clinical applications.* San Diego, CA: Academic Press.

Higgins, S. T., & Silverman, K. (1999). *Motivating behavior change among illicit-drug abusers: research on contingency-management interventions.* Washington, DC: American Psychological Association.

Higgins, S. T., Delaney, D. D., Budney, A. J., Bickel, W. K., Hughes, J. R., Foerg, F., et al. (1991). A behavioral approach to achieving initial cocaine abstinence. *American Journal of Psychiatry, 148,* 1218–1224.

Higgins, S. T., Budney, A. J., Bickel, W. K., Hughes, J. R., Foerg, F., & Badger, G. (1993). Achieving cocaine abstinence with a behavioral approach. *American Journal of Psychiatry, 150*(5), 763–769.

Higgins, S. T., Budney, A. J., Bickel, W. K., Foerg, F., Donham, R., & Badger, G. (1994). Incentives improve outcome in outpatient behavioral treatment of cocaine dependence. *Archives of General Psychiatry, 54*, 568–576.

Higgins, S. T., Wong, C. J., Badger, G. J., Ogden, D. H., & Dantona, R. (2000). Contingent reinforcement increases cocaine abstinence during outpatient treatment and 1 year follow-up. *Journal of Consulting and Clinical Psychology, 68*, 64–72.

Higgins, S. T., Sigmon, S. C., Wong, C. J., Heil, S. H., Badger, G. J., Donham, R., et al. (2003). Community reinforcement therapy for cocaine-dependent outpatients. *Archives of General Psychiatry, 60*, 1043–1052.

Hubbard, R. L. (1990). *Treating combined alcohol and drug abuse in community-based programs, recent developments in alcoholism* (Vol. 8, pp. 273–283). New York: Plenum Press.

Iguchi, M. Y., Lamb, R. J., Belding, M. A., Platt, J. J., Husband, S. D., & Morral, A. R. (1996). Contingent reinforcement of group participation versus abstinence in a methadone maintenance program. *Experimental and Clinical Psychopharmacology, 4*, 315–321.

Kamon, J., Budney, A., & Stanger, C. (2005). A contingency management intervention for adolescent marijuana abuse and conduct problems. *Journal of the American Academy of Child and Adolescent Psychiatry, 44*, 513–521.

Kandel, D., Chen, K., Warner, L. A., Kessler, R. C., & Grant, B. (1997). Prevalence and demographic correlates of symptoms of dependence on cigarettes, alcohol, marijuana and cocaine in the US population. *Drug and Alcohol Dependence, 44*, 437–442.

Kirby, K. C., Marlowe, D. B., Festinger, D. S., Lamb, R. J., & Platt, J. J. (1998). Schedule of voucher delivery influences initiation of cocaine abstinence. *Journal of Consulting and Clinical Psychology, 66*(5), 761–767.

Kirby, K. C., Amass, L., & McLellan, A. T. (1999). Disseminating contingency management research to drug abuse treatment practitioners. In S. T. Higgins, & K. Silverman (Eds.), *Motivating behavior change among illicit-drug abusers* (pp. 327–344). Washington, DC: American Psychological Association.

McLellan, A. T., Luborsky, L., Cacciola, J., Griffith, J., Evans, F., Barr, H. L., et al. (1985). New data from the Addiction Severity Index. *The Journal of Nervous and Mental Disease, 173*, 412–423.

Miller, W. A., Brown, J. M., Simpson, T. L., Handmaker, N. S., Bien, T. H., Luckie, L. F., et al. (1995). What works? A methodological analysis of the alcohol treatment literature. In R. K. Hester, & W. R. Miller (Eds.), *Handbook of alcoholism treatment approaches: effective alternatives* (pp. 12–44). Boston: Allyn and Bacon.

Moore, B. A., & Budney, A. J. (2003). Relapse in outpatient treatment for marijuana dependence. *Journal of Substance Abuse Treatment, 25*, 85–89.

National Institute on Alcohol Abuse and Alcoholism (NIAAA) (1992a). *Cognitive-behavioral coping skills therapy manual* (Vol. DHSS Publication No. ADM 92-1895). Rockville, MD: National Institute on Alcohol Abuse and Alcoholism.

National Institute on Alcohol Abuse and Alcoholism (NIAAA) (1992b). *Motivational enhancement therapy manual* (Vol. DHSS Publication No. ADM 92-1894). Rockville, MD: National Institute on Alcohol Abuse and Alcoholism.

Negrete, J. C., & Gill, K. (1999). Cannabis and schizophrenia: an overview of the evidence to date. In G. G. Nahas (Ed.), *Marihuana and medicine* (pp. 671–681). Totowa, NJ: Humana Press.

Negrete, J. C., Knapp, W. P., Douglas, D. E., & Smith, W. B. (1986). Cannabis affects the severity of schizophrenic symptoms: results of a clinical survey. *Psychological Medicine, 16*, 515–520.

Nirenberg, T. D., Celussi, T., Liepman, M. R., Swift, R. M., & Sirota, D. (1996). Cannabis vs. other illicit drug use among methadone maintenance patients. *Psychology of Addictive Behavior, 10*, 222–227.

Petry, N., & Martin, B. (2002). Lower-cost contingency management for treating cocaine and opioid abusing methadone patients. *Journal of Consulting and Clinical Psychology, 70*, 398–405.

Petry, N. M. (2000). A comprehensive guide to the application of contingency management procedures in clinical settings. *Drug and Alcohol Dependence, 58*, 9–25.

Petry, N. M., Martin, B., Cooney, J. L., & Kranzler, H. R. (2000). Give them prizes, and they will come: contingency management for treatment of alcohol dependence. *Journal of Consulting and Clinical Psychology, 68*, 250–257.

Petry, N. M., Peirce, I. M., Stitzer, M. L., Blaine, J. Roll, J. M., Cohen, A., Obert, J., Killeen, T., Saladin, M. E., Cowell, M., Kirby, K. C., Sterling, R., Royer-Malvestuto, C., Hamilton, J., Booth., R. E., Macdonald, M., Liebert, M., Rder, L., Burns, R., DiMaria, J., Copersino, M., Stabile, P. Q., Kolodner, K., Li., R. (2005). Effect of prize-based incentives on outcomes in stimulant abusers in outpatient psychosocial treatment programs: a national drug abuse treatment clinical trials network study. *Archives of General Psychiatry, 62*(10), 1148–1156.

Ries, R. K., Dyck, R. K., Short, R., Srebnik, D., Fisher, A., & Comtois, K. A. (2004). Outcomes of managing disability benefits among patient with substance dependence and severe mental illness. *Psychiatric Services, 55*, 445–447.

Roll, J., Higgins, S. T., & Badger, G. J. (1996). An experimental comparison of three different schedules of reinforcement of drug abstinence using cigarette smoking as an exemplar. *Journal of Applied Behavior Analysis, 29*, 495–505.

Roll, J. M., Higgins, S. T., Steingard, S., & McGinley, M. (1998). Use of monetary reinforcement to reduce the cigarette smoking of persons with schizophrenia: a feasibility study. *Experimental and Clinical Psychopharmacology, 6*, 157–161.

SAMHSA (2001). *Treatment episode data set (TEDS) 1996–1999: National admissions to substance abuse treatment services.* Rockville, MD: DHHS.

Saxon, A. J., Calsyn, D. A., Greenber, D., Blaes, P., Virginia, M. H., & Stanton, V. (1993). Urine screening for marijuana among methadone-maintained patients. *American Journal of the Addictions, 2*, 207–211.

Shaner, A., Eckman, T. A., Roberts, L. J., Wilkins, J. N., Tucker, D. E., Tsuang, J. W., *et al.* (1995). Disability income, cocaine use, and repeated hospitalization among schizophrenic cocaine abusers: a government-sponsored revolving door? *New England Journal of Medicine, 333*, 777–783.

Shaner, A., Tucker, D., Roberts, L. J., & Eckman, T. (1999). Disability income, cocaine use, and contingency management among patients with cocaine dependence and schizophrenia. In S. T. Higgins, & K. A. Silverman (Eds.), *Motivating behavior change in illicit-drug abusers: contemporary research on contingency-management interventions* (pp. 95–122). Washington, DC: American Psychological Association.

Sigmon, S. C., Steingard, S., Badger, G. J., Anthony, S. L., & Higgins, S. T. (2000). Contingent reinforcement of marijuana abstinence among individuals with serious mental illness: a feasibility study. *Experimental and Clinical Psychopharmacology, 8*, 509–517.

Silverman, K., Chutuape, M. A. D., Bigelow, G. E., & Stitzer, M. L. (1996). Voucher-based reinforcement of attendance by unemployed methadone patients in a job skills training program. *Drug and Alcohol Dependence, 41*, 197–207.

Sinha, R., Easton, C., & Kemp K. (2003a). Substance abuse treatment characteristics of probation-referred young adults in a community-based outpatient program. *American Journal of Drug and Alcohol Abuse, 29*(3), 585–597.

Sinha, R., Easton, C., Renee-Aubin, L., & Carrroll, K. M. (2003b). Engaging young probation referred marijuana-abusing individuals in treatment: a pilot trial. *American Journal of Addictions, 12*, 314–323.

Stephens, R. S., & Roffman, R. A. (1994). Adult marijuana dependence. In J. S. Baer, & R. J. McMahon (Eds.), *Addictive behaviors across the lifespan: prevention, treatment, and policy issues* (pp. 243–273). Newbury Park, CA: Sage Publications.

Stephens, R. S., Roffman, R. A., & Simpson, E. E. (1994). Treating adult marijuana dependence: a test of the relapse prevention model. *Journal of Consulting and Clinical Psychology, 62*, 92–99.

Stephens, R. S., Roffman, R. A., & Curtin, L. (2000). Comparison of extended versus brief treatments for marijuana use. *Journal of Consulting and Clinical Psychology, 68*, 898–908.

Sulzer-Azaroff, B., & Meyer, G. R. (1991). *Behavior analysis for lasting change.* Fort Worth, TX: Holt Rinehart and Winston.

Tidey, J. W., O'Neill, S. C., & Higgins, S. T. (1999). Effects of abstinence on cigarette smoking among outpatients with schizophrenics. *Experimental and Clinical Psychopharmacology, 7*, 347–353.

Zisook, S., Heaton, R., Moranville, J., Kuck, J., Jernigan, T., & Braff, D. (1992). Past substance abuse and clinical course of schizophrenia. *American Journal of Psychiatry, 149*, 552–553.

# 8

# The Marijuana Check-Up

ROBERT S. STEPHENS AND ROGER A. ROFFMAN

Among those in the USA who experience negative consequences from alcohol or drug use and who acknowledge a need for treatment, the number one reason given for not receiving treatment is "not being ready to stop using" (Substance Abuse and Mental Health Services, Office of Applied Sciences (SAMHSA), 2003b). The other most commonly endorsed reasons for not seeking treatment include the financial costs and stigma associated with drug abuse treatment. Embarrassment, stigma, and a negative attitude toward treatment were frequently endorsed in other studies of reasons for delaying seeking treatment (Cunningham et al., 1993; Sobell et al., 1991). Drug treatment appears to come with both social and financial costs and it is perceived as designed for those who are committed to change.

Marijuana users may be particularly unlikely to seek treatment for these very reasons. In addition, marijuana is often perceived as a "soft" drug that does not produce dependence or serious negative consequences, which may further undermine the apparent need for treatment (see Stephens & Roffman, 1993). Of those who met criteria for cannabis dependence or abuse in 2003, only 7.6% reported receiving treatment in drug treatment facilities. In contrast, 24.3% of those with cocaine abuse or dependence and 18.2% of those abusing or dependent on pain relievers reported receiving treatment (SAMHSA, 2003a). In this chapter we describe the Marijuana Check-Up (MCU), a low-cost and low-demand intervention designed to attract adult marijuana users who are experiencing some negative consequences but who are not necessarily committed to change. The philosophy, marketing, and intervention techniques of the MCU are designed to overcome barriers associated with formal treatment by reducing the demand for change, stigma, financial costs, and time demands. The MCU uses motivational enhancement therapy (MET; Miller et al., 1992) techniques to facilitate an in depth and candid "taking stock" of the positive and negative consequences of use with the goal of increasing readiness for change.

The MCU is a two-session assessment and feedback intervention that targets adult marijuana users who have questions or concerns about their use. In the initial session participants complete structured interviews and questionnaire assessments regarding their marijuana use, its consequences, and expectancies and beliefs regarding the effects of continued use versus reducing or quitting. In the second session, a therapist trained in motivational interviewing techniques (Miller & Rollnick, 1991, 2002) reviews a Personal Feedback Report (PFR) with the participant. As data collected during the assessment are presented, the therapist acknowledges the participant's reasons for continued use but attempts to elicit and focus on self-motivational statements for change. If the participant expresses interest in change, the therapist will offer a menu of treatment and self-change options and assist in developing a plan. This combination of motivational interviewing and feedback is usually referred to as MET (Miller *et al.*, 1992) and has been studied in a variety of contexts with a variety of behaviors (see Burke *et al.*, 2003, for a review).

The stages of change (SOC) model describes a series of stages through which people pass as they change behavior (Prochaska & DiClemente, 1984) and is one way of understanding where the MCU may fit into the continuum of interventions for marijuana users. Individuals with no intention of changing a behavior are described as precontemplators. Precontemplators are not a homogenous group (see DiClemente & Velasquez, 2002). They may be unaware of any reasons for changing the behavior, resist being told what to do, have rationalized why they do not need to change, or feel hopeless about the possibility of change and, hence, do not plan to try. Therefore, precontemplators need the opportunity to learn about and reflect on the effects of the behavior in their lives. Some may need help believing they could be successful. Precontemplators would not be expected to contact traditional drug abuse treatment programs where they might encounter the presumption that change is necessary. Approaches that avoid telling them what to do and help them find their own reasons for change are likely to avoid engaging reactance or outright resistance. The MCU, with its reliance on motivational interviewing techniques and feedback on personal consequences, is well matched to individuals in this stage.

Contemplators on the other hand acknowledge the need for change but are still not committed to it. DiClemente and Velasquez (2002) warn that being a contemplator is not necessarily an indication that change efforts will soon follow. Individuals in this stage are usually more open to collecting information about the behavior in question but they are also more ambivalent. Clinicians working with contemplators need to remain aware of this ambivalence and not presume that, because the person acknowledges some interest in change, they are ready to make it. Instead, the clinician's role should be to help tip the balance in favor of change. Objective, nonjudgmental feedback on the behavior and its personal risks is one strategy to shift the probabilities toward change. In the MCU, reviewing the PFR is designed to do just that while the therapist's training in motivational interviewing techniques guards against an assumption that change is imminent and a premature focus on active change therapy.

Those in the preparation, action, and maintenance SOC are ready to make changes or already have. Issues of ambivalence about change are not as great and data and theory suggest that people in these stages would profit most from action-oriented behavioral techniques designed to support self-efficacy, modify the environment and reinforce changes in behavior. Although the MCU is not specifically designed for individuals in these later SOC, they may be attracted by the opportunity to learn more about how marijuana use is affecting them. They may be seeking confirmation that their decision to reduce use is justified or they may want support in making changes. Therapists need to be able to recognize these motives and be able to shift emphasis in the feedback session away from exploring and resolving ambivalence and more toward increasing efficacy for change via treatment menu options or cognitive-behavioral techniques for change and maintenance of change.

The MCU was modeled after the Drinkers' Check-Up (DCU), a brief intervention designed to overcome the stigma of treatment and promote change in alcohol users who were not ready or likely to seek formal treatment (Miller & Sovereign, 1989). The DCU was promoted via news media as a free assessment and feedback service for drinkers who wanted to find out whether alcohol was harming them. Recruitment announcements emphasized that the DCU was confidential, not part of any treatment program, not intended for "alcoholics," and that it would be "up to the individual to decide what, if anything, to do with the feedback" (Miller *et al.*, 1993). In the initial session, alcohol use and risk factors for abuse and dependence were assessed. In the second session, a therapist provided normative and risk-related feedback to the participants using a motivational interviewing style. Those who participated in the DCU appeared to be similar to clients already in treatment on measures of alcohol use and related problems, but few had ever been in formal treatment for alcohol related problems. In two studies, these problem drinkers significantly reduced their alcohol intake and maintained changes up to 18 months after participating in the DCU (Miller *et al.*, 1988, 1993).

The efficacy of the DCU is consistent with recent reviews that have concluded that brief, motivational interviewing interventions are efficacious for a variety of drug and non-drug behavior problems (e.g., Burke *et al.*, 2002, 2003). In particular, two studies of the treatment of marijuana dependence found that 2-session, MET treatments were effective in reducing marijuana use and associated problems compared to delayed treatment controls, although the studies disagreed on whether these brief interventions were as effective as longer cognitive-behavioral treatments (see Chapter 6; Marijuana Treatment Project Research Group (MTPRG), 2004; Stephens *et al.*, 2000). Like other treatment studies of brief interventions, these studies recruited adult marijuana users who were voluntarily approaching treatment with the goal of abstinence. It might be expected that such users were more likely in preparation or action stages and more motivated to make changes in their marijuana use than the overall population of users who may be experiencing negative consequences. To our knowledge, brief MET interventions have not been tested with marijuana users who may be less motivated to make changes.

## Implementing a MCU

The DCU provided a model for the MCU, but adapting it for marijuana users required considerations on how to promote or market it, the nature of the assessment data and its presentation in the PFR, and therapeutic issues unique to marijuana. In this section we review these issues and describe the decisions made in constructing our initial version of the MCU.

### Marketing the MCU

In previous studies of the treatment of marijuana dependence (MTPRG, 2004; Stephens *et al.*, 1994, 2000), advertisements and study promotions were designed to reach a population of marijuana users who would meet diagnostic criteria for marijuana dependence and be ready to engage in treatment aimed at abstinence. Therefore, ads indicated that the project was for individuals who wanted help in quitting marijuana. In contrast, in promoting an intervention for adult marijuana users who were uninterested or who were ambivalent about making changes, the goal was to avoid arousing defensiveness while being honest and ethical regarding the nature and purpose of the project. Messages that required receivers to label themselves as substance abusers who needed treatment were avoided. Similarly, given a long history of exaggeration and misinformation regarding the negative effects of marijuana, it was important to distinguish the MCU from services intended to convince the user of the evils of marijuana use. Thus, the publicity messages described the MCU as a brief, confidential, and non-judgmental service for marijuana smokers who wanted to take a closer look at their use. It was emphasized that the MCU was not treatment, and that the educational information about marijuana would be accurate and balanced. The message additionally conveyed assurance that there would be no pressure to change, and that it would be up to the individual to decide what, if anything, to do following participation.

Two catch phrases for print media were developed with the intention of reaching users at different SOC. The phrase "Your Marijuana Use Got You Thinking?" targeted users further along in their readiness to change, i.e., people who had been actively thinking about their marijuana use, some of whom were interested in making changes. The second phrase, "Questions About Your Pot Use?" was geared to precontemplators and more ambivalent users who might have been put off by implications that they should be thinking about change. The hope was that both messages would arouse curiosity in users and prompt a contact with the research office to learn more about the project. Following Miller's earlier work with the DCU (Miller & Sovereign, 1989), we included the term "check-up" in the project name to convey the message that participants would have the opportunity to experience an assessment, but were not expected to commit themselves to either treatment or behavior change. To catch the viewer's attention as well as communicate the project's non-judgmental attitude about marijuana use, the image of a marijuana leaf was added as the backdrop behind the name. (See Figure 8.1)

A variety of media were used to reach and recruit a diverse sample of marijuana users. Print media included public service announcements, news stories about the project, and paid advertisements. While all three types of advertising channels yielded callers interested in the project, we found that display and bulletin board style ads in alternative, rather than mainstream, newspapers were particularly effective in relation to costs. Paid advertisements also allowed for a greater degree of control over the timing of the promotions that could be adjusted depending upon current rates of recruitment and staffing capabilities (see Campbell *et al.*, 2004, for a detailed presentation of the marketing strategies and analysis of the results). Radio promotions also were effective and included public service announcements, interviews with talk show hosts, and purchased advertisements (see Table 8.1). As with the print media,

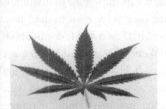

# Questions About Your Pot Use?

call

## THE MARIJUANA CHECK UP
## (206) 616-3457

www.marijuanacheckup.com
For adults who have questions.
Not a treatment program.
Free and Confidential.

Research at the UW School of Social Work

# Your Marijuana Use Got You Thinking?

# The Marijuana Check Up
## 206-616-3457

www.marijuanacheckup.com
We address concerns & questions.
No pressure to change.
Free & Confidential.

Figure 8.1 MCU display ads.

Table 8.1. *Radio advertisement for the MCU*

| Sample 60-s Radio Spot | |
|---|---|
| *Kevin* | 6 1 6-3 4 5 7, 6 1 6-3 4 5 7 |
| *Shauna* | Why do you keep repeating that number? |
| *Kevin* | I'm trying to remember it from a commercial I just heard. |
| *Shauna* | What's it for? |
| *Kevin* | It's for something called the Marijuana Check-Up, a research project through the University of Washington School of Social Work. They said they offer accurate information about marijuana and the project is strictly confidential. Not only is it free, but you get paid for participating! |
| *Shauna* | Hmmm, that sounds interesting. You know, there are so many rumors floating around these days about pot, some straight facts would be nice. |
| *Kevin* | You just have to be 18 or older. Shoot, I think I just forgot that number! |
| *Shauna* | Its 206-616-3457. |
| *Announcer* | Call the Marijuana Check-Up for more information, 206-616-3457. |

paid advertising provided the most control over content, placement, and frequency of exposure. "Classic rock" stations yielded better results than a jazz station or stations with more ethnically diverse audiences. However, these radio ads tended to generate high volumes of callers in a relatively short amount of time following their broadcast and necessitated planning for adequate project staffing.

A booth at a summer festival focusing on marijuana and hemp policies yielded a few additional participants. Efforts were made to reach a more ethnically diverse group of marijuana users through focus groups, outreach workers in ethnically rich communities, and advertisements in ethnic-specific media. Unfortunately, these efforts were not very successful and are discussed in more detail elsewhere (Campbell *et al.*, 2003).

## *The Assessment and Personal Feedback Report*

A key component of the DCU was the provision of feedback on indicators of alcohol related problems, including serum chemistry tests sensitive to alcohol's impact on physical symptoms and neuropsychological tests sensitive to the effect of chronic alcohol use on cognitive functioning (Miller & Sovereign, 1989). In addition, the participant's standings on measures of frequency and quantity of alcohol use were presented in relation to normative data from the overall population of the USA. A challenge in developing the MCU was the relative lack of similar data for marijuana use particularly in the area of quantifying the amount of marijuana consumed. Variability in the potency of marijuana preparations and methods of consuming it (e.g., joints, pipes, bongs) precluded comparisons of personal levels of use with normative data (see Stephens & Roffman, 2005 for a discussion of marijuana use assessment issues). Similarly, comparable biological assays or neuropsychological tests that would indicate the detrimental effects of chronic marijuana use on the body and brain are not available. Therefore, we modeled the assessment and subsequent PFR on the DCU when possible, but used clinical judgment in introducing additional feedback elements that we believed would provide the participant the opportunity to reflect on negative consequences and consider the impact of possible changes in marijuana use.

In order to assess the recent frequency of marijuana, alcohol, and other drug use, we modified the Time Line Follow-Back (TLFB) interview (Sobell & Sobell, 1992). The TLFB was interviewer administered and utilized calendars for the 90 days prior to the initial assessment to assess the number of days on which any marijuana, alcohol, and other drugs were used. For each day of marijuana use, participants identified the periods of the day during which they smoked (i.e., 6:00 a.m.–12:00 p.m.; 12:00 p.m.–6:00 p.m.; 6:00 p.m.–12:00 a.m.; 12:00 a.m.–6:00 p.m.). The number of days of marijuana use per month was then graphically presented on the PFR in relation to normative data from two reference groups that represent the extremes in user populations. First, we compared the participant's use to the overall population in the USA using data from the National Household Survey on Drug Abuse (now called the National Survey on Drug Use and Health). This data generally showed most participants to be part of a very small population of frequent users. Next, we compared the participant's frequency of use to data from over one thousand participants screened for participation in our previous studies of treatments for marijuana dependence. This feedback often showed the participant to be using in a manner similar to the majority of users who were actively seeking treatment for marijuana dependence. We also graphically displayed data on the periods of the day during which the participant reported using marijuana most often (i.e., mornings, afternoons, evenings, and nights) in order to promote discussion of the extent of use on a daily basis.

Trained interviewers used the Psychoactive Substance Use Disorders section of the Structured Clinical Interview for DSM-IV (SCID; First *et al.*, 1996) to assess current symptoms (past 90 days) of cannabis dependence. The PFR provided feedback on the participant's risk for dependence based on the number of seven diagnostic criteria that were met (i.e., 0–1 = Low Risk; 2–4 = Medium

Risk; 5–7 = High Risk). The number of negative consequences the participant reported resulting from marijuana use in the past 90 days was assessed with the 19-item Marijuana Problem Scale (MPS; Stephens *et al.*, 2000). The MPS assesses problems such as guilt, low energy, medical or cognitive concerns, work/school dysfunctions, financial difficulties, spouse and family conflicts, and legal problems. The number of problems reported was presented graphically on the PFR in relation to data from a previous treatment study and the specific endorsed problems were listed.

Similar data on the frequency and quantity of alcohol and other drug use, and problems associated with these drugs, were derived from the TLFB and questionnaires and presented on the PFR in absolute terms rather than as normative comparisons. The MCU specifically targeted marijuana use and those who were dependent on alcohol or other drugs were ineligible to participate (see below). However, we included these data to be sure to capture and promote discussion of any problems that might be occurring with other drugs that may affect motivation for making changes in marijuana use.

The Marijuana Effects Questionnaire (MEQ) consisted of 40 items representing commonly reported acute effects of marijuana use. Participants indicated the likelihood that each effect would occur if they smoked marijuana (1 = very unlikely; 5 = very likely). Four subscales were formed based on principal components analysis of data from a previous study of the treatment of marijuana users. Items on each subscale were averaged to indicate higher expectations of Improved Mood and Thinking (6 items), Increased Sociability (8 items), Negative Affect (13 items) and Lethargy/Procrastination (8 items). The average scores on each scale were presented graphically to facilitate discussion regarding the effects of marijuana experienced by the participant. This feedback was positioned relatively early in the PFR and immediately before the data on negative consequences of use from the MPS because of its balanced assessment of both positive and negative effects of marijuana. Including an acknowledgment of perceived positive effects of marijuana use was important to the MCU's promise of objective feedback.

In order to promote a hypothetical discussion of the costs versus benefits of making a change in marijuana use we modified the Outcome Expectancy Scale (OES; Solomon & Annis, 1989). The OES measures perceived effects of reducing alcohol use on personal, social and physical functioning. The resulting Costs and Benefits (CB) scale consisted of items tapping expected consequences of quitting or substantially reducing marijuana use. Participants answered whether each of 20 negative consequences (Costs) and 20 positive consequences

(Benefits) would occur if they reduced the amount they smoked (1 = strongly disagree; 5 = strongly agree). The total numbers of Costs versus Benefits (using only items rated 4 or 5) were presented graphically on the PFR followed by a list of the endorsed items to promote consideration of the likely effects of change.

Self-efficacy information was included in the PFR to promote consideration of the most difficult situations that would be encountered if the person chose to change their use. Depending upon the participant's level of self-efficacy for avoiding marijuana use, therapeutic interactions could shift toward supporting efficacy or remain focused on exploring motivation through consideration of the pros and cons of continued use versus change. Confidence in being able to avoid marijuana use in 19 high-risk situations was assessed using a measure of self-efficacy created for previous treatment studies (Stephens *et al.*, 1993, 1995). Confidence in being able to avoid marijuana use was rated for each item on a 7-point scale (1 = not at all confident; 7 = extremely confident), which were averaged to create a single index of self-efficacy that was graphically presented on the PFR both in absolute terms and relative to the self-efficacy data from samples of treatment seeking marijuana users. Specific situations in which the participant had higher versus lower confidence in avoiding marijuana use were listed.

## Motivational Interviewing

Therapists were trained to use motivational interviewing techniques as the PFR was reviewed with the client. These techniques are described in more detail elsewhere (Chapter 6; Miller & Rollnick, 1991, 2002; Miller *et al.*, 1992) and are based on four principles: (1) express empathy, (2) develop discrepancy, (3) roll with resistance, and (4) support self-efficacy. Open-ended questions and reflective listening are cornerstone techniques used to elicit descriptions of drug use experiences, express empathy, and emphasize particular information shared by the client. Therapists affirm and support the client whenever possible, building rapport and further encouraging exploration. Periodically, therapists summarize what the client has said in order to link ideas together and reinforce particular content. The overall goal is to elicit self-motivational statements in the form of displeasure with current drug use and perceived benefits of changes in use. Statements indicating some optimism regarding the possibility of change or direct expressions of determination to change are further indications of interest in change that are reflected and summarized by the therapist. As readiness for change becomes apparent, the therapist supports efficacy by exploring and providing strategies for change.

**Clinical and Ethical Issues**

Offering a MCU raises several clinical issues that are relatively specific to marijuana-focused interventions and a potential ethical dilemma related to "check-up" studies in general. Elsewhere we have discussed the unique aspects of treating marijuana users, some of whom have political agendas regarding the legality of the drug (see Chapter 6; Doyle *et al.*, 2003). Other users may feel that marijuana is an effective medication for them in relation to mood disorders or other illnesses and use this to justify their use. Consistent with the MET philosophy, it is important to acknowledge the individual's feelings in these matters while avoiding debate. Depending upon the clinician's own feelings, it may be useful to more generally acknowledge that there is a wide range of opinions regarding the severity and prevalence of negative consequences of use. The clinician can then state that he or she has no predetermined moral or universal judgments regarding marijuana use and is instead only interested in understanding the client's experiences. Regarding medical use issues, the clinician should acknowledge the perceived benefits while inquiring if there might also be some "not so positive" effects. Exploration of alternative ways of treating or "coping" with the medical or mood symptoms would be appropriate once a basis for considering change has been established.

Another issue that may arise in the MCU for participants who get to the point of considering change is whether they need to stop using completely or just cut back. This client-centered approach assumes that the client should make this decision. Exploring with the client the likelihood of being successful with each goal (i.e., abstinence versus moderate use) and how that success would or would not reduce any negative consequences that have been identified should help the decision process. If the client asks for advice, the clinician may want to offer the perspective that achieving and sustaining reduced use is often more difficult than achieving complete abstinence (see Chapter 6 for the rationale). If the client does not ask but the clinician feels that the client is ready to start planning for change, the clinician routinely asks about their specific goals and how they will achieve them. In offering options and advice in the planning stage, the clinician again may have opportunities to provide information on the likelihood of succeeding in moderating use versus quitting. From the motivational interviewing perspective, it is usually wise to ask permission to give such advice (e.g., "Would you like to know how I think about moderation versus abstinence?") to avoid reactance.

Some clinicians may be concerned about the brevity of the MCU intervention given what they perceive to be significant negative consequences and distress in the client. Familiarity with the brief intervention literature (e.g., Bien *et al.*, 1993; Burke *et al.*, 2003) may help assure them of the potential for meaningful change. Moreover, it is important to remind clinicians that they are reaching people who might not otherwise have approached treatment and that the intervention may increase the likelihood of future treatment seeking.

One of the issues that we have struggled with in developing and implementing the MCU applies to all interventions that attempt to reach more ambivalent users by stating that there is "no pressure to change" or it is "not treatment." This mode of marketing or advertising the MCU may raise ethical issues and concerns about deception inasmuch as MET has as its goal the enhancement of motivation for change in individuals whose drug use is causing problems. Concerns of this type are lessened when brief MET treatments are offered to those seeking support for change because there is no need to use these marketing techniques. We suspect that concerns about deception center on how one interprets terms like "pressure to change" and "treatment" and how one trains therapists to conduct the feedback sessions. Although motivational interviewing therapists systematically attempt to elicit and focus on self-motivational statements, the statements are *self*-motivational. Just as prominent in the intervention is the attempt to create a mutually respectful, safe, and supportive interaction that allows marijuana users to explore their experiences with marijuana without the need to justify their behavior. There is no pressure to change overtly imposed by the therapist, only a thorough exploration of possible reasons for change that then are reinforced by the therapist.

When clients present with suspicions regarding "ulterior motives" in the MCU, we recommend reflecting and acknowledging the concern and re-stating the rationale that the MCU provides objective feedback and what they do with it "is up to them." We believe this is the true philosophy behind the MCU and motivational interviewing with its emphasis on client responsibility for change. We have received few complaints from participants that they did not receive what they were led to expect. Interestingly, participants who received the MET intervention in the context of the MCU reported that their therapists were more likely to try to convince them to reduce use compared to participants in a purely educational comparison conditions. However, these same MET participants were more satisfied with the experience than those who got information on marijuana effects (see Stephens *et al.*, under review). Thus, clients may identify therapists' attempts to explore motivations for change, but they do not seem to perceive it as an aversive "pressure."

From the therapist training and supervision perspective, ethical concerns sometimes arise when therapists are taught the techniques that are systematically geared toward increasing motivation for change. Indeed, Miller and Rollnick (1991, 2002) describe motivational interviewing as a *directive*, client-centered therapy to distinguish it from nondirective, client-centered approaches. The motivational interviewer has an explicit goal to facilitate the clients' candid and in-depth explorations of their experiences in order to increase motivation for change in those individuals who are experiencing negative consequences related to drug use. In our training and supervision of therapists we repeatedly emphasize that their task is to use motivational interviewing techniques competently. If the client does not perceive any negative consequences or reasons for change, there can be no focus on them. Therapists create interactions with clients that maximally allow the clients to explore reasons for change, but if such reasons do not exist, they cannot create them. Therapists are given the expectation that their competence is evaluated by how well they use motivational interviewing techniques, not by their success in getting clients to change.

Yet another perspective may occur in research studies on check-ups when Institutional Review Boards (IRB) must evaluate the adequacy of how well human subjects are informed by project marketing and the informed consent process. Even if one considers the MCU marketing to be deceptive, the IRB perspective on risks and benefits is useful in evaluating the ethics of the research and intervention. Risks are minimized in the MCU by the respectful way that clients are treated and the absence of any heavy-handed tactics that would resemble what participants might consider "pressure to change." On the other hand, the potential enefits are great if individuals who are experiencing problems related to their marijuana use decide to take steps to reduce it. Our ethical standards for research generally allow for deception under such lop-sided benefit-to-risk ratios. Similarly, debriefing of deception in research studies is typically not required when the debriefing would do more harm than good. While we do not pretend that "check-up" studies do not raise some ethical issues, we believe that their intent has integrity and when conducted with primary respect for the clients they cause much less harm than good.

In summary, when questioned about the possibility that the MCU is deceptive, we respond with several points: (1) our intent is to offer helpful support to marijuana users who are experiencing problems, some of whom are struggling with competing motivations for and against change; (2) the "check-up" offers such individuals the chance to candidly "take stock" of their experiences; (3) if a client speaks of problems resulting from their marijuana smoking, the counselor offers support in further exploring these difficulties and future options for their resolution; and (4) clients who do not bring up marijuana-related problems are neither pressured to identify problems nor commit to change.

## A Controlled Trial of the MCU

A pilot study of the MCU with a single therapist (Roffman) showed promising results in being able to reach a population of marijuana users who were in the earlier SOC and who were experiencing negative consequences. Comparison of participants with those randomized to a delayed intervention control group 6 weeks after the feedback session suggested that the MCU engendered greater change in marijuana use (Stephens & Roffman, 1997). Subsequently, we were funded by the National Institute on Drug Abuse to conduct a larger trial. The MCU was hypothesized to attract users who were more ambivalent than treatment-seeking users about changing their marijuana use, yet were experiencing negative consequences of use. In order to study the efficacy of the intervention in increasing readiness for change and thereby reduce marijuana use, the study employed three conditions. A MET condition was based on feedback and motivational interviewing as described above. A delayed feedback control condition (DFC) was similar to those used in previous studies of the DCU and allowed for an assessment of short-term efficacy relative to no intervention 7 weeks later. However, because those assigned to the DFC condition were eligible to receive the feedback intervention after a 7-week delay, they could not serve as a comparison group at longer follow-up assessments. Therefore, we developed a multimedia feedback (MMF) intervention that was true to the spirit of the MCU advertisements (i.e., objective feedback about marijuana; no pressure to change), but which did not contain the proposed active ingredients of personalized and normative feedback about marijuana use delivered with a motivational interviewing style. Instead, the MMF condition provided education about the latest research on marijuana delivered in an objective, largely didactic manner. In an initial paper based on the baseline data from the project, we focused on three questions (Stephens *et al.*, 2004).

**Did the MCU reach individuals who were using marijuana in a potentially problematic pattern and who were ambivalent about making changes?**
The MCU attracted 587 adult marijuana users who expressed interest in the project and who were screened for participation by phone. The screened sample averaged 30.24 ($SD = 9.92$) years of age and was predominantly male and white. They smoked on an average of 2 out of every 3 days during the past month and they typically smoked 3 or more times per day. The majority of callers classified themselves in the precontemplation (45%) or contemplation (22%) stage of change based on an SOC algorithm included in screening interview. These data suggested high rates of marijuana use indicative of potential

problems at least in a subset of the callers. Moreover, a minority of the callers were currently planning on making changes in their use.

### Did these ambivalent marijuana using individuals actually follow through and receive the intervention?

Of those screened, 214 (36%) failed to meet one or more of the following exclusion criteria: less than 15 days of marijuana use out of the last 30 ($n = 139$; 65.0%), action or maintenance stage of change ($n = 40$; 18.7%), alcohol or other drug abuse or dependence ($n = 38$; 17.8%), currently involved in other substance abuse treatment or a self-help group ($n = 25$; 11.7%), severe psychiatric problems (e.g., psychosis, $n = 12$; 5.6%), legal status that might have interfered with treatment (e.g., mandated treatment, pending jail sentencing; $n = 9$; 4.2%), planned to move within the next 12 months ($n = 8$; 3.7%), did not live within 60 miles of the study site ($n = 5$; 2.3%), living with someone already enrolled in study ($n = 5$; 2.3%), and not fluent in English ($n = 1$; 0.5%). These eligibility criteria led to obvious differences between those who were ineligible versus eligible and no formal comparisons of those groups were conducted. In particular, those with less frequent patterns of recent use were excluded in order to increase the probability that those who participated would be experiencing some negative consequences. However, the cut-point was arbitrary and good data on the relationship between frequency of use and problem severity does not exist. Future studies might reasonably explore whether the MCU would be a useful experience for those with less regular marijuana use.

Of the 373 callers who met all eligibility criteria and were invited to participate in the randomized efficacy trial, only 188 (50%) actually attended the initial assessment session for the intervention. We compared eligible callers who did not participate with those who did in order to examine whether interested callers who were ambivalent about change would participate in the actual intervention. Attrition between screening and enrollment in treatment studies is common (e.g., Vendetti *et al.*, 2002) and we suspect often related to readiness for change. Individuals who followed through and participated were about 4 years older on average and reported slightly more drinks per typical drinking day, than those who failed to follow through. Otherwise, the groups appeared very similar demographically and particularly with regard to their recent marijuana use. The most noticeable difference between the groups was on the SOC algorithm. Whereas almost 60% of those who did not enroll were in the precontemplation stage, this proportion falls to 40% for enrolled participants. This decrease in the relative proportion of precontemplators who followed through and completed enrollment in the MCU interventions might have been expected, but even among the 188 participants randomly assigned to condition, over two-thirds still could be characterized as ambivalent about or uninterested in making changes and unlikely to seek formal treatment in the near future.

## Did the MCU reach a population of users that differed from those who voluntarily approach treatment aimed at quitting?

To answer this question we examined similarities and differences between participants in the MCU and those in a treatment-outcome study that was recruiting participants in Seattle, Washington during the same time period. The Marijuana Treatment Project (MTP; MTPRG, 2004; Stephens *et al.*, 2002) was a multi-site treatment-outcome study designed to test the efficacy of two treatments for marijuana dependence. Although comparisons across studies are difficult to interpret because of potential differences in recruitment and research procedures, several factors gave us greater confidence in the validity of these comparisons. The MCU and the MTP site we used as a comparison were supervised by the same set of investigators, employed some of the same research personnel, and used many of the same screening criteria and assessment procedures. We further restricted our comparisons to the subset of participants in each project who were screened for participation during a 6-month period in which recruitment for both projects overlapped. Advertisements for the MCU and MTP were placed in the same local print and radio media and were alternated among specific media outlets such that both projects were not advertised in the same media during the same week. In contrast to the MCU, the MTP ads invited adult marijuana users who were **interested in treatment** to phone for more information, and callers were told that the project was designed to study different ways to help people quit using marijuana (see Stephens *et al.*, 2002 for more information on the design of the MTP).

During the 6-month overlapping recruitment period, 162 callers were screened for the MCU and 124 callers were screened for the MTP. Table 8.2 compares these two samples on demographic, drug use, and treatment history variables common to the screening interviews. Callers to both projects were largely in their twenties and thirties, but those interested in the MCU tended to be somewhat younger than those who called the MTP. Callers to both projects used marijuana almost daily (i.e., 5–6 days per week), but MCU callers smoked marijuana somewhat less frequently and there was evidence of greater variability in the frequency of use in this sample. MCU callers also smoked fewer times per day than callers for the MTP, although multiple daily uses were the norm in both samples. Thus, the MCU appeared to appeal to a wider range of users in terms of age and frequency and intensity of use compared to those seeking treatment.

Table 8.2. *Comparison of MCU and MTP screened respondents*

| Variable | MCU (n = 162) | MTP (n = 124) |
|---|---|---|
| Age*** | 30.95 (9.40) | 34.89 (8.93) |
| Sex (Male) | 77.8% | 71.8% |
| Race (White) | 85.2% | 79.8% |
| Days of marijuana use in past 30 days*** | 21.17 (9.92) | 24.80 (6.60) |
| Times smoked per day in past 30 days[a]*** | 2.83 (1.60) | 3.56 (1.72) |
| Drinks per typical drinking day[b] | 2.61 (2.20) | 2.22 (2.18) |
| Used other drugs in past 30 days | 27.2% | 19.4% |
| Legal problems* | 12.3% | 4.0% |
| Currently in treatment for marijuana or other drugs | 3.7% | 5.6% |
| Currently in therapy for psychiatric problem*** | 1.2% | 12.9% |

*Note*: All values are means followed by standard deviations in parentheses unless otherwise indicated.
[a]0 = not at all; 1 = 1 time/day; 2.5 = 2–3 times/day; 4.5 = 4–5 times/day; 6 = 6 or more times a day.
[b]0 = None; 1.5 = 1–2; 3.5 = 3–4; 5.5 = 5–6; 8 = 7–9; 10 = 10 or more.
*$p < 0.05$; ***$p < 0.001$.

The findings suggest that the MCU is a promising way to reach a wider range of marijuana users.

Next we compared the subsets of participants in both projects who were eligible and completed the initial assessment which included more sensitive measures of readiness for change and problems related to marijuana use. Of the 94 eligible callers to the MCU during the six-month overlapping recruitment period, 51 (54%) gave informed consent, completed the initial assessment, and were randomized to intervention condition. Of the 92 eligible individuals in the MTP, 58 (63%) gave informed consent, completed the initial assessment, and were randomized to intervention condition. Thus, rates of enrollment among those eligible were comparable. Table 8.3 compares the enrolled participants on demographic, drug use, and motivational variables.

There were no significant differences between MCU and MTP participants on any of the demographic, marijuana use, alcohol use, or other drug use variables, but MTP participants were more likely to have received alcohol or other drug treatment in the past 90 days. On the SCID diagnostic interview, MCU participants met fewer cannabis dependence and abuse criteria than MTP participants. Whereas 100% of the MTP sample met diagnostic criteria for cannabis

Table 8.3. *Comparison of MCU and MTP enrolled participants*

| Variable | MCU ($n = 51$) | MTP ($n = 58$) |
|---|---|---|
| Age | 32.80 (10.68) | 36.00 (7.79) |
| Sex (Male) | 76.5% | 75.9% |
| Race (White) | 86.3% | 84.5% |
| Marital status (Single) | 64.4% | 58.6% |
| Highest grade completed | 13.89 (1.80) | 14.64 (2.27) |
| *Employment status* | | |
| Employed | 68.9% | 86.2% |
| Unemployed | 20.00% | 12.1% |
| Student | 11.1% | 1.7% |
| Days of marijuana use in past 90 days | 79.12 (14.38) | 76.10 (15.93) |
| Quarters smoked marijuana per smoking day | 2.12 (0.76) | 2.21 (0.87) |
| Number of times get high a day | 4.18 (5.01) | 4.97 (5.90) |
| Age when first smoked marijuana regularly (i.e., 3 or more times a week) | 17.73 (4.65) | 18.19 (4.18) |
| Age when marijuana problems first started | 24.71 (8.47) | 27.98 (8.75) |
| Number of hours feel high a day | 6.20 (4.28) | 7.16 (4.69) |
| Number of ounces smoked per week[a] | 0.21 (0.30) | 0.18 (0.19) |
| Total days of alcohol use | 23.98 (25.69) | 22.12 (24.70) |
| Average drinks per drinking day | 2.16 (1.58) | 2.05 (1.36) |
| Number of times drank 6 or more drinks per day[b] | 0.57 (0.61) | 0.41 (0.53) |
| Days of other drug use | 2.18 (5.47) | 0.95 (1.98) |
| Received alcohol or drug treatment in past 90 days* | 0.0% | 10.3% |
| How many cigarettes smoked per day[c] | 1.22 (1.40) | 0.91 (1.19) |
| Marijuana abuse symptoms*** | 1.49 (0.90) | 2.26 (0.74) |
| Marijuana dependence symptoms*** | 3.55 (2.08) | 5.88 (1.09) |
| Marijuana Problems Scale*** | 5.88 (3.62) | 9.81 (3.39) |
| *Readiness to Change* | | |
| Precontemplation*** | −0.27 (0.86) | −1.14 (0.66) |
| Contemplation*** | 0.25 (1.07) | 1.29 (0.59) |
| Action*** | −0.33 (0.99) | 0.48 (0.98) |
| Self-Efficacy | 3.24 (1.25) | 3.21 (1.15) |

*Note*: All values are means followed by standard deviations in parentheses unless otherwise indicated.
[a] 0.01 represents less than 0.06 ounces; 2.00 represents more than 1.00 ounce.
[b] 0 = Never; 1 = Less than weekly; 2 = Weekly; 3 = Less than daily; 4 = Daily or almost daily.
[c] 0 = None; 1 = Less than 10; 2 = About 1/2 pack; 3 = About 1 pack; 4 = More than a pack.
*$p < 0.05$; *** $p < 0.001$.

dependence, 63% of MCU participants were dependent. Similarly, MCU participants endorsed fewer problems related to their marijuana use on the MPS than MTP participants. MCU participants scored higher on the precontemplation scale and lower on the contemplation and action scales of the RTC measure, indicating lower acknowledgement of problems and less readiness to make changes. There were no differences in MCU and MTP participants in their confidence that they could avoid marijuana use on the self-efficacy scale. These findings held in several subsequent analyses designed to control for differences in the eligibility criteria between projects (Stephens *et al.*, 2004). Thus, as with the DCU (Miller & Sovereign, 1989), participants enrolled in the MCU appeared fairly similar to those in treatment studies in terms of the extent of marijuana use and the presence of at least some negative consequences. However, as a group they experienced fewer problems related to marijuana use and were less ready for change.

### Did the MET condition increase readiness to change and reduce marijuana use?

In order to evaluate the efficacy of the MCU we compared outcomes for those randomly assigned to the MET ($n = 62$), MMF ($n = 62$) and DFC ($n = 64$) conditions (see Stephens *et al.*, under review). The MET condition consisted of one 90-min session in which the therapist reviewed a PFR with the participant using motivational interviewing as described earlier in the chapter. The MMF condition involved the use of video and therapist-delivered computer presentations on research findings on marijuana during a single 90-min individual session. No feedback regarding the participant's personal use of marijuana was provided. Participants in the DFC conditions were assessed at baseline, but received no further intervention until after the completion of a 7-week follow-up for all participants. Those in the MET and MMF condition also completed follow-up assessments at 6 and 12 months after randomization to condition.

Three masters-level therapists with previous experience in behavioral therapies conducted the feedback sessions. The therapists received approximately 20 hours of training from the supervisor (Roffman) over a 2-month period. The training included several components: (1) knowledge of the effects of marijuana on health and behavior; (2) motivational interviewing skills; and (3) cognitive-behavioral counseling skills. In addition, the therapists were trained to follow a detailed treatment manual that prescribed the content and technique of the feedback sessions for each condition. As part of their training, therapists role-played sessions with each other and with mock clients, and then conducted audio-taped counseling sessions with pilot participants that were reviewed by the supervisor. Therapists were assigned actual study participants only after they were judged competent in conducting the interventions. All feedback sessions were audio-taped and therapists participated in weekly group supervision sessions throughout the study period. Checklists and ratings of adherence were completed by therapists following each feedback session and suggested good adherence to protocols. Coding of a subset of the audiotapes by independent evaluators showed differences between the MET and MMF conditions that were consistent with the intended style and content of the interventions.

At the 7-week follow-up, those participants who received personalized feedback with motivational interviewing reduced their frequency of marijuana use and the number of periods of the day during which they smoked more than those in either the delayed feedback or educational comparison conditions (see Table 8.4 and Figure 8.2). The reductions in marijuana use corresponded to reductions in the number of dependence symptoms. However, the magnitude of the reduction was on the order of about 1 day less per week of use and an average of about one-half fewer periods of use per day of use. Given that participants were averaging 6 days of use per week and 2 periods of use per day at baseline, these reductions left them as fairly heavy users who still met an average of 2 dependence symptoms and self-reported almost 4 problems related to use. More encouraging were the findings that reductions in the frequency of use and dependence symptoms were sustained for the most part throughout the 12-month follow-up period. Although reductions in use by the participants in the MMF condition had nearly caught up at the 6-month follow-up, the groups had diverged again by 12 months on the measure of frequency of use but not periods smoked per day. This pattern suggests that the effect was not transient and was more robust for days of any use relative to intensity or duration of use per day.

Significant differences between conditions were not found on self-reported marijuana-related problems even though there were significant reductions in dependence symptoms at all follow-ups for those in the MET condition. The meaning of this pattern is not clear and may relate to greater variability in the acknowledgement of problems or to the differences between dependence symptoms and other negative consequences. Dependence symptoms were assessed by trained interviewers using a structured set of questions and probes with guidelines for scoring the presence or absence of the symptom. The MPS measure of self-reported problems required participants to make more subjective judgments regarding the presence or absence of specific negative consequences

Table 8.4. Adjusted means, standard errors (SE), and confidence intervals (CI) for marijuana use and related consequences assessed at baseline, 7 weeks, 6 months and 12 months by treatment conditions

| Measure | Assessment | Personalized feedback (n = 62) | | | Multi-media feedback (n = 62) | | | Delayed feedback (n = 64) | | |
|---|---|---|---|---|---|---|---|---|---|---|
| | | M | (SE) | 95% CI | M | (SE) | 95% CI | M | (SE) | 95% CI |
| Days of marijuana use per week | Baseline | 5.82[a] | (0.15) | [5.52; 6.12] | 5.80[a] | (0.15) | [5.49; 6.10] | 6.00[a] | (0.15) | [5.70; 6.29] |
| | 7 weeks | 4.83[a] | (0.24) | [4.35; 5.32] | 5.46[b] | (0.25) | [4.98; 5.94] | 5.64[b] | (0.24) | [5.17; 6.11] |
| | 6 months | 4.92[a] | (0.27) | [4.39; 5.45] | 5.21[a] | (0.27) | [4.68; 5.73] | | | |
| | 12 months | 4.65[a] | (0.28) | [4.10; 5.20] | 5.58[b] | (0.28) | [5.03; 6.12] | | | |
| Periods smoked per day | Baseline | 2.06[a] | (0.10) | [1.87; 2.25] | 2.01[a] | (0.10) | [1.81; 2.20] | 2.17[a] | (0.09) | [1.98; 2.36] |
| | 7 weeks | 1.69[a] | (0.11) | [1.48; 1.90] | 1.91[b] | (0.11) | [1.70; 2.11] | 2.18[b] | (0.10) | [1.97; 2.38] |
| | 6 months | 1.84[a] | (0.11) | [1.61; 2.06] | 2.02[a] | (0.11) | [1.79; 2.24] | | | |
| | 12 months | 1.79[a] | (0.11) | [1.56; 2.02] | 1.96[a] | (0.11) | [1.74; 2.19] | | | |

| Measure | Assessment | Personalized feedback (n = 62) | | | Multi-media feedback (n = 62) | | | Delayed feedback (n = 64) | | |
|---|---|---|---|---|---|---|---|---|---|---|
| | | X | (SE) | 95% CI | X | (SE) | 95% CI | X | (SE) | 95% CI |
| Dependence symptoms | Baseline | 3.69[a] | (0.22) | [3.27; 4.12] | 3.50[a] | (0.22) | [3.07; 3.93] | 3.16[a] | (0.21) | [2.74; 3.57] |
| | 7 weeks | 2.34[a] | (0.21) | [1.92; 2.76] | 2.91[b] | (0.21) | [2.49; 3.33] | 2.88[b] | (0.21) | [2.48; 3.29] |
| | 6 months | 2.59[a] | (0.22) | [2.15; 3.03] | 3.27[b] | (0.22) | [2.83; 3.71] | | | |
| | 12 month | 2.42[a] | (0.19) | [2.04; 2.81] | 2.88[b] | (0.19) | [2.50; 3.23] | | | |
| Number of problems | Baseline | 5.76[a] | (0.39) | [4.99; 6.54] | 5.98[a] | (0.39) | [5.20; 6.76] | 6.25[a] | (0.39) | [5.49; 7.01] |
| | 7 weeks | 3.91[a] | (0.45) | [3.03; 4.79] | 5.07[a] | (0.45) | [4.19; 5.96] | 4.77[a] | (0.44) | [3.91; 5.62] |
| | 6 months | 4.14[a] | (0.44) | [3.26; 5.01] | 5.38[a] | (0.44) | [4.51; 6.25] | | | |
| | 12 months | 4.02[a] | (0.42) | [3.19; 4.84] | 5.14[a] | (0.42) | [4.32; 5.97] | | | |

Note: Data are adjusted for baseline scores on the SOC algorithm and the Precontemplation scale of the RTC and baseline values were substituted for missing data at follow-ups. Means in the same row with different superscripts differ significantly at $p < 0.05$.

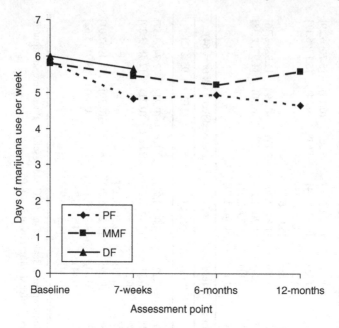

Figure 8.2  Days of marijuana use per week by treatment condition and assessment point.

described by a few words. The MPS has been sensitive to much greater reductions in use in prior studies (MTPRG, 2004; Stephens *et al.*, 2000), but may not be able to capture subtler changes. On the other hand, most of the DSM-IV dependence symptoms tend to assess impairments in self-control that may be affected by even small changes in use that signal a new degree of control. The MPS taps into more objective sequelae of use that may only change with larger reductions in use.

We also were unable to detect any influence of the MET intervention on changes in motivation, self-efficacy for avoiding use, or expectancies associated with either the effects of marijuana or reductions in use. The measures of expectancies in the current study were created primarily for the purpose of generating feedback and had not been validated. However, the self-efficacy and readiness to change measures have been used to predict or assess change in prior studies, but failed to be systematically affected by the intervention conditions. Again, it may be that the magnitude of the effect in the current study was insufficient to be manifest in measures that lack perfect construct validity.

However, other studies of motivational interviewing-based interventions have also failed to detect changes in similar measures of proposed mediating processes (see Burke *et al.*, 2002, for review). Paper and pencil measures simply do not seem to be able to capture the processes that mediate the effects of these interventions.

## Conclusions and Future Directions

It seems clear that the MCU was effective in reaching a population of marijuana users who, on average, were less ready for change than those in treatment studies. Of course, it is likely that these populations are not independent and overlap such that some MCU participants might have approached treatment and some treatment seekers would likely be interested in the MCU. This low-burden intervention holds potential for attracting users, screening for problem use, resolving ambivalence about change, and providing information on self-change and treatment options. Addressing these needs in a population unlikely to approach treatment in the near future could meaningfully add to the continuum of care for drug users (Humphreys & Tucker, 2002; Sobell & Sobell, 2000).

The effect sizes for reductions in frequency of use and dependence symptoms tended to fall in the small to medium range and were generally consistent with those found in other studies of motivational interviewing interventions (Burke *et al.*, 2003). On the other hand, the effects for problems related to use were smaller and non-significant. Thus, it is unclear whether the present findings represent clinically meaningful change. However, it may not be appropriate to use the same definition of clinically significant change in check-up studies. Any change might be considered meaningful if it occurs with a very brief intervention in a population unlikely to approach any other programs. It also may be that the effects of a check-up are delayed and will emerge in form of greater readiness to consider the pros and cons of continued use as time goes on. Although we did not find much formal treatment seeking during the follow-up period, positive experiences with drug professionals engendered by interventions that show respect for the individual and that do not impose dogmatic views regarding drug use may increase the probability of treatment seeking in the future. This may be particularly true if, unlike the present study, the MCU were offered as part of a continuum of care in an integrated, comprehensive treatment facility where clients could return to a similar staff with similar training and treatment philosophy. On the other hand, placement of a check-up intervention in treatment facilities may detract from its ability to attract those who want to avoid the stigma of substance abuse treatment or may decrease the perceived likelihood that the check-up would actually be an "objective" look at one's marijuana use with "no pressure" to change. The ultimate impact of check-up interventions may be dependent on tailored and easily accessed subsequent supports for those individuals who have become more ready for change. Research in these different types of settings and contexts (e.g., free standing, primary care, drug abuse treatment agencies) with larger samples and longer follow-ups would be needed to resolve these issues.

It also seems reasonable to suspect that the length or dose of the intervention in the present study was inadequate to promote change in truly ambivalent individuals. In the present study, therapists had 90 min to review a PFR, elicit self-motivational statements, and support change via goal setting and strategizing (provided the participant indicated an interest in change). Anecdotally, our therapists told us it was a lot to expect with the current sample. Most motivational interviewing studies have been conducted in treatment facilities where many participants already have either intrinsic or extrinsic reasons for wanting to change. More ambivalent individuals may profit from the opportunity to return to a motivational interviewer on multiple occasions to continue weighing the pros and cons of change. Therefore, future studies should compare longer and briefer versions of the MCU to determine optimal dosages. Although questions remain about the magnitude and long term meaningfulness of the change that was produced, the MCU may help reduce barriers to engagement in drug abuse services, opening doors to reaching marijuana users that do not currently exist in our treatment system.

## References

Bien, T. H., Miller, W. R., & Tonigan, J. S. (1993). Brief interventions for alcohol problems: a review. *Addiction, 88,* 315–336.

Burke, B. L., Arkowitz, H., & Dunn, C. (2002). The efficacy of motivational interviewing and its adaptations: what we know so far. In W.R. Miller, & S. Rollnick (Eds.), *Motivational interviewing: preparing people to change addictive behavior* (2nd ed., pp. 217–250). New York: Guilford Press.

Burke, B. L., Arkowitz, H., & Menchola, M. (2003). The efficacy of motivational interviewing: a meta-analysis of controlled clinical trials. *Journal of Consulting and Clinical Psychology, 71,* 843–861.

Campbell, A. N. C., Fisher, D. S., Picciano, J. F., Orlando, M. J., Stephens, R. S., & Roffman, R. A. (2004). Marketing effectiveness in reaching non-treatment-seeking marijuana smokers. *Journal of Social Work Practice in the Addictions, 4,* 39–59.

Cunningham, J. A., Sobell, L. C., Sobell, M. B., Agrawal, S., & Toneatoo, T. (1993). Barriers to treatment: why alcohol and drug abusers delay or never seek treatment. *Addictive Behaviors, 18*, 347–353.

DiClemente, C. C., & Velasquez, M. M. (2002). Motivational interviewing and the stages of change. In W.R. Miller, & S. Rollnick (Eds.), *Motivational interviewing: preparing people to change addictive behavior* (2nd ed., pp. 201–216). New York: Guilford Press.

Doyle, A., Swan, M., Roffman, R., & Stephens, R. (2003). The Marijuana Check-Up: a brief intervention tailored for individuals in the contemplation stage. *Journal of Social Work Practice in the Addictions, 3*, 53–71.

First, M. B., Spitzer, R. L, Gibbon, M., & Williams, J. B. (1996). *Structured clinical interview for DSM-IV, axis I disorders – patient edition* (SCID-I/P, Version 2.0). Biometrics Research Department, New York State Psychiatric Institute, NY.

Humphreys, K., & Tucker, J.A. (2002). Towards more responsive and effective intervention systems for alcohol-related problems (Editorial). *Addiction, 97*, 127–132.

Marijuana Treatment Project Research Group (MTPRG) (2004). Brief treatments for cannabis dependence: findings from a randomized multisite trial. *Journal of Consulting and Clinical Psychology, 72*, 455–466.

Miller, W. R., & Rollnick, S. (1991). *Motivational interviewing: preparing people to change addictive behavior*. New York: Guilford Press.

Miller, W. R., & Rollnick, S. (2002). *Motivational interviewing: preparing people to change addictive behavior* (2nd ed.). New York: Guilford Press.

Miller, W. R., & Sovereign, R. G. (1989). The check-up: a model for early intervention in addictive behaviors. In T. Loberg, W. R. Miller, P. E. Nathan, & G. A. Marlatt (Eds.), *Addictive behaviors: prevention and early intervention* (pp. 219–231). Amsterdam, Holland: Swets & Zeitlinger.

Miller, W. R., Sovereign, R. G., & Krege, B. (1988). Motivational interviewing with problem drinkers: II. The Drinker's Check-Up as a preventive intervention. *Behavioural Psychotherapy, 16*, 251–268.

Miller, W. R., Zweben, A., DiClemente, C. C., & Rychtarik, R. G. (1992). *Motivational enhancement therapy manual: a clinical research guide for therapists treating individuals with alcohol abuse and dependence* (DHHS Publication No. ADM 92-1894). Washington, DC: U.S. Government Printing Office.

Miller, W. R., Benefield, G. S., & Tonigan, J. S. (1993). Enhancing motivation for change in problem drinking: a controlled comparison of two therapist styles. *Journal of Consulting and Clinical Psychology, 61*, 455–461.

Prochaska, J. O., & DiClemente, C. C. (1984). *The transtheoretical approach: crossing the traditional boundaries of therapy*. Malabar, FL: Krieger.

Sobell, L. C., & Sobell, M. B. (1992). TimeLine Follow-Back, a technique for assessing self-reported alcohol consumption. In R. Litten, & J. Allen (Eds.), *Measuring alcohol consumption*. New Jersey: The Humana Press Inc.

Sobell, M. B., & Sobell, L. C. (2000). Stepped care as a heuristic approach to the treatment of alcohol problems. *Journal of Consulting and Clinical Psychology, 68,* 573–579.

Sobell, L. C., Sobell, M. B., & Toneatto, T. (1991). Recovery from alcohol problems without treatment. In N. Heather, W. R. Miller, & J. Greeley (Eds.), *Self-control and the addictive behaviours.* Botany, Australia: Maxwell Macmillan Publishing.

Solomon, K. E., & Annis, H. M. (1989). Development of a scale to measure outcome expectancy in alcoholics. *Cognitive Therapy & Research, 13,* 409–421.

Stephens, R. S., & Roffman, R. A. (1993). Adult marijuana dependence. In J. S. Baer, G. A. Marlatt, & J. McMahon (Eds.), *Addictive behaviors across the lifespan: prevention, treatment, and policy issues* (pp. 202–218). Newbury Park, CA: Sage.

Stephens, R. S., & Roffman, R. A. (1997). The Marijuana Check-Up: motivating change in ambivalent marijuana users. Poster presented *31st Annual Conference of the Association for Advancement of Behavior Therapy,* Miami Beach, Florida.

Stephens, R. S., & Roffman, R. A. (2005). Assessment of cannabis use disorders. In D. M. Donovan, & G. A. Marlatt (Eds.), *Assessment of addictive behaviors* (2nd ed., pp. 248–273). New York: Guilford.

Stephens, R. S., Wertz, J. S., & Roffman, R. A. (1993). Predictors of marijuana treatment outcomes: the role of self-efficacy. *Journal of Substance Abuse, 5,* 341–354.

Stephens, R. S., Roffman, R. A., & Simpson, E. E. (1994). Treating adult marijuana dependence: a test of the relapse prevention model. *Journal of Consulting and Clinical Psychology, 62,* 92–99.

Stephens, R. S., Wertz, J. S., & Roffman, R. A. (1995). Self-efficacy and marijuana cessation: a construct validity analysis. *Journal of Consulting and Clinical Psychology, 63,* 1022–1031.

Stephens, R. S., Roffman, R. A., & Curtin, L. (2000). Comparison of extended versus brief treatments for marijuana use. *Journal of Consulting and Clinical Psychology, 68,* 898–908.

Stephens, R. S., Babor, T. F., Kadden, R. A., Miller, M., & Marijuana Treatment Project Research Group (2002). The marijuana treatment project: rationale, design, and participant characteristics. *Addiction, 97,* 109–124.

Stephens, R. S., Roffman, R. A., Fearer, S. A., Williams, C., Picciano, J. F., & Burke, R. S. (2004). The Marijuana Check-Up: reaching users who are ambivalent about change. *Addiction, 99,* 1323–1332.

Stephens, R. S., Roffman, R. A., Fearer, S., & Williams, C., & Burke, R. S. (under review). The Marijuana Check-Up: promoting change in ambivalent marijuana users. *Journal of Consulting and Clinical Psychology.*

Substance Abuse and Mental Health Services Administration, Office of Applied Sciences (SAMHSA) (2003a). *Results from the 2002 National Survey on Drug Use and Health: Detailed Tables.* Retrieved on January 3, 2005 from http://oas.samhsa.gov/nhsda.htm

Substance Abuse and Mental Health Services Administration, Office of Applied Sciences (SAMHSA) (2003b). *Reasons for not receiving substance abuse treatment. The NSDUH Report*. Retrieved on January 3, 2005 from http://oas.samsha.gov/factsNHSDA.htm

Vendetti, J., McRee, B., Miller, M., Christiansen, K., Herrell, J., & The Marijuana Treatment Project Research Group (2002). Correlates of pre-treatment drop-out among people with marijuana dependence. *Addiction, 97*, 125–134.

# 9

# Guided Self-Change: A Brief Motivational Intervention for Cannabis Abuse

LINDA C. SOBELL, MARK B. SOBELL, ERIC F. WAGNER, SANGEETA AGRAWAL AND TIMOTHY P. ELLINGSTAD

Studies of treated cannabis abusers (Ellingstad *et al.*, 2002; Sobell *et al.*, 1990; Stephens *et al.*, 2000) and those who have recovered without treatment (L. C. Sobell *et al.*, 2000) are few in number compared with studies of other drug abusers. Since national surveys have repeatedly shown that cannabis is the most widely used illicit drug (Substance Abuse and Mental Health Services Administration, 1997, 1998, 2000a, b) this finding is somewhat counterintuitive. In fact, a recent review of drug treatment studies found that only 8% (2 of 28) that met review criteria included primary cannabis abusers in their treatment samples (Ellingstad *et al.*, 2002). Further, a review of natural recovery studies found that only 1 of 40 reported data from cannabis abusers (L. C. Sobell *et al.*, 2000).

## Prevalence

Given cannabis' popularity, an interesting question is why only about half a million of the 6.8 million frequent cannabis users (defined as using cannabis ⩾50 times) enter treatment (Substance Abuse and Mental Health Services Administration, 2000a). One possible reason is that compared with other illicit drugs, the negative consequences of cannabis use are fewer, and if they occur, are much less severe. For example, most of those who initiate abstinence from cannabis do not report severe withdrawal symptoms (Budney *et al.*, 2001; Wiesbeck *et al.*, 1996; Zimmer & Morgan, 1995) and the most frequently reported problems appear more related to personal dissatisfaction with drug use rather than objective negative consequences (Stephens *et al.*, 1994, 2000). In contrast, withdrawal from cocaine and heroin can be very serious and negative consequences often involve other negative health effects, unemployment, and legal difficulties. Thus, there may be less of a perceived need to study treatment or recovery from cannabis use disorders because (a) a large number of users do not abuse the drug and/or (b) compared with alcohol and other illicit drugs, cannabis use is associated with a much lower level of clinical severity.

In this chapter, we describe guided self-change (GSC) treatment as applied to cannabis users. The brief motivational nature of this intervention may be particularly appropriate for cannabis users who approach treatment with less severe problems and ambivalence about reducing use, and who may be reluctant to accept a goal of complete abstinence from marijuana use. First, we review the rationale for and fundamental techniques of GSC treatment. Studies of brief treatment, natural recovery, and unsolicited help seeking among marijuana users are then reviewed to support the application of GSC to the population of cannabis-dependent adults. Finally, we report outcome data from a trial of GSC treatment that included a small sample of marijuana users.

## GSC Treatment

### *Background and Development of the Approach*

Before describing the GSC treatment approach and findings, it will be helpful for readers to understand the rationale for the GSC treatment and why it was viewed as a potentially effective approach for treating cannabis problems. GSC treatment was developed in the early 1980s as a brief treatment for persons with low severity alcohol problems (M. B. Sobell & L. C. Sobell, 1993). Studies have found that persons who overcome their problems without the benefit of treatment or self-help groups generally have less serious problems than those in treatment (M. B. Sobell & L. C. Sobell, 1993; L. C. Sobell *et al.*, 1992, 2000). It has also been suggested that natural recoveries are the most common pathway to recovery from alcohol (L. C. Sobell *et al.*, 1996a) and other drug problems (Cunningham, 1999; Klingemann *et al.*, 2001). The fact that many people resolve substance use problems without formal help or treatment suggests that in many cases the key issues in recovery are motivational rather than a skills deficit. Natural recovery research, therefore, has been one line of work suggesting that interventions focusing on enhancing motivation for change might be particularly appropriate for individuals with low-level substance use problems.

Another important influence on the development of the GSC treatment was the purported efficacy of brief treatments for alcohol problems, especially less severe problems. Seminal to the development of such treatments was the well-known clinical trial of treatment versus advice by Edwards *et al.* (1977) in England. That study found that the treatment outcomes of male alcohol abusers who were randomly assigned to a standard treatment program (individualized care that could have included inpatient and outpatient treatment and Antabuse®)

were no different than for those who had been randomly assigned to a single session of advice/counseling. A corollary finding was that participants whose problems were less severe did better during their second year of follow-up if they had been treated by the single session of advice/counseling, while participants whose problems were more severe did better if they had received the standard treatment (Orford *et al.*, 1976). The efficacy of a single session of advice and counseling squarely put the spotlight on motivation as the facilitator of change. A reasonable explanation of the findings was that the single advice/counseling session had enhanced participants' commitment to change and their confidence that they could change with minimal help. Therefore, this second line of research also suggested that problem drinkers, individuals with less severe alcohol problems, would do well in a brief motivational intervention.

Adding further strength to the utility of motivational interventions was work by Prochaska and colleagues on stages of change (DiClemente & Prochaska, 1982; Prochaska *et al.*, 1992), and Miller's formulation of motivational interviewing as a focus of treatment (Miller, 1983, 1985). This research suggested that a valuable focus of treatment could be on increasing an individual's motivation to change, especially for individuals who were ambivalent about changing. This would include those with lower severity alcohol and drug problems, because in most cases their substance use would not yet have yielded major adverse consequences.

Finally, the development of GSC treatment was greatly influenced by research on alcohol treatment goals, and the formulation by Bandura (1986) of a social learning theory that hypothesized that allowing goal choice could be important for increasing an individual's commitment to a goal. As discussed elsewhere (M. B. Sobell & L. C. Sobell, 1995), findings related to alcohol treatment goals and outcomes can be summarized as: (a) severely dependent alcohol abusers recover predominantly through abstinence; (b) alcohol abusers not severely dependent on alcohol recover predominantly through moderation; and (c) outcome type and dependence severity appear to be independent of treatment advice. Thus, not only is severity of dependence (rather than treatment goal advice) the best predictor of whether one will achieve an abstinence or moderation recovery, but goal advice seems to have little relevance. If goal assignment makes no difference and allowing choice increases commitment to change, an important component of a brief motivational treatment would be to allow clients to select their own goals.

## *Major Principles and Techniques of GSC*

These influences formed the basis for the development of the GSC treatment, a brief motivational intervention tailored to increase and maintain commitment to change and to help empower clients to use their own resources to change. Based on the literature, the treatment included a strong emphasis on choice and on the provision of personalized feedback and advice so that clients had a basis for making informed decisions about their future. The approach encourages clients to take an active role in the change process.

Several types of cognitive-behavioral and motivational interventions and strategies are used in the GSC treatment approach. The major elements include the following: (a) Clients are introduced to the GSC treatment and encouraged to assume an active role in their own change process (M. B. Sobell & L. C. Sobell, 1993). (b) To increase clients' commitment to change, advice/feedback materials based on their assessment are used (for examples of such materials see Substance Abuse and Mental Health Services Administration, 1999). (c) Therapists provide feedback of assessment findings to clients (i.e., extent of use, problem severity) to help identify problem areas and bolster motivation for change. (d) A decisional balance homework exercise was given to clients to help them cognitively appraise the pros and cons of continuing to abuse drugs or alcohol and the pros and cons of not abusing (Sobell *et al.*, 1996b; Substance Abuse and Mental Health Services Administration, 1998). (e) Treatment goal advice (abstinence versus moderation) is typically given but clients select their own goal (M. B. Sobell & L. C. Sobell, 1987, 1993). (f) Clients were asked to keep self-monitoring logs throughout treatment to evaluate the extent and pattern of their substance use and urges. The use of such self-feedback is consistent with a motivational approach (Substance Abuse and Mental Health Services Administration, 1998). (g) Clients were provided with short readings and homework assignments to guide them through a functional analysis of individual high-risk situations/triggers related to drug use. The intent was then to develop a general problem-solving strategy that could be used during treatment and in the future to deal with high-risk situations (M. B. Sobell & L. C. Sobell, 1993; M. B. Sobell *et al.*, 1976). (h) To provide a realistic perspective on recovery, a cognitive perspective on relapse prevention is built into the readings and discussed in treatment (i.e., intervening early if a relapse occurred, viewing a slip as a learning experience that identified unrecognized high-risk situations or inadequate methods of coping, and attributing the slip to situational factors rather than personal failings). (i) To monitor clients' post-treatment substance use and functioning, telephone aftercare calls are scheduled to be completed by therapists 1 and 3 months after clients have completed treatment. Aftercare contacts also provide an opportunity for therapists to help clients with other concerns and to schedule additional appointments, if necessary (Breslin *et al.*, 1996).

As should be evident, the GSC approach incorporates several motivational and cognitive-behavioral strategies in a single brief treatment. It is relatively unique in explicitly allowing clients to choose their outcome goal (M. B. Sobell & L. C. Sobell, 1987, 1993, 1995) and in routinely using self-monitoring logs (Korotitsch & Nelson-Gray, 1999; L. C. Sobell & M. B. Sobell, 1973; M. B. Sobell & L. C. Sobell, 1990; Sobell *et al.*, 1989) for data collection and for comparative feedback in terms of changes in drug use (i.e., changes from pre-treatment to end of treatment). It has been evaluated in group and individual formats and been found to be effective in both modalities (M. B. Sobell & L. C. Sobell, 1998; Walters *et al.*, 2002). GSC treatment utilizes a flexible approach to the number of sessions offered. After an assessment and four semi-structured sessions, clients are given an opportunity to request additional sessions (M. B. Sobell & L. C. Sobell, 1993, 1998, 2005). Telephone contact is often included 1 month after the last session to evaluate clients sooner after treatment and allows for reinitiation of treatment services if needed.

## Applying GSC Treatment to Cannabis Users

Evidence for the applicability of GSC treatment to cannabis users comes from a recent study of natural recovery in cannabis users, controlled studies of brief treatments with this population, and the characteristics of clients seeking treatment for cannabis problems.

### Cannabis-Specific Natural Recovery Studies

In contrast to other illicit drugs, studies of naturally recovered cannabis abusers are rare (reviewed in Klingemann *et al.*, 2001; L. C. Sobell *et al.*, 2000). In a review of studies of naturally recovered substance abusers (L. C. Sobell *et al.*, 2000) only 1 of 40 studies included individuals who had recovered from cannabis problems, and this study involved only one or two respondents (Copeland, 1997). Recently, we recruited cannabis abusers who had stopped using without treatment (Ellingstad, 2001; Ellingstad *et al.* 2001) in order to examine the factors that contributed to successful recovery. In that study, 25 cannabis users who recovered without treatment from South Florida ($n = 12$) and San Diego, California ($n = 13$) were recruited through advertisements in local newspapers. The advertisements read as follows: HAVE YOU SUCCESS-FULLY STOPPED USING MARIJUANA WITHOUT TREATMENT?

All participants had to meet the following criteria: (a) daily cannabis use for $\geq 12$ consecutive months prior to their recovery date; (b) current abstinence from cannabis for $\geq 12$ months; (c) $\geq 18$ years of age; (d) never received formal substance abuse treatment for cannabis, defined as a specific intervention (i.e., professional or self-help) with the purpose of facilitating a reduction in cannabis use; (e) attended no more than two self-help group meetings (e.g., *Cannabis Anonymous, Narcotics Anonymous*) for cannabis; (f) no known history of head injury with loss of consciousness or other significant neurological condition; and (g) ability to understand and write English. The decision to allow no more than two self-help meetings was based on previous studies (Klingemann, 1991; L. C. Sobell *et al.*, 1992; 1993; Solomon, 1993; Tucker *et al.*, 1994) that allowed for brief exposure to self-help groups as long as the substance use recoveries did not coincide with self-help group attendance, and respondents did not attribute their recoveries to the influence of the self-help group.

On average, at the time of their recovery, participants were 29.6-year old, 84% were white, 64% were male, 16% were married, and all had completed high school or its equivalent (mean years of education = 15.4). At the time of their recovery, 60.0% were employed, and of those in the workforce, 36% held blue-collar jobs. In terms of their cannabis use, the average age at marijuana use initiation was 16, and they had used for an average of 13.7 years before quitting. On average respondents had been abstinent for 6.1 years. The majority (76.0%) reported $\leq 1$ quit attempt before successfully quitting. In terms of lifetime use, respondents reported using cannabis for an average of 5.0 days per week and averaged 2.7 joints per day when they used. Very few respondents reported past cannabis-related arrests (mean = 0.7) and only one respondent had ever been hospitalized for cannabis use.

In terms of a DSM-IV-TR diagnosis (American Psychiatric Association, 2000) respondents endorsed significantly more criteria for a lifetime cannabis-dependence diagnosis [$M$ (SD) = 3.7 (1.8)] than for the year before their recovery [$M$ (SD) = 2.9 (2.0), $t$ (24 = 3.6, $p$ < 0.01)]. Likewise, 72.0% met DSM-IV-TR criteria for a lifetime cannabis dependence diagnosis compared to 56.0% for the year before their recovery. Respondents' mean (SD) score on the 10-item Drug Abuse Screening Test (Skinner, 1982) for the year before their recovery [$M$ (SD) = 4.5 (2.2)] was significantly lower [$t$ (24 = 3.57, $p$ < 0.01)] than their mean lifetime score [$M$ (SD) = 5.4 (2.2)]. These findings suggest that cannabis users who recover on their own have started to reduce their use in the year prior to recovery as the severity of their problem appears less compared to similar measures of lifetime use.

The most frequent reason for quitting was reported as a change in the way cannabis was viewed, with 76% reporting that they saw cannabis and its effects as less positive. Two-thirds (64.0%) reported that cannabis use had a negative personal effect (i.e., respondents viewed themselves as less positive), and 52% reported social pressure to quit. Health concerns were reported by less than half (44.0%) the sample. The most frequently reported factors that helped respondents maintain their resolutions were the development of or return to interests or activities not related to cannabis (72.0%), avoidance of trigger people or situations to use (72.0%), and changes in lifestyle (e.g., diet, exercise; 72.0%). More than half of the sample reported support from a spouse/significant other/family member (60.0%) and a change in or support from a social group (56.0%) as helpful.

Most respondents (80.0%) reported that a factor that acted as a barrier to treatment seeking was the belief that their cannabis use was not a problem or at least not enough of a problem to warrant treatment. The majority (76.0%) also reported that they wanted to quit on their own. Slightly less than half of the sample listed stigma or negative labels associated with treatment (48.0%) as a barrier. Both "barriers" and "wanting to quit on their own" have been reported by many naturally recovered alcohol and drug abusers as major reasons for avoiding treatment (Klingemann *et al.*, 2001; L. C. Sobell *et al.*, 1993). These findings suggest that a brief motivational intervention where the client sets the goals and actively participates in the change process may be particularly appealing to the population of adult cannabis users.

### Efficacy of Brief Treatments for Cannabis Users

Controlled treatment outcome studies have shown that adult, chronic marijuana smokers can be successfully recruited into treatment programs and that their recovery rates parallel those of other drug treatment studies (e.g., Stephens *et al.*, 1994a, 2000). At least two of these studies suggest that brief interventions may be particularly appropriate with cannabis users. Stephens and his colleagues (Stephens *et al.*, 2000) compared the efficacy of (a) a two-session motivational interviewing individual treatment, (b) a 14-session cognitive-behavioral group treatment, and (c) a delayed treatment control. The two active interventions (cognitive-behavioral group treatment and motivational interviewing individual treatment) performed significantly better than the delayed treatment control. Furthermore, there were very few outcome differences between the group and brief motivational treatments over the 16 months of follow-ups suggesting that a brief treatment is as effective as a longer treatment for cannabis abusers.

Lang *et al.* (2000) found that regular cannabis users following a single session of "accelerated empathic therapy" that included feedback, self-monitoring, and a cognitive-behaviorally oriented self-help booklet reported reductions in use at 1- and 3-month post-treatment. Although there was no control group, this study also suggests that a brief intervention may be sufficient to reduce cannabis use for many problem users. Thus, brief treatments may be effective for cannabis use disorders.

*Help Seeking Among an Outpatient Sample of Cannabis Users*

Much of what is known about treated cannabis users derives from research studies. In preparing to extend the GSC treatment to cannabis users, we decided to review the clinical files of clients who had voluntarily sought treatment for a primary cannabis problem at the Addiction Research Foundation (ARF) in Toronto, Ontario, Canada from April 1993 through March 1994. At that time, the ARF was the largest provider of outpatient substance abuse services in Toronto. Over a 12-month time period, 151 clients were identified as having a primary cannabis problem. The vast majority (87%) were male, and nearly half (47.1%) were married or living in a common-law relationship. Their mean (SD) age was 31.5 (5.8) years, 60% were employed, and 18% had a family income of $60,000 Canadian dollars or more.

These 151 clients reported using cannabis for a mean (SD) of 14.3 (5.8) years and they considered their use have been a problem for a mean (SD) of 9.8 (7.0) years. Almost three-quarters (71%) reported no prior drug treatment. They also reported having spent a mean (SD) of 9.0 (17.5) months thinking about entering treatment before doing so, had made a mean (SD) of 5.6 (19.9) prior attempts to quit using cannabis (range = 0–100), and 95% reported that cannabis was their only drug of concern. Clients were also asked to describe their major reason(s) for seeking treatment. The reason most commonly reported by clients was considering the pros and cons of changing which in turn led to a decision to seek treatment (87%). This reason was reported twice as frequently compared to all other reasons. Other frequently reported reasons for seeking treatment included being warned by a spouse (41%), changing one's lifestyle (38%), seeing someone else high (36%), hitting rock bottom (34%), and experiencing a traumatic event (30%). Reports of health concerns were infrequent (13%). In summary, these clients were largely male, young, had a long history of cannabis use, were not polydrug abusers, and most reported that what led to their seeking treatment was weighing the pros and cons of using and not using cannabis (i.e., cognitive appraisal). Thus, a motivational intervention that would help clients examine the pros and cons of using appeared appropriate.

## A Controlled Treatment Trial Using GSC with Cannabis Users

In order to evaluate the efficacy of the GSC approach with cannabis users, we used data from a randomized controlled trial comparing an individual and group format of GSC treatment. Participants were either referred to the study from the central intake service at the ARF or had responded to newspaper advertisements. A joint ethics committee at the University of Toronto/ARF approved the study.

## Participants

Clients at the ARF were eligible to participate if they: (1) were ≥18 and ≤70 years of age; (2) voluntarily entered treatment (i.e., not mandated by courts or employers); (3) were not currently receiving psychotherapy elsewhere; (4) reported no current injection drug use; (5) were not currently using heroin; (6) provided the name of at least one collateral informant who could be contacted to corroborate their self-reports of post-treatment functioning; and (7) had a zero blood alcohol level at assessment. Participants were also screened to have adequate reading ability, a stable housing situation, and the absence of organic brain damage. In this chapter, we focus on the 17 participants who met these criteria and who had a primary cannabis problem. Following an initial assessment, participants were randomly assigned to receive GSC treatments either individually or in small groups.

## Assessment

All participants first participated in an individual assessment that took about 2 h to complete. Assessment data included demographic and substance abuse history data, identification, and classification of potential high-risk situations for drug use (Annis *et al.*, 1997; Sklar *et al.*, 1997), the Drug Abuse Screening Test (DAST-20: Skinner, 1982), and subjective evaluation of the severity of drug problems. Drug goal statements were given to clients on four occasions (assessment; fourth treatment session; 6- and 12-month follow-ups). These goal statements parallel those that have been used with alcohol abusers except that they asked about a client's primary drug problem (M. B. Sobell & L. C. Sobell, 1993, 1998, 2005).

The primary outcome measure assessing drug use at baseline and over the 1-year follow-up was the TimeLine FollowBack (TLFB: Smith *et al.*, 1983; L. C. Sobell & M. B. Sobell, 1995; L. C. Sobell *et al.*, 1996). The TLFB method, originally developed as a research tool for use with alcohol abusers, has been adapted for use in clinical settings as well as with drug abusers, including cannabis users (L. C. Sobell & M. B. Sobell, 1996, 2000; L. C. Sobell *et al.*, 1996). Using a calendar and other memory aids to enhance recall at each assessment, clients were asked to provide retrospective estimates of their daily cannabis use (e.g., number of joints or equivalent per day) and abstinent days (Budney *et al.*, 1999, 2001; Sobell *et al.*, 1997; Waldron *et al.*, 2001).

At the end of the assessment interview, each client was given an envelope and advised that it contained, the following materials: (a) description of the treatment program; (b) three readings and homework exercises; (c) self-monitoring logs including an explanation how to fill them out; and (d) instructions that the homework exercises and self-monitoring logs, needed to be completed prior to their assigned treatment session.

### *Treatment Description for Individual and Group Treatment Formats*

Both treatment conditions consisted of an assessment and four sessions. Typically, the sessions were scheduled to occur weekly for 4 weeks. At the end of the four treatment sessions, clients could request further sessions if they wished. Clients were told that from a feasibility standpoint it would not be possible to make up missed group sessions. Group participants could request additional group sessions if there were enough members to constitute a group. Individual treatment sessions were 60 min each and run by one therapist, while group sessions lasted 90 to 120 min and had two therapists. All groups were closed with anywhere from four to eight clients per group.

Regardless of their treatment condition assignment, clients were treated using largely the same GSC procedures described earlier in this chapter. However, the group condition promoted and used group processes in that therapists were facilitators of social interaction, encouraging group members to share their views and plans (e.g., discussing their homework assignments with the group) and to provide feedback to other group members. This approach was in contrast to what could be viewed as providing individual treatment in a group setting (i.e., a therapist works with a client while other group members observe). This latter style was avoided, as the strength of the group treatment procedure lies largely in the social influence process (Dies, 1994). Thus, the conditions differed in that for those in the group format many of the procedures (e.g., review of homework answers) were conducted in a round robin fashion, with feedback and advice largely coming from the group members rather than the therapists.

All drug abusers in the study were instructed that abstinence from drugs was the best way to avoid harmful drug consequences, but we recognized that many drug abusers are not abstinent from treatment entry, but rather reduce their use over time (Simpson *et al.*, 1999; Simpson & Curry, 1997). Further, some drug abusers have chosen to resolve their drug problems through a harm reduction approach (Denning, 1998; Desmond *et al.*, 1995; MacCoun, 1998; Marlatt *et al.*,

1997; Swift *et al.*, 2000). Cannabis abusers in the group treatment condition were in groups with clients who had primary alcohol as well as primary drug problems. All clients shared their goals with the group as a topic of group discussion. Thus, they received feedback from their peers concerning the viability of their goal choice, whereas in the individual treatment condition, clients discussed their goal choice with their therapist.

To achieve consistency across sessions and therapists, detailed clinical guidelines outlining session content and procedures were developed and used throughout the study (copies of the protocol are available from the senior author). Pilot sessions were conducted for several months prior to the actual study. Sessions were taped and a random portion was evaluated for adherence to the protocol. Therapists' professional degrees ranged from bachelor's, to master's, to doctoral degrees in psychology or related fields (e.g., social work, nursing, mental health).

Regardless of their group assignment clients were treated using the same GSC procedures. The conditions differed in that for those in the group format many of the procedures (e.g., review of homework answers) were conducted in a round robin fashion, with feedback and advice largely coming from the group members rather than the therapists.

To allow flexibility of the treatment program aftercare contacts were scheduled at 1 and 3 months after clients completed treatment. The therapist conducted aftercare contacts by telephone to monitor clients' post-treatment substance use and problem perception. Aftercare contacts also provided the opportunity for therapists to help clients with other concerns and to schedule additional appointments, if necessary (Breslin *et al.*, 1996).

## Within Treatment Data, Retention Rates, and Follow-up

Of the 17 cannabis users, only seven (41.7%) completed all four sessions. This figure is lower than for other drug (74.3%; 26/35) and alcohol (89.4%; 180/212) abusers in this study. Evaluations of all alcohol and drug clients' outcomes indicated no significant differences whether participants completed one or four sessions.

Participants were followed up 6 and 12 months after their last treatment session. Follow-up measures were similar to those used at the assessment. As participants self-monitored their substance use during treatment, it was possible to compare their daily reports of cannabis use pre-treatment, during treatment, and post-treatment. Data for both the pre-treatment and post-treatment interval were for 12 months, while the data during treatment were limited to the number of days from the time of the assessment to the client's last treatment session (typically this was 5 weeks). Follow-up rates at 6 and 12 months were 88.2% (15/17) and 82.4% (14/17), respectively. These rates are comparable to other substance abuse studies (Brown *et al.*, 1993; Project MATCH Research Group, 1998; Wutzke *et al.*, 2000). The 12-month follow-up rate for cannabis abusers (82.4%) was slightly higher than that for other drug abusers in the study (71.4%), but slightly lower than that for alcohol abusers (89.6%).

### Cannabis Abuser Characteristics at Pre-treatment

As there were no pre-treatment or post-treatment differences in terms of drug and alcohol treatment outcomes between the group and individual treatment conditions, data will be presented for all cannabis participants combined for this chapter. The pre-treatment characteristics of the 17 participants with a cannabis problem are shown in Table 9.1. As can be seen, the cannabis abusers who participated in the controlled trial were very similar to those in the voluntary sample of ARF clients described earlier, except for a slightly higher employment rate and fewer past quit attempts. Most clients were young males (mean age = 30.4 years) who had some college education (mean = 13.8 years), and were employed (82.4%). They considered their cannabis use to be problem for nearly a decade (mean = 8.4 years), and reported using cannabis on average 82.2% of all days in the 3 months prior to the assessment. Most (82.4%) had never been in treatment for a drug problem. Lastly, all clients were asked to provide a subjective evaluation of their drug use problem at assessment. The fact that only one-half (50.1%) of the cannabis users evaluated their problem as major to very major suggests that many of them did not view their problem as very serious. Lastly, at the assessment, almost two-thirds of the cannabis abusers (64.7%; 11/17) chose a reduced cannabis use goal rather than abstinence.

### GSC Treatment Outcomes

Outcome data are presented for the 14 cannabis abusers followed-up for 12 months. These 14 clients significantly ($p < 0.001$) increased their mean (SD) percentage of abstinence days five-fold from 10.7% pre-treatment to 54.5% (33.6%) over the course of treatment. However, they also showed a decrease in abstinent days to a mean (SD) frequency of 39.6% (37.4%) of days over the follow-up year. Although this difference was not statistically significant ($p = 0.21$), the small size had limited power to detect a difference in rates (the pre-treatment to within treatment difference was very large), especially given the amount of variance in the data. Despite the fact that the percentage of days

Table 9.1. *Pre-treatment characteristics of 17 participants in the GSC treatment who had a primary cannabis problem*

| Variable | Mean (SD) or % |
| --- | --- |
| *Demographic* | |
| Male | 76.5% |
| Marital status (single) | 41.2% |
| Current occupation status (white collar) | 47.1%[a] |
| Current employment status (full or self) | 82.4% |
| Satisfied/very satisfied with current lifestyle | 47.1% |
| Education (years) | 13.8 (2.5) |
| Age (years) | 30.4 (5.1) |
| Employed current job (years) | 4.3 (3.2)[b] |
| *Drug use history* | |
| DAST-20 score[c] | 7.1 (3.9) |
| Years cannabis a drug problem | 8.4 (7.5) |
| Years used cannabis[a] | 14.4 (5.8) |
| Cannabis-related consequences past 6 months | 2.8 (1.8) |
| DSM-III-R (cannabis dependent) | 70.1% |
| Drug-related hospitalizations | 0.2 (0.8) |
| Drug-related arrests | 0.4 (1.2) |
| Days used cannabis past 90 days | 82.2 (19.0) |
| Prior quit attempts | 2.8 (3.2) |
| Reported daily cannabis use over past 90 days | 82.4% |
| Typical route of use (smoking/oral) | 100% |
| Longest consecutive abstinence period (months) | 2.3 (2.7) |
| No prior drug treatment | 82.4% |
| Cannabis use evaluation past year "major/very major" | 50.1%[a] |
| Reduced cannabis use goal at assessment[d] | 64.7% |

[a]$N = 16$. [b]$N = 15$. [c]Scores range from 0 to 20. [d]Other goal choice was abstinence ($N = 6$; 35.3%).

abstinent decreased from within treatment to 12-month post-treatment, the difference between percent days abstinent 12-month pre- and 12-month post-treatment was still significant ($p < 0.01$).

Figure 9.1 shows the mean percent days abstinent for 12-month pre-treatment, within treatment, and 12-month post-treatment for three groups of clients in this study: (a) cannabis abusers ($n = 14$); (b) cocaine abusers ($n = 22$); and (c) alcohol abusers ($n = 176$). An interesting outcome finding for the cannabis abusers was that while all groups demonstrated an increase in abstinent days from

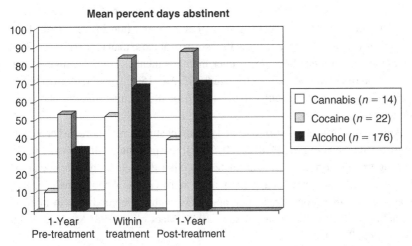

Figure 9.1 Mean percent days abstinent.

pre-treatment to the end of treatment, the cannabis abusers showed a decrease of abstinent days following treatment suggesting a tailing off of treatment effects.

**Conclusions and Recommendations**

In summary, although the number of cannabis abusers who participated in the GSC controlled trial of individual versus group treatment was small relative to alcohol abusers and even to other drug abusers (the primary other drug of abuse was cocaine), the study demonstrated that such individuals can be attracted to a brief motivational intervention. The fact that these results' parallel findings from three other recent studies with cannabis abusers (Copeland *et al.*, 2001; Lang *et al.*, 2000; Stephens *et al.*, 2000) suggests that a brief motivational intervention is a good first treatment of choice for cannabis abusers. In the context of a stepped care model of treatment, for individuals where the treatment is not effective, the treatment can be stepped up (Breslin *et al.*, 1999; M. B. Sobell & L. C. Sobell, 2000). Furthermore, we found that a group intervention compared to individual treatment can be delivered effectively for alcohol and drug abusers, including cannabis abusers, and with a significant cost reduction over individual treatment (M. B. Sobell & L. C. Sobell, 1998, 2005). In a day and age of health care cost containment, this is an important finding (Seelye, 1979; Steenberger & Budman, 1996).

The cannabis abusers in the GSC treatment were somewhat less likely to complete the treatment and more likely to see their problems as less severe at the outset than the other alcohol and drug abusers in the study. Cannabis users very substantially decreased their frequency of use while in treatment. This seems consistent with the fact that at the assessment close than two-thirds (64.7%; 11/17) chose a reduced use goal rather than abstinence. This is similar to the proportion of alcohol abusers in this study (75.2%; 156/210) who chose a moderation goal. In contrast, only 16.9% (5/30) of the cocaine abusers choose a reduced use goal.

Although several abstinence-oriented treatment studies have attracted cannabis abusers (Stephens *et al.*, 1994b, 2000, 2002), the percentage of cannabis users seeking treatment remains low in relation to other drugs (e.g., heroin, cocaine). The fact that the majority of cannabis abusers in the GSC trial chose a reduced use goal suggests that a harm reduction approach might be a good way to involve cannabis abusers in treatment (Kalant, 1999; MacCoun, 1998; Marlatt, 1998; Swift *et al.*, 2000).

In previous GSC clinical trials with alcohol abusers, positive effects produced during treatment were maintained over the course of a 1-year follow-up (Ayala *et al.*, 1998a, b; Breslin *et al.*, 1999; L. C. Sobell & M. B. Sobell, 1998; L. C. Sobell *et al.*, 1995, 2000; M. B. Sobell *et al.*, 1995, 2000). However, in this study this pattern was not found for the cannabis abusers. The decrease in the abstinent days over follow-up suggests an atrophy of treatment effects, a finding similar to the majority of drug treatment outcome studies. Despite the reduction in the frequency of abstinent days over follow-up, post-treatment abstinence was still nearly four times that of the year before treatment. Overall, the results of the GSC intervention for cannabis abusers were very positive with the suggestion that further treatment may be warranted to maintain the treatment gains (M. B. Sobell & L. C. Sobell, 2000).

Finally, taken as a whole, the evidence presented in this chapter suggests that a motivational enhancement approach may be a good match for cannabis abusers entering treatment. Although confrontational approaches have not been evaluated with cannabis abusers, the relatively low rates of such individuals considering their cannabis use to constitute a major problem suggests that they would react to confrontational approaches with resistance, similar to the reaction of problem drinkers (Miller *et al.*, 1993; Substance Abuse and Mental Health Services Administration, 1999).

### References

American Psychiatric Association (2000). *Diagnostic and statistical manual of mental disorders* (4th ed. revised). Washington, DC: American Psychiatric Association.

Annis, H. M., Sklar, S. M., & Turner, N. E. (1997). *Drug taking confidence questionnaire: user's guide*. Toronto, Ontario: Addiction Research Foundation.

Ayala, H. E., Echeverría, L., Sobell, M. B., & Sobell, L. C. (1998a). Una alternativa de intervencin breve y temprana parabebedores problema en México [An early and brief intervention alternative for problem drinkers in Mexico]. *Acta Comportamentalia, 6,* 71–93.

Ayala, H. E., Lopez, G. C., Echeverria, L., & Lara, M. (1998b). *Manual de autoayuda para personas con problemas en su forma de beber*. Mexico City, Mexico: National University of Mexico.

Bandura, A. (1986). *Social foundations of thought and action: a social cognitive theory*. Englewood Cliffs, NJ: Prentice-Hall.

Breslin, C., Sobell, L. C., Sobell, M. B., Buchan, G., & Kwan, E. (1996). Aftercare telephone contacts with problem drinkers can serve a clinical and research function. *Addiction, 91,* 1359–1364.

Breslin, F. C., Sobell, M. B., Sobell, L. C., Cunningham, J. A., Sdao-Jarvie, K., & Borsoi, D. (1999). Problem drinkers: evaluation of a stepped care approach. *Journal of Substance Abuse, 10,* 217–232.

Brown, T. G., Seraganian, P., & Tremblay, J. (1993). Alcohol and cocaine abusers 6 months after traditional treatment: do they fare as well as problem drinkers. *Journal of Substance Abuse Treatment, 10,* 545–552.

Budney, A. J., Novy, P. L., & Hughes, J. R. (1999). Marijuana withdrawal among adults seeking treatment for marijuana dependence. *Addiction, 94*(9), 1311–1322.

Budney, A. J., Hughes, J. R., Moore, B. A., & Novy, P. L. (2001). Marijuana abstinence effects in marijuana smokers maintained in their home environment. *Archives of General Psychiatry, 58*(10), 917–924.

Copeland, J. (1997). A qualitative study of barriers to formal treatment among women who self-managed change in addictive behaviours. *Journal of Substance Abuse Treatment, 14*(2), 183–190.

Copeland, J., Swift, W., & Rees, V. (2001). Clinical profile of participants in a brief intervention program for cannabis use disorder. *Journal of Substance Abuse Treatment, 20*(1), 45–52.

Cunningham, J. A. (1999). Untreated remissions from drug use: the predominant pathway. *Addictive Behaviors, 24*(2), 267–270.

Denning, P. (1998). Therapeutic interventions for individuals with substance use, HIV, and personality disorders: harm reduction as a unifying approach. *In Session: Psychotherapy in Practice, 4*(1), 37–52.

Desmond, D. P., Maddux, J. F., Johnson, T. H., & Confer, B. A. (1995). Obtaining follow-up interviews for treatment evaluation. *Journal of Substance Abuse Treatment, 12*(2), 95–102.

DiClemente, C. C., & Prochaska, J. O. (1982). Self-change and therapy change of smoking behavior: a comparison of processes of change in cessation and maintenance. *Addictive Behaviors, 7,* 133–142.

220                                                          *Linda C. Sobell* et al.

Dies, R. R. (1994). The therapist's role in group treatments. In H. S. Bernard, & K. R. MacKenzie (Eds.), *Basics of group psychotherapy* (pp. 60–99). New York: Guilford Press.

Edwards, G., Orford, J., Egert, S., Guthrie, S., Hawker, A., Hensman, C., *et al.* (1977). Alcoholism: a controlled trial of "treatment" and "advice." *Journal of Studies on Alcohol, 38*, 1004–1031.

Ellingstad, T. P. (2001). *Natural recovery from cannabis abuse.* Unpublished Dissertation, Nova Southeastern University, Ft. Lauderdale, FL.

Ellingstad, T. P., Venner, K., Sobell, L. C., Sobell, M. B., & Eickleberry-Goldsmith, L. (2001). Factors associated with cannabis self-resolution and barriers to treatment seeking. Poster presented at the *Association for the Advancement of Behavior Therapy*, Philadelphia, PA.

Ellingstad, T. P., Sobell, L. C., Sobell, M. B., & Planthara, P. (2002). Drug treatment outcome methodology (1993–1997): strengths, weaknesses, and a comparison to the alcohol field. *Addictive Behaviors, 27*, 319–330.

Kalant, H. (1999). Differentiating drugs by harm potential: the rational versus the feasible. *Substance Use and Misuse, 34*(1), 25–34.

Klingemann, H. (1991). Coping and maintenance strategies of spontaneous remitters from problem use of alcohol and heroin in Switzerland. Poster presented at the *17th Annual Alcohol Epidemiological Symposium*, Sigtuna, Sweden.

Klingemann, H. K., Sobell, L. C., Barker, J., Blomqvist, J., Cloud, W., Ellingstad, T. P., *et al.* (2001). *Promoting self-change from problem substance use: implications for policy, prevention and treatment.* Boston, MA: Kluwer Academic Publishers.

Korotitsch, W. J., & Nelson-Gray, R. O. (1999). An overview of self-monitoring research in assessment and treatment. *Psychological Assessment, 11*(4), 415–425.

Lang, E., Engelander, M., & Brooke, T. (2000). Report of an integrated brief intervention with self-defined problem cannabis users. *Journal of Substance Abuse Treatment, 19*(2), 111–116.

MacCoun, R. J. (1998). Toward a psychology of harm reduction. *American Psychologist, 53*(11), 1199–1208.

Marlatt, G. A. (Ed.) (1998). *Harm reduction: pragmatic strategies for managing high-risk behaviors.* New York: Guilford.

Marlatt, G. A., Tucker, J. A., Donovan, D. A., & Vuchinich, R. E. (1997). Help-seeking by substance abusers: the role of harm reduction and the role of behavioral-economic approaches to facilitate treatment entry and retention. In L. S. Onken, J. D. Blaine, & J. J. Boren (Eds.), *Beyond the therapeutic alliance: keeping the drug-dependent individual in treatment (Research Monograph No. 165)* (pp. 44–84). Rockville, MD: National Institute of Drug Abuse.

Miller, W. R. (1983). Motivational interviewing with problem drinkers. *Behavioural Psychotherapy, 11*, 147–172.

Miller, W. R. (1985). Motivation for treatment: a review with special emphasis on alcoholism. *Psychological Bulletin, 98*, 84–107.

Miller, W. R., Benefield, R. G., & Tonigan, J. S. (1993). Enhancing motivation for change in problem drinking: a controlled comparison of two therapist styles. *Journal of Consulting and Clinical Psychology, 61*, 455–461.

Orford, J., Oppenheimer, E., & Edwards, G. (1976). Abstinence or control: the outcome for excessive drinkers two years after consultation. *Behaviour Research and Therapy, 14*, 409–418.

Prochaska, J. O., DiClemente, C. C., & Norcross, J. C. (1992). In search of how people change. *American Psychologist, 47*, 1102–1114.

Project MATCH Research Group (1998). Matching alcoholism treatments to client heterogeneity: project MATCH three-year drinking outcomes. *Alcoholism: Clinical and Experimental Research, 22*, 1300–1311.

Seelye, E. E. (1979). Relationship of socioeconomic status, psychiatric diagnosis and sex to outcome of alcoholism treatment. *Journal of Studies on Alcohol, 40*, 57–62.

Simpson, D. D., Joe, G. W., Fletcher, B. W., Hubbard, R. L., & Anglin, M. D. (1999). A national evaluation of treatment outcomes for cocaine dependence. *Archives of General Psychiatry, 56*(6), 507–514.

Simpson, D. W., & Curry, S. J. (Eds.) (1997). Drug abuse treatment outcome study (DATOS) [special issue]. *Psychology of Addictive Behaviors, 11*(4).

Skinner, H. A. (1982). The Drug Abuse Screening Test. *Addictive Behaviors, 7*, 363–371.

Sklar, S. M., Annis, H. M., & Turner, N. E. (1997). Development and validation of the Drug-Taking Confidence Questionnaire: a measure of coping self-efficacy. *Addictive Behaviors, 22*(5), 655–670.

Smith, E. M., Cloninger, C. R., & Bradford, S. (1983). Predictors of mortality in alcoholic woman: a prospective follow-up study. *Alcoholism: Clinical and Experimental Research, 7*, 237–243.

Sobell, L. C., & Sobell, M. B. (1973). A self-feedback technique to monitor drinking behavior in alcoholics. *Behaviour Research and Therapy, 11*, 237–238.

Sobell, L. C., & Sobell, M. B. (1995). Alcohol consumption measures. In J. P. Allen, & M. Columbus (Eds.), *Assessing alcohol problems: a guide for clinicians and researchers* (pp. 55–73). Rockville, MD: National Institute on Alcohol Abuse and Alcoholism.

Sobell, L. C., & Sobell, M. B. (1996). *Alcohol TimeLine FollowBack (TLFB) users' manual*. Toronto, Canada: Addiction Research Foundation.

Sobell, L. C., & Sobell, M. B. (2000). Alcohol TimeLine FollowBack (TLFB). In American Psychiatric Association (Ed.), *Handbook of psychiatric measures* (pp. 477–479). Washington, DC: American Psychiatric Association.

Sobell, L. C., Sobell, M. B., & Toneatto, T. (1992). Recovery from alcohol problems without treatment. In N. Heather, W. R. Miller, & J. Greeley (Eds.), *Self-control and the addictive behaviours* (pp. 198–242). New York: Maxwell MacMillan.

Sobell, L. C., Sobell, M. B., Toneatto, T., & Leo, G. I. (1993). What triggers the resolution of alcohol problems without treatment? *Alcoholism: Clinical and Experimental Research, 17*, 217–224.

222                                                                Linda C. Sobell et al.

Sobell, L. C., Sobell, M. B., Brown, J., & Cleland, P. A. (1995). A randomized trial comparing group versus individual guided self-change treatment for alcohol and drug abusers. Poster presented at the 29th Annual Meeting of the Association for Advancement of Behavior Therapy, Washington, DC.

Sobell, L. C., Cunningham, J. A., & Sobell, M. B. (1996a). Recovery from alcohol problems with and without treatment: prevalence in two population surveys. American Journal of Public Health, 86(7), 966–972.

Sobell, L. C., Cunningham, J. A., Sobell, M. B., Agrawal, S., Gavin, D. R., Leo, G. I., et al. (1996b). Fostering self-change among problem drinkers: a proactive community intervention. Addictive Behaviors, 21(6), 817–833.

Sobell, L. C., Sobell, M. B., Buchan, G., Cleland, P. A., Fedoroff, I., & Leo, G. I. (1996). The reliability of the TimeLine FollowBack method applied to drug, cigarette, and cannabis use. Poster presented at the 30th Annual Meeting of the Association for Advancement of Behavior Therapy, New York, NY.

Sobell, L. C., Agrawal, S., & Sobell, M. B. (1997). Factors affecting agreement between alcohol abusers' and their collaterals' reports. Journal of Studies on Alcohol, 58(4), 405–413.

Sobell, L. C., Ellingstad, T. P., & Sobell, M. B. (2000). Natural recovery from alcohol and drug problems: methodological review of the research with suggestions for future directions. Addiction, 95(5), 749–764.

Sobell, L. C., Leo, G. I., Agrawal, S., Johnson-Young, L., Sobell, M. B., & Cunningham, J. (2000). Fostering self-change: one year outcome results from a large scale community intervention for alcohol abusers. Poster presented at the 34th Annual Meeting of the Association for Advancement of Behavior Therapy, New Orleans, LA.

Sobell, M. B., & Sobell, L. C. (Eds.) (1987). Conceptual issues regarding goals in the treatment of alcohol problems. New York: Haworth Press.

Sobell, M. B., & Sobell, L. C. (1990). Problem drinkers and self-control treatments: a closer look. Poster presented at the Fifth International Conference on Treatment of Addictive Behaviors, Sydney, Australia.

Sobell, M. B., & Sobell, L. C. (1993). Problem drinkers: guided self-change treatment. New York: Guilford Press.

Sobell, M. B., & Sobell, L. C. (1995). Moderation, public health and paternalism. Addiction, 90(9), 1175–1177.

Sobell, M. B., & Sobell, L. C. (1998). Guiding self-change. In W. R. Miller, & N. Heather (Eds.), Treating addictive behaviors (2nd ed., pp. 189–202). New York: Plenum.

Sobell, M. B., & Sobell, L. C. (2000). Stepped care as a heuristic approach to the treatment of alcohol problems. Journal of Consulting and Clinical Psychology, 68(4), 573–579.

Sobell, M. B., & Sobell, L. C. (2005). Guided self-change treatment for substance abusers. Journal of Cognitive Psychotherapy, 19, 199–210.

Sobell, M. B., Sobell, L. C., & Sheahan, D. B. (1976). Functional analysis of drinking problems as an aid in developing individual treatment strategies. Addictive Behaviors, 1, 127–132.

Sobell, M. B., Bogardis, J., Schuller, R., Leo, G. I., & Sobell, L. C. (1989). Is self-monitoring of alcohol consumption reactive? *Behavioral Assessment, 11*, 447–458.

Sobell, M. B., Wilkinson, D. A., & Sobell, L. C. (1990). Alcohol and drug problems. In A. S. Bellack, M. Hersen, & A. E. Kazdin (Eds.), *International handbook of behavior modification and therapy* (2nd ed., pp. 415–435). New York: Plenum.

Sobell, M. B., Sobell, L. C., & Gavin, D. R. (1995). Portraying alcohol treatment outcomes: different yardsticks of success. *Behavior Therapy, 26*(4), 643–669.

Sobell, M. B., Sobell, L. C., & Leo, G. I. (2000). Does enhanced social support improve outcomes for problem drinkers in guided self-change treatment? *Journal of Behavior Therapy and Experimental Psychiatry, 31*(1), 41–54.

Solomon, S. D. (Ed.) (1993). *Individual versus group therapy: evaluation of drug treatment programs.* New York: Haworth Press.

Steenberger, B. T., & Budman, S. H. (1996). Group psychotherapy and managed behavioral health care: current trends and future challenges. *International Journal of Group Psychotherapy, 46*, 297–309.

Stephens, R. S., Curtin, L., Simpson, E. E., & Roffman, R. A. (1994a). Testing the abstinence violation effect construct with marijuana cessation. *Addictive Behaviors, 19*, 23–32.

Stephens, R. S., Roffman, R. A., & Simpson, E. E. (1994b). Treating adult marijuana dependence: a test of the relapse prevention model. *Journal of Consulting and Clinical Psychology, 62*, 92–99.

Stephens, R. S., Roffman, R. A., & Curtin, L. (2000). Comparison of extended versus brief treatments for marijuana use. *Journal of Consulting and Clinical Psychology, 68*(5), 898–908.

Stephens, R. S., Babor, T. F., Kadden, R., Miller, M., & The Marijuana Treatment Project Research Group (2002). The Marijuana Treatment Project: rationale, design, and participant characteristics. *Addiction, 97*, 109–124.

Substance Abuse and Mental Health Services Administration, Office of Applied Studies (1997). *National household survey on drug abuse: population estimates 1996.* Rockville, MD: US Department of Health and Human Services.

Substance Abuse and Mental Health Services Administration, Office of Applied Sciences (1998). *National household survey on drug abuse: main findings 1996.* Rockville, MD: US Department of Health and Human Services.

Substance Abuse and Mental Health Services Administration, Office of Applied Studies (1999). *Enhancing motivation for change in substance abuse treatment (Treatment improvement protocol series).* Rockville, MD: US Department of Health and Human Services.

Substance Abuse and Mental Health Services Administration, Office of Applied Studies (2000a). *National household survey on drug abuse: main findings 1998.* Rockville, MD: US Department of Health and Human Services.

Substance Abuse and Mental Health Services Administration, Offices of Applied Studies (2000b). *Summary of findings from the 2000 national household survey on drug abuse.* Rockville, MD: US Department of Health and Human Services.

Swift, W., Copeland, J., & Lenton, S. (2000). Cannabis and harm reduction. *Drug and Alcohol Review, 19*(1), 101–112.

Tucker, J. A., Vuchinich, R. E., & Gladsjo, J. A. (1994). Environmental events surrounding natural recovery from alcohol-related problems. *Journal of Studies on Alcohol, 55*, 401–411.

Waldron, H. B., Slesnick, N., Brody, J. L., Turner, C. W., & Peterson, T. R. (2001). Treatment outcomes for adolescent substance abuse at 4-month and 7-month assessments. *Journal of Consulting and Clinical Psychology, 69*, 802–813.

Walters, S. T., Ogle, R. O., & Martin, J. E. (2002). Perils and possibilities of group-based motivational interviewing. In W. R. Miller, & S. Rollnick (Eds.), *Motivational interviewing: preparing people to change* (2nd ed., pp. 377–390). New York: Guilford.

Wiesbeck, G. A., Schuckit, M. A., Kalmijn, J. A., Tipp, J. E., Bucholz, K. K., & Smith, T. L. (1996). An evaluation of the history of a marijuana withdrawal syndrome in a large population. *Addiction, 91*(10), 1469–1478.

Wutzke, S. E., Conigrave, K. M., Kogler, B. E., Saunders, J. B., & Hall, W. D. (2000). Longitudinal research: methods for maximizing subject follow-up. *Drug and Alcohol Review, 19*(2), 159–163.

Zimmer, L., & Morgan, J. P. (1995). Exposing marijuana myths: a review of the scientific evidence. New York: Open Society Institute.

# 10

# Supportive–Expressive Psychotherapy for Cannabis Dependence

BRIN F. S. GRENYER AND NADIA SOLOWIJ

Supportive–expressive (SE) dynamic psychotherapy forms one variation of a number of psychotherapies that emphasize the importance of effective interpersonal relationships for psychological health (Grenyer, 2002a). The overall goal of SE psychotherapy is to help the client achieve mastery over their difficulties, gain self-understanding, and practice self-control over habitual drug use and related problems. From this framework, cannabis dependence is understood within the context of the client's interpersonal relationships, work, and social problems. The theory behind the SE approach emphasizes the formative influence of life experiences on the development of personality and on the genesis of problems, including habitual cannabis use. Change is brought about through mastering (understanding and controlling) relationship conflicts and problems with a focus on the role of drug use within these interpersonal patterns. The therapist establishes a firm, consistent, and predictable therapeutic framework to strengthen the helping alliance between client and therapist. The therapist maintains this framework by focusing on the client's goals and fostering an understanding of relationship conflicts as they interact with conditions for drug abuse.

There is evidence that supports the SE approach to understanding and treating cannabis dependence. Cannabis dependence may adversely affect interpersonal relationships (Solowij & Grenyer, 2002a). Heavy use during adolescence may produce a developmental lag, entrenching adolescent styles of thinking and coping which can impair one's ability to form adult interpersonal relationships (Baumrind & Moselle, 1985; Kandel & Logan, 1984; Kandel et al., 1986). A high rate of relationship failure is predicted by a strong correlation between drug use, precocious sexual activity, and early marriage. Studies have shown that a high degree of involvement with cannabis predicts a reduced probability of marriage or an increased probability of early marriage, an increased rate of cohabiting, an increased risk of divorce or terminated de facto relationships, and a higher rate of unplanned parenthood and pregnancy termination

(Fergusson & Horwood, 1997; Newcombe & Bentler, 1988). It has been suggested that heavy cannabis users "tend to bypass or circumvent the typical maturational sequence of school, work and marriage, and become engaged in adult roles of jobs and family prematurely without the necessary growth and development to enhance success with these roles ... [developing] a pseudomaturity that ill prepares them for the real difficulties of adult life" (Newcombe & Bentler, 1988, pp. 35–36). In addition, habitual users are more likely to have a social network in which friends and partners are also cannabis users. Many chronic cannabis users appear socially and occupationally functional on the surface. Upon cessation, however, reports of increased anxiety in social situations, interpersonal problems, and difficulty in controlling anger suggest that cannabis may have been used in a self-medicating or adaptive manner (Haas & Hendin, 1987; Hall & Solowij, 1997). This suggests the need for a treatment approach that not only focuses on modifying drug use, but also on the interpersonal sequelae in relation to psychosocial development (Solowij & Grenyer, 2002b).

A study of 150 adult heavy cannabis users (Hendin *et al.*, 1987) found that approximately two-thirds of the sample was in a steady relationship, but only half of these were described as satisfactory. Difficulties in relationships with parents were also apparent. Cannabis users' most frequently reported psychological problems concerned feelings of insecurity, low self-image, extreme introversion, depression, and relationship problems. The latter were described variously as serious dissatisfaction with their current relationships, fears of intimacy and commitment, and a lack of meaningful relationships. Less than 5% saw drugs as the primary cause of their problems. The elevated levels of depression and anxiety among cannabis users may increase during the course of withdrawal from cannabis (Kouri & Pope, 2000). The focus of SE psychotherapy on the whole person's personal and interpersonal functioning, including the role of drug use, makes this approach particularly suitable for the cannabis user.

## Empirical Bases

SE dynamic therapy originated in Freud's papers on technique (e.g., Freud, 1914/1958), and was developed in the late 1940s and 1950s at the Menninger Foundation and Clinic, Menninger School of Psychiatry, Topeka, Kansas. The treatment is systematically documented in a manual (Luborsky, 1984) that includes methods for evaluating adherence to the technique. A number of specialized versions of the main SE manual are tailored towards specific drug dependence disorders (Barber & Crits-Christoph, 1995) including the following: opiate dependence (Luborsky *et al.*, 1995); cocaine dependence (Mark & Faude, 1995);

and cannabis dependence (Grenyer *et al.*, 1995). In addition to the manuals, a number of therapist training resources are also available, including a monograph on the clinical application of SE psychotherapy (Book, 1998).

This approach has been repeatedly and successfully evaluated over the past 30 years (Crits-Christoph & Connolly, 1998). For example, the Penn Psychotherapy Project (Luborsky *et al.*, 1988) evaluated the treatment on 73 mixed-diagnosis clients, and found a mean effect size of 1.05. It has been incorporated in the treatment of chronic and major depression with mean effect sizes of 1.80 and 2.75, respectively, on the Global Assessment Scale (Diguer *et al.*, 1993). It was a key component of the VA-Penn psychotherapy study of treatment for opioid dependence (Woody *et al.*, 1983, 1987), one of the largest and most successfully conducted studies of its type. In this study, SE psychotherapy plus drug counseling (DC) was compared to cognitive-behavioral therapy (CBT) plus DC, and DC alone. At 1 and 12 months, SE and CBT were essentially equivalent in effectiveness, and both were significantly superior to DC alone. A later validation study found SE to be more effective than DC for opiate-dependent clients receiving methadone in the community (Woody *et al.*, 1995). SE has also been compared to CBT in a large-scale collaborative study of cocaine abuse treatment (Crits-Christoph *et al.*, 1999). Again, there was no difference in effectiveness between SE and CBT, although neither treatment was as effective for this population as DC. To date, the literature suggests that SE dynamic psychotherapy is effective for treating some drug problems, and at least equivalent in efficacy to CBT. Its emphasis on interpersonal functioning suggests that it would be useful for treating cannabis dependence.

**SE Psychotherapy Techniques**

The term "supportive–expressive" refers to the two main treatment techniques of this approach. The therapist develops supportive techniques to create a positive, helpful, and empathic relationship with the client. The therapist uses expressive techniques to help the client express and understand problems, and ultimately effect changes. Sessions focus on identifying and interpreting the client's recurring problematic interpersonal relationship themes as they occur (a) with the therapist (transference), (b) in relationships with other people (e.g., partners, family, friends, and parents), and (c) around specific behaviors (e.g., drug taking), in order to find solutions to life problems. The Core Conflictual Relationship Theme (CCRT) method is used to help identify the recurring relationship patterns. The CCRT method (Book, 1998; Luborsky & Crits-Christoph, 1998) summarizes the client's core relationship problems, and guides the expressive component of

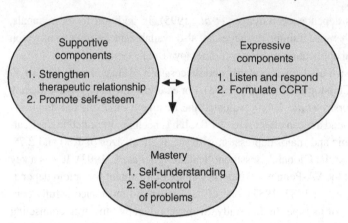

Figure 10.1  Components of SE treatment and outcome in terms of augmented mastery.

treatment. Helping the client understand the relationship between CCRT patterns and their drug use is a central technique of this method, and this promotes mastery (self-understanding and self-control) over their problems (Grenyer, 2002a). Figure 10.1 overviews the basic components of treatment – the supportive and expressive components, and the outcome in terms of mastery.

## Supportive Techniques

The supportive techniques create a strong working relationship between client and therapist upon which the success of the treatment rests. Support refers to the establishment of a working relationship that is focused on helping the client strengthen competence, bolster esteem, achieve goals, and solidify their grip on reality. Support requires sensitivity, patience, and a genuine wish to help. The helping alliance reflects the degree to which the client experiences the relationship with the therapist as helpful in achieving therapeutic goals. The client's feelings of optimism and confidence that therapy and the therapist are being helpful constitute part of the therapeutic alliance. There is now a considerable body of research indicating that the quality of the helping alliance predicts therapy outcome (Martin *et al.*, 2000). Research suggests that, in particular, therapist respect, accurate empathy, warmth, and genuineness are necessary ingredients in forming a helping alliance (Beutler *et al.*, 1994). In short, the therapist must convey hope and optimism for their work, and show respect and an affinity for the client. Luborsky (1984) suggests that a "we" bond is fostered, and that it is helpful to refer to the experiences that the client and therapist have shared to underscore the theme of therapy as a shared collaboration.

## Expressive Techniques

In contrast to the supportive techniques, expressive techniques are focused on understanding the client and helping them change. The four phases of the expressive task are outlined by Luborsky (1984) as (a) listening, (b) understanding, (c) responding, and (d) listening again. Listening can be seen as having three phases: (a) open inquiring listening, (b) listening to form hypotheses, and (c) listening to check the accuracy of formed hypotheses (Schlesinger, 1994). Listening allows the therapist to better understand the client, and in turn, governs how the therapist responds to the client. Via responding, the therapist communicates to the client information that has been understood through listening (e.g., "it sounds like your problems with your Dad really made you mad and it seems like smoking dope was a way of switching off from all that").

## Identifying CCRTs

Formulating the main problematic relationship theme and its connection to cannabis use should be accomplished relatively early in therapy, as this forms a focal point for the remaining sessions. Also, it is particularly important to maintain a therapeutic focus in short-term therapy, and this focus should be centered around the CCRT. Research has shown that treatment outcomes improve when appropriate CCRT-focused interpretations are used judiciously in therapy sessions (Crits-Christoph & Luborsky, 1998; Crits-Christoph *et al.*, 1988). The CCRT technique (Luborsky, 1977; Luborsky & Crits-Christoph, 1998) involves the analysis of narratives told by the client which detail relationship interactions with close relatives or friends, the therapist, or the self. Within the narratives, one can find the "transference template"; that is, the client's regular characteristic conflictual personality style. The CCRT has three components: (a) the wish, (b) the response of other, and (c) the response of self. "The wish" refers to the person's needs and desires (e.g., to obtain love and nurturing). "The response of other" refers to others' reactions to the client (e.g., hostility or aggression). "The response of self" refers to how the client responds to others (e.g., withdrawing and becoming intoxicated with cannabis). The three elements of the CCRT influence the dynamics of therapeutic interactions, and illustrate the basic means by which clients attempt to satisfy their needs. They narrate the expression of a wish, how this was received and responded to by another person, and how the response of this other person, in turn, affected them. Research corroborates the frequently observed phenomenon that clients often repeat similar relationship patterns (CCRTs) with different people in their life, including the therapist.

Helping the client realize these patterns is the first step in teaching the client to take charge of their interpersonal interactions, and ultimately, to institute adaptive goal fulfillment strategies in place of the initial, less effective techniques. This process inspires clients to work towards achieving their goals and fulfilling needs in more effective and adaptive ways.

A therapist can deduce clients' central problems by observing repetitions of similar themes in different contexts, charting the relationship between one set of conditions and a corresponding set of predictable reactions, and constructing an exemplar of these sequences over multiple sessions. For example, a client may feel enraged and complain that one of his friends always takes advantage of him by smoking more than his share of the cannabis. At another time, the client may discuss how he is expected to visit his grandparents much more than his brothers and sisters. Later, he may talk about how the psychotherapy sessions are never long enough, and he feels like he is not getting the help that he deserves. These examples manifest the same CCRT pattern, which the therapist could illuminate by saying, "it seems like at many different times you have wished to be treated fairly, but you feel others have not done so, and you feel enraged and cheated by these things which has lead you to continue smoking." Helping the client see these patterns' roles in their life is a substantial step towards engendering adaptive responses (i.e., responses that do not incorporate drug use) to similar situations. The basic principles of the scientific method – observing causes and effects – informs the structure of listening and the ways to respond after listening. Responses by SE psychotherapists typically concern an aspect of the CCRT pattern, and when possible, relate this element to the emergence of a chief symptom (e.g., drug use, feelings of anger, states of helplessness). Within psychotherapy sessions, the therapist continually relates drug-using themes to the interpersonal context. The therapist educates the client about how difficulties in fulfilling their needs and wishes can reinforce drug use. Early in therapy, the therapist explains to the client that this treatment will emphasize not only ceasing cannabis use, but also helping the client more effectively handle interpersonal and personal triggers. The sessions, therefore, focus on the clients' current and past relationships, their CCRT patterns, and the role drug use plays in helping and hindering their goal attainment.

### *Dealing with Cognitive Deficits from Long-Term Use*

Cannabis use does not result in any severe cognitive deficits, but long-term or heavy use may produce subtle impairments in higher cognitive functions such as memory, attention, and the organization and integration of complex information

(Solowij, 1998; Solowij *et al.*, 2002). While subtle, these impairments can affect day-to-day functioning. The longer and more frequently that cannabis has been used, the more pronounced are the cognitive impairments. Some long-term heavy users may complain of memory- or concentration-related problems. Others may not be aware of any cognitive impairment. The therapist should be aware that these subtle cognitive impairments, particularly attentional dysfunction, are not always accessible to the user's conscious awareness. Difficulty in maintaining focus and high levels of distractibility may affect the therapeutic process and developments that should occur between sessions. Impaired memory function may result in forgetting information that was covered in previous sessions. Presenting information in a clear fashion and repeating material across sessions may obviate some of the difficulties clients can run into when trying to integrate the therapeutic process while they are still using (Lundqvist, 1995). It is recommended that more in depth expressive techniques proceed only after the user has quit or reduced considerably for a few weeks.

### *Typical Sequencing of Treatment Components*

Treatment can be either time limited (with a set termination date) or unlimited. The typical recommendation is for 4–6 months (16–24 sessions) of treatment. Brief treatments may also be suitable, depending on the severity of the client's problems and the availability of interpersonal support aside from drug-using companions. Following an assessment in which the clients' drug use and other psychosocial strengths and problems are reviewed, a plan for treatment should be presented. This plan should focus on client-identified goals, and be structured around assessable milestones. Before commencing therapy, it is helpful to conduct a "socialization interview," which introduces the client to the ins and outs of psychotherapy. The format for a socialization interview is given in Orne and Wender (1968).

The relationship between the client and therapist is a special one. Goals define and prescribe this relationship, and maintain its focus on the tasks of therapeutic change. A common goal is to alter or cease cannabis use, while other goals may include improving relationships or professional endeavors. Particularly in time-limited therapy, goals (if they are reasonably achievable) modulate the breadth of material that can be covered during the sessions. A client's goals should be elicited with a statement such as, "what are the three main goals that you want to achieve in these sessions?" The overall goal of SE therapy is to integrate these goals with skills of self-understanding and self-control, in order to help the client achieve mastery over their problems. For purposes of evaluation, it is helpful to have clients rate the severity of their target complaints at the beginning of treatment, so they can be re-evaluated and compared at the completion (Deane & Spicer, 1998).

It is important to pace therapy sessions so that they proceed smoothly and have a natural beginning, middle, and end. The first 10 min should be left empty for the client to express their immediate concerns and recollections with minimal therapist commentary. The next 30 min contain the therapeutic work: the expressive components and the joint search for understanding. The final 10 min should be spent disengaging from the intensity of the material, and should gradually progress towards more general work. A frequent error of inexperienced therapists is interpreting too soon and for too long. In these cases, the client is abruptly cut off when the 50 min are up, and there is no time for reflection or strengthening the therapeutic alliance. Another error of inexperienced therapists occurs when they operate in the supportive mode for the whole session, which can deter progress and exploration.

Based on our treatment-outcome experience, a sample 16-week treatment would proceed as follows. Following the assessment and socialization interview, the first session should involve eliciting goals and establishing therapeutic arrangements (e.g., discussing the time limit). Sessions 2–4 should focus on inaugurating and nurturing a strong therapeutic alliance in preparation for the client's upcoming task of reducing or ceasing cannabis use. It is recommended that the client have a trial abstinence from cannabis before setting a quit date. The 4th session of therapy is generally a good time period to coincide with the client's quit date. Also in the 4th session, the major features of the client's interpersonal functioning and the role of cannabis within their life are assessed to derive a preliminary CCRT formulation. Sessions 5–6 involve monitoring the client's withdrawal from cannabis, using mainly supportive techniques. Sessions 7–12 typically focus on the client's core problems and CCRT patterns, and use mainly expressive techniques. Sessions 13–16 continue the exploration of interpersonal issues, but introduce preparation for termination as an increasing priority. Reinforcing mastery and its preventive role in averting relapse becomes helpful in the final phase of treatment.

### Therapist Training

Any qualified mental health practitioners such as social workers, psychologists, or psychiatrists, can be trained to use this approach. In order to adequately deliver this psychotherapy, the trainee should meet the following three criteria. First, the trainee should have a general orientation to the dynamic psychotherapy approach, as based on psychoanalytic tradition (e.g., Gabbard, 1990). Second, the trainee should be conversant with the specific SE dynamic techniques (Barber & Crits-Christoph, 1995; Book, 1998; Grenyer *et al.*, 1995; Luborsky, 1984). Third, the trainee should receive individual clinical supervision of their casework by an experienced practitioner. In addition, if possible, audio recordings of the trainee's psychotherapy sessions should be checked for treatment fidelity using an adherence scale (Luborsky, 1984).

## Studies of SE Psychotherapy with Cannabis Users

As reviewed above, there are a number of treatment-outcome trials that have evaluated the utility of SE psychotherapy for drug dependence. With regards to cannabis, only one outcome trial to date has been conducted using this approach. A brief overview of this study is presented here. In addition, further work has been done on investigating additional processes in the application of SE therapy for cannabis dependence and this work is also reviewed below.

The aim of the outcome study was to compare a 16-session time-limited version of SE dynamic therapy for cannabis dependence with a brief self-help intervention (Grenyer *et al.*, 1996a), following a successful pilot study (Solowij *et al.*, 1995). Participants ($n = 100$, 79 males, mean age 32.7 years, SD 7.7, range 20–56) with a primary DSM-IV diagnosis of cannabis dependence were recruited through local media and treatment agencies. Participants were required to have used cannabis for at least 5 years, and to have used daily or nearly daily use within the past 30 days. Participants were excluded if they had other drug abuse or dependence. Following confirmation of entry criteria, participants were assigned to groups of 50 using an adaptive or quasi-randomization procedure (Pocock, 1975). As individuals were recruited, their duration of cannabis use was monitored and balanced between groups since cognitive impairments which might impact on treatment have been shown to develop with increasing years of cannabis use (Solowij, 1998; Solowij *et al.*, 2002). There were no differences between groups on intake drug use or clinical variables.

The psychotherapy group received 16 sessions of manual-driven SE dynamic psychotherapy. Adherence to the protocol was monitored through weekly supervision sessions, and independently verified for adherence and competence using a random subset of therapy audiotapes. Participants in the brief self-help group received a single session of brief advice and self-help materials, including a self-help guide to quitting (Grenyer *et al.*, 1996b). This guide contained sections on health information about cannabis, and instructed readers on topics such as: how to assess the pros and cons for quitting (e.g., health, financial, social, and legal issues); how to make a contract to quit; how to deal with withdrawal symptoms; how to cope with lapses and maintain change; and finally, the guide addressed situations that might reinforce drug use. After discussing the participants' history of cannabis use and their current problems, the clinician provided brief motivational advice to reinforce the participants' personal choice in quitting, oriented them to the use of the self-help guide, and then discharged them from treatment. Participants in the SE psychotherapy group also received a copy of the self-help guide to quitting, but this material was not incorporated within therapy. Seven trained dynamic psychotherapists (5 female, mean age 40.1 years, range 29–48) conducted the SE psychotherapy, and two trained graduate psychologists (2 females, aged 26 and 27 years) conducted the brief intervention. The primary outcome variables were: (1) reported abstinence from cannabis and recent frequency and quantity of use; (2) severity of psychiatric symptoms measured by the Global Assessment of Functioning Scale (GAF – Axis V of DSM-IV; American Psychiatric Association, 1994) and the Beck depression inventory (BDI; Beck *et al.*, 1961); and (3) consumer outcome and satisfaction ratings.

Results found that the whole sample achieved significant reductions in cannabis use at 4 and 12 months. At the 4-month follow-up, a significant difference between the groups emerged in terms of self-reported abstinence – 58% of the psychotherapy participants were abstinent compared to 16% of the brief intervention participants (Chi-square $= 18.92$, $p < 0.001$). Urinalyses were available for 41% of the sample that self-reported abstinence at 4 months, and confirmed abstinence in 93% of cases. By the 12-month follow-up, the difference between the two groups in terms of self-reported abstinence was no longer significant: 28% of psychotherapy participants were abstinent compared to 14% of the brief intervention participants (Chi-square: $2.95$, $p = 0.09$). Analyses of quantity and frequency of cannabis use showed essentially the same results, with a significant difference favoring the psychotherapy group at 4 months, but a non-significant trend by 12 months. With respect to improvements in psychiatric symptoms, both groups improved significantly in the first 4 months of treatment on both the GAF and BDI, but there were no additional gains from 4 to 12 months. The psychotherapy group improved significantly more compared to the brief group at 4 months and this superiority was maintained at 12-month follow-up. Consumer outcome and satisfaction ratings significantly favored the psychotherapy group compared to the brief self-help group, with participants in the psychotherapy group rating being more satisfied (78.6% versus 63.5%, respectively), and more likely to recommend the treatment to a friend (90.2% versus 65.9%).

To summarize, the SE psychotherapy was more effective than the brief self-help intervention over the 4-month treatment study period in achieving abstinence, reductions in cannabis use and improvements in mood and general psychiatric functioning. Participants in the psychotherapy group were more satisfied with the treatment received. By the 12-month follow-up, both groups had significant reductions in cannabis use with a non-significant trend favoring the psychotherapy group. The psychotherapy group also maintained superior gains in general psychiatric functioning and reductions in symptoms. While the results of the study support the notion that psychotherapy leads to better outcomes than self-help treatment, what remains unclear is whether these results can be explained by particular features of the SE technique, or more non-specific effects such as the cumulative effect of attention from a trained counselor. In addition, the therapists conducting the brief intervention were slightly younger and had different training experience than the dynamic psychotherapists, which may also have contributed to differences in outcomes. To further investigate these questions, a process study was conducted to examine the relationship between clinical gains and changes brought about by the SE techniques.

The process study explored the mode of action of SE psychotherapy, and helped to articulate how its application could assist the long-term habitual user. This study investigated changes in a clinically relevant concept: the client's mastery (self-understanding and self-control), scored from the verbatim transcripts of interviews at the beginning of treatment and at the 4-month follow-up of 43 long-term cannabis users (Grenyer, 2002b). The participants were a representative subsample of the 100 from the outcome study (23 in the psychotherapy group, 20 from the brief intervention group). Each participant was asked to speak for 5 min about "your life at the moment – the good things and the bad – what it is like for you" following the instructions by Viney (1983). Although the instructions specify 5 min (as a guide), many spoke for longer than 5 min. The verbatim transcripts were then scored using the Mastery Scale (Grenyer, 1994), which involves content analysis of claused speech by assigning mastery scale scores to scorable clauses. The Mastery Scale is a reliable and valid research instrument (Grenyer & Luborsky, 1996), and has six levels: (1) lack of impulse control (e.g., being overwhelmed, extreme defensiveness, regression, and ego-boundary ruptures); (2) introjection and projection of negative affects (e.g., paranoia, sadistic and rageful feelings, helplessness, and interpersonal withdrawal); (3) difficulties in understanding and control (e.g., cognitive confusion, ambivalence, partial awareness, and struggling with change); (4) interpersonal awareness (e.g., questioning the self and others' points of view, and interpersonal assertion); (5) self-understanding (e.g., having insight into repeating personality patterns of the self and others in the present and past); and (6) self-control (e.g., being able to analyze emotional conflicts and show emotional self-control over them). For each level, the manual specifies 3–4 typical categories of statements indicative of that level, making a total of 23 categories (from A–W) for the whole scale. Statements in client speech that corresponded to one of the 23 types of categories were assigned the corresponding mastery level score independently by two trained judges with high inter-rater reliability. These scores were averaged for each sample (deriving a mastery score between 1 and 6) and used in the analysis.

Initial mastery scores between the two groups were not significantly different ($F = 0.17$, $p = 0.68$), with the psychotherapy group averaging a mastery score of 2.98 (SD 0.92) and the brief self-help group 3.18 (SD 0.71). By the 4-month evaluation, analyses of covariance of mastery scores controlling for initial intake scores significantly favored the psychotherapy group (mean 4.61; SD 0.77 versus 3.13; SD 0.92, respectively, $F = 24.6$, $p < .001$). At 4 months, 87% of the SE group were abstinent, compared with 20% of the brief self-help group. Those who were abstinent had significantly higher mastery scores than those who were not abstinent (mean 4.52; SD 0.76 versus 3.09; SD 1.00, respectively, $F = 28.14$, $p < 0.001$). These data support the view that the SE psychotherapy techniques contributed to augmented mastery, and that these gains were associated with a greater likelihood of abstinence from cannabis.

Figure 10.2 illustrates differential changes in the six mastery levels at the 4-month evaluation, as made by the psychotherapy group in comparison to the brief self-help group. Given that there were few changes in mastery for the brief self-help group, this group's 4-month mastery data was used as a quasi-baseline from which to contrast the changes found in the psychotherapy group. We calculated proportions of scorable clauses (indicative of each level of mastery) from the transcripts for the psychotherapy group, and subtracted the proportions found in the brief self-help group. This yielded a graphic representation that showed the largest increase and the largest decrease in levels of mastery among members of the psychotherapy group, with respect to levels found in the brief self-help group.

The psychotherapy group had reductions in the lower level mastery scores compared to the brief intervention group, as indicated by the negative percent change in levels 1 (lack of impulse control) and 2 (introjection and projection of negative affects) categories. Conversely, there were gains in levels 4–6, which are indicative of higher mastery. In particular, for this sample of cannabis users, SE psychotherapy particularly improved level 4 (interpersonal awareness; 37% gain), and level 6 (self-control; 46% gain). These changes are

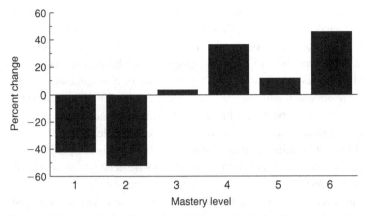

Figure 10.2 Percentage of frequency of Mastery Scale levels appearing in transcripts at 4-month follow-up for the SE psychotherapy group, expressed as percentage change from 4 months brief self-help transcripts. *Note*: $N = 43$. Dimensions indicative of poor mastery (levels 1–3) show a reduction or little difference in appearance in narratives in the psychotherapy group compared to the brief intervention group; dimensions indicative of good mastery (levels 4–6) show a corresponding increase in the psychotherapy group compared to the brief intervention group.

consistent with the SE model of therapy, which involves a focus on interpersonal functioning through mastery of the CCRTs, leading to greater self-control over drug use and the interpersonal problems associated with this use. In particular, the participants in this sample evidenced greater self-assertion and greater understanding of their repeating personality traits. This helped them overcome helpless and hopeless feelings associated with their cannabis use, which were evident at the beginning of treatment. Psychotherapy provided an escape from the feeling of being interpersonally trapped and conflicted within their relationships, and lead to a greater sense of self-control.

### Illustrative Case Study

The following brief case study illustrates some of the SE psychotherapy processes, and how they and how they lead to positive change. John, aged 47 years and married with three children, had been smoking cannabis continuously since he was 16 years. He came to treatment concerned that his life was stagnating, his relationships were suffering due to his drug use, and cannabis was adversely affecting his memory and ability to complete tasks at work. At intake, his GAF score was 56 and his BDI score was 22, indicating moderate to severe symptoms and impact on life functioning. He met 5 of the 7 DSM-IV criteria for cannabis dependence. Early measures of therapeutic alliance indicated that he had formed a positive relationship bond with his therapist, who focused on being supportive of John's struggle to change his drug use and overcome his feelings of depression. John's goals were to quit cannabis use, to improve his relationship with his wife, and to improve his functioning at work. He commented that "dope covers up my feelings, my despair inside, it keeps my worries and feelings away and allows me to float off." He reported considerable problems with relating to his partner, which he attributed partly to his tendency to procrastinate, and partly to his explosive feelings of anger. He would typically arrive home from work angry and frustrated, and to counter these feelings, he would sit in front of the television and "smoke dope and withdraw from the world and my worries." This enraged his wife, who constantly complained that his life was going nowhere and that he was not talking to her or helping with the children. He reported feeling trapped in a vicious circle – dope was helping him overcome his feelings of stress in the short term, yet was significantly impacting his ability to achieve at work and maintain personal relationships.

During the early phase, the therapist found it difficult to keep John focused on his goals, as he would frequently divert the conversation to superficial topics. Eventually, the therapist became aware that the client was struggling with intimacy, keeping his wife, relationships with his work colleagues, and keeping his therapist at a safe distance to prevent a deeper relationship from forming. Cannabis was being used to block out intimate relationships and his conflicted emotions. The therapist chose to use an expressive technique to interpret these feelings for the client by stating, "I keep getting this feeling that the relationship you are in is very detached and that there is a sadness about the detachment." The client broke down crying, admitting, "I never talk to anybody about myself, how I feel, because they might take advantage of me. People take advantage of your vulnerabilities." His use of cannabis as a crutch to cope with these feelings was explored. With the therapist's support, John was able to quit cannabis after the first month of treatment and work on his ability to relate to others in the new drug-free state. Over the middle phase of therapy, a number of strikingly similar relationship themes emerged and were further explored. John related being teased at school and being dismissed by his father when approached for help. These and other experiences lead him to bottle up his feelings and withdraw, resulting in having no friends and feeling unable to talk to his parents about his feelings. A strong CCRT pattern had been established – a wish to reach out and communicate with others, and an experience of others responding to him by taking advantage, ridiculing or dismissing him. John's characteristic response was to withdraw and avoid others in order to feel safe. The therapist helped him become aware of this pattern, and see how it was pervasive in his relationships and tied to the core of his difficulties and goals. At the end of therapy, he stated that "feeling safe with my therapist has really helped me to see beyond what I was feeling and get to the roots of it … I realize that marijuana was blocking a lot of issues inside me that needed to be discussed, and through therapy I feel I now understand myself more and feel I have grown in my emotional development." His GAF score at follow-up was 71 and his BDI score was 3, indicating mild to minimal symptoms.

### Conclusion and Future Directions

SE dynamic psychotherapy offers one potentially useful approach to help cannabis users who want to change their drug use. As interpersonal, social, intimacy, and work difficulties are often reported by cannabis users, this approach may be particularly salient as it focuses not only on drug use, but also on the relationship between use and interpersonal problems. It is useful due to its focus on the meaning of drug use within the context of the client's life. The therapy is structured to allow these holistic links to be formed and understood. It is respectful of the client because it allows them to freely discuss their current goals, concerns, and difficulties, and takes these as the primary material upon which to work within the sessions. Previous studies with other drugs of abuse have compared SE psychotherapy with CBT, and found the two therapies to be of equivalent effectiveness. For cannabis dependence, the evidence to date suggests that in addition to eliciting significant reductions in cannabis use, SE psychotherapy is particularly effective at dealing with comorbid depression, anxiety, and other symptoms.

Future research needs to further investigate the application of this approach to different client populations, such as adolescent cannabis users or those with more pronounced polysubstance abuse. Further clinical trials are needed to compare it to another standard treatment delivered over an equal number of sessions. To date, evidence in the psychotherapy field suggests that longer treatment leads to better outcomes. Some evidence proposing that the optimum cost-benefit occurs at approximately 26 weeks of treatment (Howard *et al.*, 1986). It remains to be seen whether better outcomes may be achieved for cannabis dependence by extending therapy duration. Community validation studies are required to assess its utility within community clinics, and it would be valuable to assess the utility of an SE group therapy format with cannabis users.

## References

American Psychiatric Association (1994). *Diagnostic and statistical manual of mental disorders* (4th ed.). Washington, DC: American Psychiatric Association.

Barber, J. P., & Crits-Christoph, P. (1995). *Dynamic therapies for psychiatric disorders (Axis 1)*. New York: Basic Books.

Baumrind, D., & Moselle, K. A. (1985). A developmental perspective on adolescent drug abuse. *Advances in Alcohol and Substance Abuse, 5*, 41–67.

Beck, A. T., Ward, C. H., Mendelson, M., Mock, J., & Erbaugh, J. (1961). An inventory for measuring depression. *Archives of General Psychiatry, 4*, 561–571.

Beutler, L. E., Machado, P. P. P., & Neufeldt, S. A. (1994). Therapist variables. In A. E. Bergin, & S. L. Garfield (Eds.), *Handbook of psychotherapy and behaviour change* (4th ed., pp. 229–269). New York: John Wiley and Sons.

Book, H. E. (1998). *How to practice brief psychodynamic psychotherapy: the Core Conflictual Relationship Theme method*. Washington, DC: American Psychological Association.

Crits-Christoph, P., & Connolly, M. B. (1998). Empirical basis of supportive–expressive psychodynamic psychotherapy. In R. F. Bornstein, & J. M. Masling (Eds.), *Empirical studies of the therapeutic hour. Empirical studies of psychoanalytic theories* (Vol. 8, pp. 109–151). Washington, DC: American Psychological Association.

Crits-Christoph, P., & Luborsky, L. (1998). Self-understanding of the CCRT. In L. Luborsky, & P. Crits-Christoph (Eds.), *Understanding transference: the Core Conflictual Relationship Theme method* (2nd ed., pp. 213–220). Washington, DC: American Psychological Association.

Crits-Christoph, P., Cooper, A., & Luborsky, L. (1988). The accuracy of therapist's interpretations and the outcome of dynamic psychotherapy. *Journal of Consulting and Clinical Psychology, 56*, 490–495.

Crits-Christoph, P., Siqueland, L., Blaine, J., Frank, A., Luborsky, L., Onken, L. S., *et al.* (1999). Psychosocial treatments for cocaine dependence. National Institute on Drug Abuse Collaborative Cocaine Treatment Study. *Archives of General Psychiatry, 56*, 493–502.

Deane, F. P., & Spicer, J. (1998). Validity of a simplified target complaints measure. *Assessment, 4*, 119–130.

Diguer, L., Barber, J., & Luborsky, L. (1993). Three concomitants: personality disorders, psychiatric severity, and outcome of dynamic psychotherapy of major depression. *American Journal of Psychiatry, 150*, 1246–1248.

Fergusson, D. M., & Horwood, L. J. (1997). Early onset cannabis use and psychosocial adjustment in young adults. *Addiction, 92*, 279–296.

Freud, S. (1914/1958). Remembering, repeating and working-through (Further recommendations on the technique of psycho-analysis II). In J. Strachey (Ed.), *Standard edition of the complete psychological works of Sigmund Freud* (Vol. 12, pp. 145–156). London: Hogarth Press and The Institute of Psycho-Analysis.

Gabbard, G. O. (1990). *Psychodynamic psychiatry in clinical practice.* Washington, DC: American Psychiatric Association.

Grenyer, B. F. S. (1994). *Mastery Scale I: a research and scoring manual.* Wollongong: University of Wollongong.

Grenyer, B. F. S. (2002a). *Mastering relationship conflicts: new discoveries in theory, research and practice.* Washington, DC: American Psychological Association Books.

Grenyer, B. F. S. (2002b). Mastery and different client presentations: depression, personality disorders, and substance dependence. In B. F. S. Grenyer (Ed.), *Mastering relationship conflicts: discoveries in theory research and practice* (pp. 169–193). Washington, DC: American Psychological Association.

Grenyer, B. F. S., & Luborsky, L. (1996). Dynamic change in psychotherapy: mastery of interpersonal conflicts. *Journal of Consulting and Clinical Psychology, 64,* 411–416.

Grenyer, B. F. S., Luborsky, L., & Solowij, N. (1995). *Treatment manual for supportive–expressive dynamic psychotherapy: special adaptation for treatment of cannabis(marijuana) dependence.* Sydney: National Drug and Alcohol Research Centre.

Grenyer, B. F. S., Solowij, N., & Peters, R. (1996a). A comparison of brief versus intensive treatment for cannabis dependence. *Australian Journal of Psychology, 48* (Suppl.), 106.

Grenyer, B. F. S., Solowij, N., & Peters, R. (1996b). *Marijuana: a guide to quitting.* Sydney: National Drug and Alcohol Research Centre.

Haas, A. P., & Hendin, H. (1987). The meaning of chronic marijuana use among adults: a psychosocial perspective. *Journal of Drug Issues, 17,* 333–348.

Hall, W., & Solowij, N. (1997). Long term cannabis use and mental health. *British Journal of Psychiatry, 171,* 107–108.

Hendin, H., Haas, A. P., Singer, P., Ellner, M., & Ulman, R. (1987). *Living high: daily marijuana use among adults.* New York: Human Sciences Press.

Howard, K. I., Kopta, S. M., Krause, M. S., & Orlinsky, D. E. (1986). The dose-effect relationship in psychotherapy. *American Psychologist, 41,* 159–164.

Kandel, D. B., & Logan, J. A. (1984). Patterns of drug use from adolescence to young adulthood. I. Periods of risk for initiation, continued use and discontinuation. *American Journal of Public Health, 74,* 660–666.

Kandel, D. B., Davies, M., Karus, D., & Yamaguchi, K. (1986). The consequences in young adulthood of adolescent drug involvement. *Archives of General Psychiatry, 43,* 746–754.

Kouri, E. M., & Pope, H. G. (2000). Abstinence symptoms during withdrawal from chronic marijuana use. *Experimental & Clinical Psychopharmacology, 8,* 483–492.

Luborsky, L. (1977). Measuring a pervasive psychic structure in psychotherapy: the Core Conflictual Relationship Theme. In N. Freedman, & S. Grand (Eds.), *Communicative structures and psychic structures* (pp. 367–395). New York: Plenum Press.

242 *Brin F. S. Grenyer and Nadia Solowij*

Luborsky, L. (1984). *Principles of psychoanalytic psychotherapy: a manual for supportive–expressive treatment.* New York: Basic Books.

Luborsky, L., & Crits-Christoph, P. (1998). *Understanding transference: The Core Conflictual Relationship Theme method* (2nd ed.). Washington, DC: American Psychological Association.

Luborsky, L., Crits-Christoph, P., Mintz, J., & Auerbach, A. (1988). *Who will benefit from psychotherapy? Predicting therapeutic outcomes.* New York: Basic Books.

Luborsky, L., Woody, G. E., & Hole, A. V. (1995). Supportive–expressive dynamic psychotherapy for treatment of opiate dependence. In J. P. Barber, & P. Crits-Christoph (Eds.), *Dynamic therapies for psychiatric disorders (Axis 1)* (pp. 225–293). New York: Basic Books.

Lundqvist, T. (1995). *Cognitive dysfunctions in chronic cannabis users observed during treatment.* Stockholm: Almqvist & Wiksell International.

Mark, D., & Faude, J. (1995). Supportive–expressive therapy of cocaine abuse. In J. P. Barber & P. Crits-Christoph (Eds.), *Dynamic therapies for psychiatric disorders (Axis 1)* (pp. 294–331). New York: Basic Books.

Martin, D. J., Garske, J. P., & Davis, M. K. (2000). Relation of the therapeutic alliance with outcome and other variables: a meta-analytic review. *Journal of Consulting and Clinical Psychology, 68,* 438–450.

Newcombe, M. D., & Bentler, P. (1988). *Consequences of adolescent drug use: impact on the lives of young adults.* Newbury Park: Sage Publications.

Orne, M., & Wender, P. (1968). Anticipatory socialization for psychotherapy: method and rationale. *American Journal of Psychiatry, 124,* 88–98.

Pocock, S. J. (1975). Sequential treatment assignment with balancing for prognostic factors in the controlled clinical trial. *Biometrics, 31,* 103–115.

Schlesinger, H. J. (1994). How the analyst listens: the pre-stages of interpretation. *International Journal of Psychoanalysis, 75,* 31–37.

Solowij, N. (1998). *Cannabis and cognitive functioning.* Cambridge, UK: Cambridge University Press.

Solowij, N., & Grenyer, B. F. S. (2002a). The long term effects of cannabis on psyche and cognition. In F. Grotenhermen (Ed.), *Cannabis and cannabinoids: pharmacology, toxicology and therapeutic potential* (pp. 325–338). London: Haworth Press.

Solowij, N., & Grenyer, B. F. S. (2002b). Are the adverse consequences of cannabis use age dependent? *Addiction, 97,* 1083–1086.

Solowij, N., Grenyer, B. F. S., Chesher, G., & Lewis, J. (1995). Biopsychosocial changes associated with cessation of cannabis use: A single case study of acute and chronic cognitive effects, withdrawal and treatment. *Life Sciences, 56,* 2127–2134.

Solowij, N., Stephens, R. S., Roffman, R. A., Babor, T., Kadden, R., Miller, M., et al. for the Marijuana Treatment Project Research Group (2002). Cognitive functioning of long term heavy cannabis users seeking treatment. *Journal of the American Medical Association, 287,* 1123–1131.

Viney, L. L. (1983). The assessment of psychological states through content analysis of verbal communications. *Psychological Bulletin, 94,* 542–563.

Woody, G. E., Luborsky, L., McLellan, T., O'Brien, C. P., Beck, A. T., Blaine, J., *et al.* (1983). Psychotherapy for opiate addicts: Does it help? *Archives of General Psychiatry, 40,* 639–645.

Woody, G. E., McLellan, T. A., Luborsky, L., & O'Brien, C. P. (1987). Twelve month follow-up of psychotherapy for opiate dependence. *American Journal of Psychiatry, 144,* 590–596.

Woody, G. E., McLellan, T. A., Luborsky, L., & O'Brien, C. P. (1995). Psychotherapy in community methadone programs: a validation study. *American Journal of Psychiatry, 152,* 1302–1308.

# Part III
## Interventions with Cannabis-Dependent Adolescents and Young Adults

# 11

# The Cannabis Youth Treatment Study: The Treatment Models and Preliminary Findings

GUY DIAMOND, JODI LECKRONE, MICHAEL L. DENNIS AND
SUSAN H. GODLEY

## Introduction

Marijuana is the most prevalent psychoactive substance used by adolescents in the US and in many other countries (Office of Applied Studies, 2000; World Health Organization (WHO), 1997). Though the rates of use have leveled off recently, adolescents in the US still report more past month cannabis use than all other illicit substances combined and more daily use of cannabis than alcohol (Monitoring the Future (MTF), 2000). Moreover, while the age of first use has been declining during the past two decades (Bureau of Justice Statistics (BJS), 2000), the potency of cannabis has increased threefold (El Sholy *et al.*, 2000). By 1999, 6.8% of US 18-year-old met criteria for past year cannabis dependence. Cannabis is now the leading illicit substance reported in adolescent arrests, emergency room admissions, autopsies, and treatment admissions (Office of Applied Studies, 2000).

While many adolescents use cannabis without serious problems, it is estimated that half of weekly users develop both behavior and physiological problems (Dennis *et al.*, 2002a). A variety of psychiatric conditions precede or are co-morbid with marijuana abuse and dependence including conduct disorder, attention deficit/hyperactivity disorder, depression, and anxiety (Crowley & Riggs, 1995; Hofler *et al.*, 1999; Robins & McEvoy, 1990). Adolescent cannabis use is also associated with increased problems at school (Fergusson *et al.*, 1996; Newcomb & Bentler, 1988), health problems such as sexually transmitted diseases, and delinquency (National Institute of Justice, 2001). Complicating matters further, over 90% of adolescents who use cannabis also engage in binge drinking, a combination that is associated with more health and behavioral problems than either alone (Bukstein *et al.*, 1992; Dennis *et al.*, 1999; Newcomb *et al.*, 1986; Siemens, 1980).

Concurrent with the increased incidence of cannabis use among adolescents, demand for cannabis treatment has also increased. From 1992 to 1998, the

247

number of adolescents with primary, secondary, or tertiary problems related to cannabis who presented to the US public treatment system grew 115% from 51,081 to 109,875 (Dennis *et al.*, 2003). In 1998, over 80% of these adolescents received treatment in an outpatient setting.

Given the high prevalence of cannabis use during adolescence, its associated problems and the increasing demand for services, there is a critical need for the health care system to develop effective cannabis interventions. Relatively few clinical trials of interventions for adolescents with substance abuse problems have been conducted and none have evaluated interventions specifically designed to address cannabis abuse or dependence (Ozechowski & Liddle, 2000; Williams & Chang, 2000). Findings from existing studies have demonstrated mixed results (Gerstein & Johnson, 1999; Grella *et al.*, 2001; Hser *et al.*, 2001; Simpson *et al.*, 1978). No studies have even approached the rigorous standards established for a therapy to be considered efficacious (Chambless & Hollon, 1998) and therefore ready for exportation into the community.

Recognizing the need for more scientifically supported interventions for adolescents with cannabis abuse and dependence, the Center for Substance Abuse Treatment (CSAT) funded the Cannabis Youth Treatment (CYT) study, the first multi-site randomized field trial ever conducted with this population. The trial included five interventions that mirrored some of the most effective existing practice models. The five interventions incorporated some treatments that were already in existence, some that were modified from successful adult models, and some that were adapted from other adolescent treatment modalities. Each intervention had varying theoretical and empirical support from the adolescent or adult substance abuse treatment literature.

This chapter outlines the clinical approaches tested and preliminary findings from the CYT study (Dennis *et al.*, 2002b, 2004; Diamond *et al.*, 2002). CYT was a cooperative agreement sponsored by SAMHSA's CSAT under the Department of Health and Human Services Secretary's Youth Initiative to address the lack of adequate treatments for adolescents being treated in outpatient settings for marijuana abuse or dependence (ASAM levels I and II). The purpose of CYT was to test the clinical and cost-effectiveness of a variety of interventions targeted at reducing or eliminating marijuana use and associated problems in adolescents. The five brief (5 or 12 weeks) interventions were selected because they represented current practice models in the field and could be manualized and easily disseminated. Motivational Enhancement Therapy/Cognitive Behavioral Therapy (MET/CBT5) is a five session treatment, consisting of two individual MET and three CBT group sessions. Motivational Enhancement

Therapy/Cognitive Behavioral Therapy-12 (MET/CBT12) consists of MET/CBT5 with seven additional CBT group sessions (12 total sessions). Family Support Network (FSN) added six sessions of parent education classes, four home visits, family sessions, and case management to MET/CBT12 for a potential total of 22 sessions. Adolescent Community Reinforcement Approach (ACRA) (14 sessions) consists of 10 individual sessions and four parent or family sessions. Multidimensional Family Therapy (MDFT) consists of a flexible mixture of 12–15 individual, family, and parent-alone sessions. This chapter begins by presenting each treatment's theoretical foundation, goals and proposed mechanisms, and structure and content. Subsequently, the empirical support for these treatments, based on the findings from the CYT study, is briefly reviewed.

## Description of the Interventions

### MET/CBT5 (Sampl & Kadden, 2001)

*Theory*

MET is an application of Motivational Interviewing and was developed to enhance client motivation to change. It is based on the hypothesis that individuals will achieve greater change when motivation comes from within themselves rather than when others attempt to impose it (Miller & Rollnick, 1991). MET adapts Prochaska and DiClemente's (1984) five stages of change model to help assess and guide the client. These stages include precontemplation, contemplation, determination, action, and maintenance. The CBT component focuses on helping adolescents develop the coping skills needed to recognize and manage common risk situations that typically lead to drug use. Within this model, skill deficits are viewed as a primary cause of relapse. Therefore, group process focuses on teaching and rehearsing these skills.

*Goals and Treatment Mechanisms*

Five core principles are hypothesized to enhance motivation (Miller & Rollnick, 1991). First, in contrast to a confrontational agenda, the therapists use empathy and empathetic listening to make the adolescent feel understood and accepted. Second, the therapist highlights discrepancies between the adolescent's stated life goals and the adolescent's own concerns about problems related to marijuana (e.g., school failure, legal consequences, etc.). Third, the therapist avoids arguments in order to avoid provoking resistance. Fourth, therapists "roll with resistance" by responding to resistant verbal statements with empathy rather than confrontation. Fifth, the therapist bolsters the adolescent's self-efficacy (i.e., confidence in his/her ability to stop using marijuana) by identifying past successes with reducing drug use or mastering other life problems, and by praising current progress toward change.

The CBT component provides alternative skills for coping with situations that might otherwise lead to marijuana use (Monti *et al.*, 1989). The group CBT format provides a context for behavioral modeling, rehearsal, and feedback, as well as habituation to social anxiety. Group discussions provide opportunities for therapists to normalize individual members' struggles with avoiding use and/or relapse and for participants to practice new social behaviors. Ideally, group members become part of a recovery network for each other.

### Treatment Structure and Content

Treatment begins with two individual MET sessions. The first session focuses on building rapport, explaining treatment expectations, assessing and building motivation, and reviewing the adolescent's Personalized Feedback Report (PFR). The PFR presents information from the intake assessment that outlines the adolescent's substance use, related problems, and reasons for quitting. Therapists use this information to develop the adolescent's motivation for change. The adolescent's frequency of use is compared to national norms in order to provide a new perspective on his or her level of use. During the second session, the adolescent completes a personal goal worksheet related to quitting marijuana. Therapists conduct a functional analysis of marijuana to help the adolescent identify triggers, thoughts, and feelings, behaviors, and consequences from use. Finally, the therapist prepares the adolescent for the group CBT sessions that will follow.

In sessions three through five, CBT skills training is provided to groups of five to six adolescents. To teach these skills, therapists use brief didactic presentations, modeling, role-playing, and homework exercises. The first CBT session (treatment session 3) focuses on developing skills for refusing offers to buy or use marijuana. During a discussion of social pressure, participants learn how to say "no" quickly and convincingly, suggest an appropriate alternative activity, and avoid using excuses. Role-plays are used to demonstrate passive, aggressive, passive–aggressive, and assertive ways of responding. The fourth session focuses on enhancing the participant's positive social support network and reducing associations with substance-using peers. Participants identify the kinds of support needed to live a drug-free lifestyle, and specific people who could assist in this challenge. Methods for increasing social supports and pro-social activities are reviewed. The last meeting (session 5) concentrates on planning for unanticipated high-risk situations and coping with relapse. Participants identify events that could precipitate marijuana use and learn coping strategies to avoid or manage these high-risk situations.

## MET/CBT12 (Webb et al., 2002b)

The background, underlying theory, and hypothesized treatment mechanisms are the same as MET/CBT5. However, MET/CBT12 provides additional relapse coping skills training by adding seven more CBT sessions.

### Treatment Structure and Content

The sixth session (after MET/CBT5) focuses on effective problem-solving skills that serve as the basis for the remainder of the program. A five stage problem-solving model is presented consisting of:

(a) general orientation,
(b) problem identification,
(c) generating alternatives,
(d) decision-making,
(e) verification.

The seventh and eighth sessions focus on anger management. Initially, the group focuses on anger awareness skills, highlighting both internal and external cues, and triggers. The focus then shifts to techniques for managing anger. The group leader teaches different strategies including the use of calm-down phrases and anger reducing thoughts. The ninth session concentrates on communication skills. Participants learn techniques for active listening, assertiveness and positive ways of responding to criticism. The tenth session offers a menu of coping options for cravings and urges for marijuana. Participants are encouraged to keep a daily log of the intensity, length, and source of urges, and alternative ways to resist them. The eleventh session focuses on managing depressed feelings. Participants learn about the impact of negative emotions and the role of negative automatic thoughts. Techniques for substituting positive for negative thoughts are then reviewed and rehearsed. The last session (treatment session 12) returns to the primary focus of managing thoughts about marijuana. In this session, the group leader reviews the 12 most common excuses for relapse and discusses termination.

## FSN plus MET/CBT12 (Hamilton et al., 2001)

### Background and Rationale

FSN was designed as an adjunct to the 12-week MET/CBT12. FSN is based on the belief that a single treatment modality, possibly regardless of duration, is neither intensive nor comprehensive enough to reduce a persistent and multifaceted problem such as adolescent substance use disorders. Instead, a multi-component treatment package is needed for maximum treatment effectiveness (CSAT, 1993). Earlier randomized clinical trials have demonstrated that family involvement could enhance patient retention and outcomes (Henggeler *et al.*, 1991; Liddle *et al.*, 2001). In addition, case management has been strongly recommended for adult substance abusers (McLellan *et al.*, 1999; Siegal & Rapp, 1996) and a model has been proposed for adolescent substance abusers (Godley *et al.*, 1994). These recommendations were incorporated by adding a family-based component (parent psychoeducation and family therapy) as well as case management for the parents while the adolescent participates in MET/CBT12. The rationale for including these components is twofold: (1) ideally, parental involvement will help promote the adolescents' engagement and retention in treatment; and (2) case managers can facilitate family engagement in the treatment process by reducing barriers to treatment participation (e.g., transportation, childcare, etc.).

### Treatment Goals and Mechanisms

The treatment goals and mechanisms of MET/CBT12 remain the same as described above. There are four general goals related to the family components. Therapists seek to:

(a)  include family members in the recovery process,
(b)  enhance family communication and general relationship quality,
(c)  improve parents' behavioral management skills,
(d)  increase adolescents' and parents' commitment to the recovery process.

The parent education sessions are intended to build a support system for parents and educate them about adolescent development, adolescent drug use patterns, and family management. Home visits are intended to enhance commitment to treatment and help adolescents and their families individualize skills learned in the parent education, and MET/CBT12 sessions to their specific needs and family dynamics.

*Treatment Structure and Content*

Each of the parent education sessions are didactic, highly structured, and focus on specific topics. During the first session, the therapist presents information about normal and deviant adolescent development and how parents might influence this trajectory. For example, parents learn the importance of balancing their adolescent's need for autonomy and their connection to the family. During session two, the therapist defines adolescent substance abuse and dependency and discusses how family and peer pressures can contribute to these problems. Parents are encouraged to stay involved in the treatment process and provide support for recovery. Session three focuses on relapse signs and recovery, emphasizing the role that parents can play in detecting and preventing relapse. Session four focuses on family functioning and the importance of parents' rules and expectations. Session five addresses family communication and conflict resolution. Group leaders review techniques for active listening, reducing criticism, and remaining focused on one problem at a time. The final parent group provides information about family systems principles (e.g., how rigid family roles may contribute to family conflict).

On the first home visit, therapists assess the family environment and encourage parental participation in the family education classes and home visit components. During the second visit, therapists lead a discussion about family rules, roles, and routines. The third and fourth visits are less structured and are used to assess and reinforce treatment progress and commitment. Every session focuses on strengthening the alliance between the family members and the FSN treatment providers/program.

Case managers focus on maintaining treatment participation using activities such as weekly phone calls to discuss attendance or helping with transportation and childcare. Families with multiple or complex needs are provided more intensive case management for 2 months that includes connecting the adolescent or caregivers to other support services in the community (e.g., housing, school, work programs, etc.). After 2 months of intensive case management, families are stepped down to regular case management focused on support and barrier reduction.

## *ACRA (Godley et al., 2001a)*

*Treatment Rationale*

ACRA is a behavioral therapy that focuses on rearranging environmental contingencies such that non-using (substance) behavior is more rewarding than using behavior. ACRA is an adaptation of the Community Reinforcement Approach that was initially developed for the treatment of adult alcoholics (Meyers *et al.*, 1999; Meyers & Smith, 1995). In a number of studies by Azrin and colleagues, CRA and its various components were found to be superior to standard inpatient and outpatient approaches for adults (e.g., Azrin, 1976), and one study was promising for adolescents (Azrin *et al.*, 1994).

*Theory*

ACRA integrates an operant conditioning model with skills training and a social systems approach to increase the adolescent's likelihood of engaging in alternative, positive behaviors as a replacement for behaviors that increase the likelihood of marijuana use. ACRA therapists help adolescents recognize that their drug use is incompatible with other short- or long-term reinforcers (e.g., parental approval, staying out of the criminal justice system, having a girl/boy friend). Therapists also work to increase alternative positive, non-drug-related social/recreational activities, while teaching social skills (e.g., problem-solving, drug refusal, etc.) that will increase the likelihood of success in these endeavors.

*Goals and Treatment Mechanisms*

In individual sessions with the adolescent, the therapist has several objectives. Therapists promote abstinence from marijuana and other drugs, participation in pro-social activities, and positive relationships with friends and caregivers. The Functional Analysis of Substance Use helps isolate internal and external triggers that lead to substance abuse, and identify consequences of these behaviors, while the Functional Analysis of Pro-social Behavior helps identify current or desired pro-social activities. This information is combined with other procedures to motivate increased participation in pro-social behaviors. Skills training in relapse prevention, communication, and problem-solving offers additional techniques that can be used to address the treatment goals.

One of the adaptations of the model for adolescents has been the addition of parent/caregiver involvement in four treatment sessions. These sessions focus on motivating caregiver participation in the treatment and promoting parenting practices that can help reduce adolescent risk of relapse. For example, caregivers are educated about the impact of their own substance use on the adolescent's recovery process, and the value of parental monitoring, positive communication, and encouragement of pro-social activities. Parents are also taught communication and problem-solving strategies, and are encouraged to practice these skills with their adolescents. In addition to individual and family goals, therapists focus on improving adolescents' circumstances in the larger social system. Essentially, therapists serve as advocates in resolving problems and increasing resources in the community (e.g., school, mental health, probation, employment, etc.).

*Treatment Structure and Content*

The treatment is composed of 10 sessions with the adolescent alone and four sessions with caregivers. Two sessions are with the caregivers alone and two include the adolescent and caregivers together. While the manual recommends a sequencing of procedures, the order of delivery is flexible and based on individual needs of the adolescents. Three procedures make up the unique core of the model, each of which are revisited and updated frequently throughout the treatment. Functional Analysis of Substance Use teaches adolescents to avert relapse by controlling antecedent behaviors that have led to substance use before. Similar attention is given to results of the Functional Analysis of Prosocial Behavior. Second, adolescents regularly complete a Happiness Scale rating their degree of happiness with 14 different life domains (e.g., drug use, school, peers, etc.). Therapists use this tool to guide conversations about the adolescent's satisfaction with life, and to monitor treatment progress. Third, based on information from the Functional Analyzes and the Happiness Scale, therapists and adolescents formulate the ACRA Treatment Plan. This tool identifies specific treatment goals and concrete plans for achieving them. Due to all 14 areas of the Happiness Scale are discussed, this process expands the focus of treatment beyond the use of marijuana and other drugs.

Once these core procedures have been completed, sessions focus on assessing progress and skill building. With the adolescent, skill-building focuses on pro-social recreation, relapse prevention, communication, and problem-solving skills. With the caregivers, skill-building focuses on rapport building, motivation, communication, and problem-solving.

## MDFT (Liddle, 2002)

*Background and Rationale*

MDFT is family-based, multi-systems, multi-component, developmentally and ecologically oriented approach specifically designed for the treatment of adolescents with substance abuse and related problems (Liddle & Hogue, 2000). The approach has been tested in several randomized trials, is manualized, and has a published treatment adherence scale (Hogue *et al.*, 1998; Liddle & Hogue, 2000; Liddle *et al.*, 2001; Rowe *et al.*, in press). Several studies of the therapeutic process have illuminated core aspects of MDFT including changes in parenting practices (Schmidt *et al.*, 1996), improving poor therapist–adolescent alliance (Diamond *et al.*, 2000), engaging African American males in therapy (Jackson-Gilfort & Liddle, 1999), gender-based treatment issues (Dakof, 2000), and parent–adolescent conflict resolution (Diamond & Liddle, 1996, 1999).

*Theory*

The theoretical bases of MDFT reside in several areas (Liddle, 1999). First adolescent drug abuse is understood as a multidimensional phenomenon. Individual, family, social, and environmental risk and protective factors are considered as contributing to or buffering against substance use (Liddle & Hogue, 2000). Second, developmental psychology and developmental psychopathology provide important conceptual and practical foci for assessment and intervention (Liddle *et al.*, 2000). Third, structural and strategic family therapy provides some of the clinical strategies for this modality (Minuchin, 1974; Stanton & Todd, 1982). In general, treatment focuses on four areas:

1. individual characteristics of the adolescent (e.g., perceptions about drugs, drug taking behaviors, and emotion regulation processes);
2. the parent(s) (e.g., parenting practices and personal problems not related to parenting);
3. family interaction patterns;
4. extra-familial sources of influence (e.g., school, juvenile justice, medical, and legal systems).

*Goals and Treatment Mechanisms*

The overarching goal of treatment is to re-establish normative developmental processes and challenges in an adolescent's life. Goals and focal areas with the adolescents include building competency, reducing involvement with a deviant peer network, increasing participation in pro-social activities, and developing better coping skills regarding affective regulation and problem-solving. For the parent(s), goals include reducing psychiatric distress, drug use, and economic stress, and improving social support and parenting practices. At the family level, treatment focuses on rekindling developmentally appropriate parental connection and commitment to the adolescent, and increasing family organization, warmth and emotional investment. These goals should lead to the re-establishment of the family as a developmentally facilitative context.

## Treatment Structure and Content

The first phase of treatment emphasizes three areas. First, the therapist works to establish therapeutic alliances with all relevant participants in the system: the adolescent, parent(s), other family members, and other providers (e.g., teachers, probation officers, etc.). This is essential to creating conditions conducive to change. Second, using the broadly informed MDFT framework and information shared by participants, therapists make a comprehensive, multi-systemic assessment of each area of the adolescent's life. Direct observation of interactions between adolescents, parents, and other individuals generally provides the richest source of information. Phase one should conclude with a strong therapist-system alliance, clear and mutually acceptable treatment goals, and a commitment to repairing the parent–adolescent connection.

The mid-phase of treatment builds upon the clinical themes identified in phase one. Sessions with the adolescent alone identify and attack barriers to participation in normative developmental activities. These sessions focus on imparting new motivation, ideas, and problem-solving skills that will facilitate a decrease in drug using and antisocial activities and an increase of pro-social behaviors at home and socially. Discussions can focus on drug use history, motivation, patterns, urges, circumstances, and perceived benefits and disadvantages of drug use. Therapists also teach communication, problem-solving, and relationship skills, support job or vocational training, or facilitate the pursuit of a General Educational Development (GED). In addition, therapists help adolescents address the conflictual issues that stand between them and their parents. These may include conflicts over autonomy, long standing family disagreements, or crises (Diamond & Liddle, 1999). Sessions alone with the parents focus on the self-of-the-parent, apart from their parental role, including motivations, social supports, and psychiatric distress. These sessions must also examine parenting philosophy and styles (Schmidt *et al.*, 1996). Parents learn to distinguish influence from control, and to develop realistic expectations about change. During this second phase, the therapist becomes more action-oriented than reflective, seeking to prompt new transactional alternatives (e.g., enactments) between the adolescent and his/her family, and social world. The final phase of treatment focuses on generalization and maintenance of change with a special focus on establishing specific and overt new ways of thinking, responding, and interacting.

Table 11.1. *Comparison of intended treatment modality and dosage by condition*

|  | Treatment condition | | | | |
|---|---|---|---|---|---|
| Study arm<br>Type of service | Both arms<br>MET/CBT5 | Arm 1<br>MET/CBT12 | Arm 1<br>FSN | Arm 2<br>ACRA | Arm 2<br>MDFT |
| Individual adolescent sessions | 2 | 2 | 2 | 10 | 6 |
| CBT group sessions | 3 | 10 | 10 | | |
| Individual parent sessions | | | | 2 | 3 |
| Family sessions/home visits | | | 4 | 2 | 6 |
| Parent education sessions | | | 6 | | |
| Total formal sessions | 5 | 12 | 22 | 14 | 15 |
| Case management/other contacts | | | As needed | As needed | As needed |
| Total expected contacts | 5 | 12 | 22+ | 14+ | 15+ |

Table 11.1 provides a summary of the intended treatment duration and component parts. Although many of the theories and interventions strategies described above are quite distinct in terms of treatment modality (individual, group, family, parent, case management), many treatments share common elements. Moreover, every intervention used at least two modalities, indicative of the need to target a range of domains when treating this complex patient population. This multi-component, multi-targeted structure of all the treatments may contribute to the treatment effectiveness described below, and may help explain the lack of differential outcomes between the treatments.

**Overview of CYT Study**

*Study Design*

The five treatment models were evaluated in two research arms (see Table 11.1). Each arm was replicated in two sites: a community-based program and an academic medical center. The first study arm evaluated the hypothesis that there would be an "incremental" or dose-response effect of providing increasingly more and varied treatment. Conducted at Operation PAR in St. Petersburg, Fl and the University of Connecticut Health Center (UCHC), the "incremental arm" compared MET/CBT5, MET/CBT12, and the multiple component FSN intervention. This comparison included differences in planned number of sessions

(5 versus 12 versus 20) and weeks of treatment (6 versus 12) and the addition of family and case management services in the FSN intervention. Conducted at Chestnut Health Systems (CHS) in Madison County, Illinois and Children's Hospital of Philadelphia (CHOP), the "alternative arm" compared MET/CBT5, ACRA, and MDFT. This study arm evaluated the relative impact of three distinct intervention strategies based on different theoretical approaches and varied percentages of group, individual, and family therapy sessions. Replication of the MET/CBT5 intervention across all four sites made it possible to study site differences and conduct quasi-experimental comparisons of the interventions across study arms.

Within each site, eligible adolescents were randomly assigned to one of the three local interventions. Intake and 3-, 6-, 9-, and 12-month follow-up interviews were conducted by independent research staff who were trained and certified by the coordinating center. Data were collected from several sources including participant interviews, collateral interviews, urine tests, services logs, and other process measures. The primary assessment tool was the Global Appraisal of Individual Needs (GAIN) (Dennis, 1999). This comprehensive, structured interview has eight main sections: background; substance use; physical health; risk behaviors; mental health; environment; legal; and vocational. The primary dependent measures were changes in the days of cannabis use and the number of substance-related problems reported in the previous month. The GAIN's Substance Problem Index (SPI) is composed of 16 recency items (e.g., "When was the last time you ... ?") based on the seven DSM-IV criteria for dependence, four assessing abuse criteria, two for substance-induced health and psychological problems, and three on lower severity symptoms of use (hiding use, people complaining about use, weekly use). Items were summed to create a total score ranging from 0–16. Secondary dependent measures include days of behavioral problems, family problems, anger/violence, illegal activity, and school and work attendance.

### Analytic Procedure

All analyzes were conducted with an "intent-to-treat" approach. The baseline clinical measures (days of abstinence or percent in recovery) were included as covariates to allow for individual differences. Within each trial, site differences were modeled with a dummy variable. Reflecting the randomized block design, conditions were modeled as nested within site, which produces a statistic for the significance of site effects, conditions across site effects, and conditions within site effects. Logistic regression was used to analyze differences for the percent in recovery at 12 months, as this is a dichotomous outcome. Where there were significant differences by condition, Tukey multiple range tests were conducted to verify which condition or conditions were different in pair-wise comparisons. Statements about the size of an effect or trends are based on Cohen's (1988) effect size $f$ (for multiple groups), with 0.10 being considered small, 0.20 moderate, and 0.40, or more large.

### *Participants*

Participants were eligible for CYT if they were between the ages of 12–18, reported one or more DSM-IV criteria for cannabis abuse or dependence, used cannabis in the past 90 days (or 90 days prior to being in a controlled environment), and were appropriate for outpatient or intensive outpatient treatment (American Society of Addiction Medicine, 1996). Participants were not eligible if they:

(a)  reported use of alcohol 45 or more of the 90 days prior to intake;
(b)  reported use of other drugs 13 or more of the 90 days prior to intake;
(c)  reported an acute medical or psychological problem that was likely to prohibit full participation in treatment;
(d)  had insufficient mental capacity to understand the consent procedure or participate in treatment;
(e)  lived outside of the program's catchment area; or
(f)  had a history of repeated, violent behavior, or severe conduct disorder that might put other participants at risk.

### *Characteristics of Adolescents Presenting for Outpatient Cannabis Treatment*

Consistent with the prior evaluations of outpatient treatment outlined above and the profile of adolescents presenting for treatment in the nation, the majority of the 600 participating adolescents were male (83%), in school (87%), started using under the age of 15 (85%), were currently over the age of 15 (85%), white (61%), had a history of victimization (57%), and/or from single parent families (50%). Approximately 62% were involved in the criminal justice system at the time of intake, including 42% who were on probation, 21% awaiting a trial, 17% assigned to Treatment Assessment screening (TASC) or other diversion program, and 7% awaiting sentencing. Many were also employed (47%), coming from a controlled environment (25%), or had recently been homeless/a runaway (7%). Most faced one or more potential negative environmental influences on recovery, including regular peer use of drugs (89%) or alcohol (64%), weekly use in the home of alcohol (23%) or drugs (11%). In addition, 72% were sexually active in the past 90 days including 39% with multiple sexual partners, and 23% without any kind of protection. Relative to patients in publicly funded outpatient treatment programs, the adolescents seen in CYT were much more likely to be going to treatment for the first time (74% versus 50%). Seventy-one percent of the sample reported weekly marijuana, 17% reported weekly alcohol consumption (17%), only 1% reported weekly use of other drugs. Lifetime injection drug use was less than 1%. Though only 20% saw their marijuana use as a problem, 96% self reported sufficient symptoms to meet criteria for abuse (50%) and/or dependence (48%). Most of those meeting criteria for dependence reported the physiological symptom of tolerance (i.e., needing more to get the same high). Though there are a few minor differences within arm, they are less than would be expected by chance. The most notable of which is that the adolescents in the alternative arm, and particularly in Philadelphia, were more likely to be African American, female, and to be sexually active, as well as less likely to be employed.

*Co-morbidity*

Along with their substance use, most adolescents also had one or more co-occurring problems. Overall, the most common co-occurring past year problems were related to conduct disorder (53%), attention deficit/hyperactivity disorder (38%), acute emotional (27%) or memory distress (27%), acute health problems (26%), and/or pregnancy (11% of females). The rate of these problems is higher among those with past year dependence (48%). These co-occurring problems, including violence and illegal activity, come together to form a common dimension of global individual severity that we expected to interact with treatment effectiveness. Both substance use and global severity were also generally higher for females and those under 15 who we believe have to reach a higher problem threshold in order for their families, schools, or the courts to refer them to treatment. There were no differences between intervention groups within arms on any of these variables.

*Comparison with Family or other Collateral Reports*

During the past 90 days, adolescents were more likely than family members or other collaterals to report days of any substance use (39 versus 31 days, $r = 0.46$, $p < 0.0001$) and marijuana use (37 versus 30, $r = 0.46$, $p < 0.0001$). They reported about the same number of days of alcohol use (7 versus 8, $r = 0.24$,

$p < 0.0001$), and symptoms of substance abuse/dependence during the past month (2.4 versus 2.6 of 11 symptoms, $r = 0.27$, $p < 0.0001$), past year (4.6 versus 4.6 symptoms, $r = 0.21$, $p < 0.0001$), and their lifetime (5.1 versus 5.2 symptoms, $r = 0.27$, $p < 0.0001$). Though these overall rates are very similar, the correlations show that family members and other collaterals are often reporting different information for a given individual. While over 70% of the family members or other collaterals were unable to report on all of the GAIN's 16 past-month substance problems, on average they reported more total problems of abuse or dependence than the adolescent (8 versus 7). In particular, they were more likely to report role failure, tolerance, and substance induced psychological problems. Using the combined adolescent–family/collateral information raised the average number of past month problems from 7 to 11. This suggests the importance of assessing both adolescents and their collaterals and the need to look at their combined reports.

## Clinical Procedures

### Therapist Selections

Therapists were hired at each site by the site principal investigator and the treatment model developer. MDFT and FSN family therapy providers were required to have at least a master's degree while MET/CBT, and ACRA therapists were required to have at least a bachelor's degree. Preference was given to therapists who had experience working with adolescents with drug and alcohol problems and therapists who agreed to use a manual-guided intervention (Godley *et al.*, 2001b).

### Therapist Training and Supervision

Each treatment site had a local therapist coordinator to monitor therapist activities, caseloads, and record keeping in addition to providing onsite support and management of cases. Each treatment also had a cross-site clinical supervisor with expertise in their respective models. Clinical supervisors oversaw the therapist certification process, provided weekly supervision, and conducted regular adherence monitoring. After attending a 2-day training session in their respective model, each therapist began treating cases with every session being reviewed either through live observation or via video/audio tape. Therapists were certified after the clinical supervisor judged their work to be sufficiently faithful to the model. To maintain treatment fidelity, therapists received at least 2 h a week of supervision (for caseloads of 8–12 cases), and supervisors rated two sessions for each therapist per month on intervention specific adherence measures.

## Results

### Retention

Of the 600 adolescents randomized, 98% completed follow-up interviews at 3 months, with similar rates at 6 and 12 months. On average, adolescents completed 71% of their prescribed sessions, 22% received partial dosages, and 5% were randomized but never received treatment. Of the adolescents assigned to one of the 12-week treatments, 81% completed 2 or more months of treatment with a mean of 80 days from intake to last formal session. The comparable number of days was 43 for the adolescents assigned to the 5-week treatments.

### Overall outcomes

The days of abstinence increased from 52 (of 90) in the 90 days before intake to an average of 65 days across the four follow-up periods. The overall change occurred during active treatment (from intake to month 3) and was stable across follow-up, though individuals did vary (intraclass correlation coefficient (ICC) = 0.47). The percent of adolescents in recovery at each interview increased from 3% at intake to an average of 24% across the four follow-up periods. Again, across conditions and sites, change occurred during active treatment, was stable across follow-up waves, and individual adolescents continued to move in and out of recovery (ICC = 0.33). Abstinence is summed across the four follow-up waves and the percent in recovery at the end of the study in month 12.

In Trial 1, the total days of abstinence (summed across the four follow-up waves) was not significantly different by site or condition (within or across sites). The percent in recovery at the end of the study was significantly different by condition overall (Cohen's $f = 0.12$, $p < .05$) with MET/CBT5 (27%) having the highest percent in recovery, followed by FSN (22%) and MET/CBT12 (17%). However, the pair-wise differences were not large enough to reach significance using a Tukey multiple range test. These findings held both across and within sites.

In Trial 2, the total days of abstinence were not significantly different by site or condition (within or across sites). The percent in recovery was not significantly different by condition across sites, though there was a small trend (Cohen's $f = 0.16$) for ACRA (34%) to have a slightly higher percent of participants in recovery than MET/CBT5 (23%) and MDFT (19%). This finding was driven by Site 3 (CHS), where within site there was a moderate-sized significant difference by condition (Cohen's $f = 0.20$, $p < 0.05$) with ACRA (40%) having a higher percent in recovery than MDFT (22%) and MET/CBT5 (18%). However, the pair-wise differences were not large enough to reach significance using a Tukey multiple range test.

*Subsequent Treatment*

While the 6–12 week CYT treatments appear to be effective on average, there is a very important qualification to make. Approximately 21% of the adolescents went on to get additional treatment in the 3 months "after" CYT. On average this subset of adolescents got another 22 days of treatment (more than the initial dosage). This suggests that while effective, the kind of short-term (6–12 week) approaches used here are not sufficient for all adolescents. While subsequent treatment was not correlated with CYT treatment assignment, it presumably helps to explain at least some part of the additional gains across treatments at the 6-month follow-up.

*Who Will Benefit from Treatment?*

Given the relative efficacy of each treatment, we became interested in exploring more generally, what patient characteristics might predict who benefits from treatment. Babor *et al.* (2002[AQ3]) looked at whether six key patient characteristics had any association with patient dysfunction and whether these characteristics predicted outcome. These characteristics included gender, temperament, age of onset, externalizing distress, internalizing distress, and family history of drug or alcohol dependence. Results indicated that all these patient characteristics, or subtypes, were associated with more dysfunction in a number of domains even when controlling for demographic factors (age and ethnicity). When examining all these characteristics simultaneously (as covariates), externalizing disorder, age of onset, temperament and internalizing disorders continued to add unique variance to discriminating patients with more severe problems. Of all the patient characteristics, only severe externalizing and internalizing distress was associated with poorer outcomes, but only on one of the two dependent measures. Webb *et al.* (2002a) found that involvement in the juvenile justice systems was also associated with more severe drug use and associated problems, but did not mitigate against treatment benefits. Among other things, these findings suggest that greater attention to assessing and treating co-occurring psychiatric distress may potentate treatment and certainly would help with the most severe cases. More importantly, brief outpatient treatment can be effective for substance abusing delinquent teens and should be made more available to this population.

## Treatment Costs

Since this was an effectiveness study designed to provide clinically relevant knowledge, we also evaluated the "economic" cost of each intervention episode (French *et al.*, 2002). In the incremental arm the average cost per episode was $1089 for MET/CBT5, $1256 for MET/CBT12, and $3920 for FSN. In the alternative arm the average cost per episode was $1445 for MET/CBT5, $1459 for ACRA, and $2105 for MDFT. (The time needed to coordinate the groups (MET/CBT5) with low income patients at CHOP increased the over all cost of this condition in this arm.) This gradual increase in cost reflects the gradual increase in patient contact hours and actual staff time. Most importantly, the weekly cost of all five interventions was below the average weekly cost ($267 adjusted to 1999 dollars) reported by directors of outpatient programs in a national survey (Gerstein & Johnson, 1999). It is, therefore, likely that these interventions are economically feasible for behavioral health and substance abuse treatment providers to implement. The cost comparisons are confounded with the unique characteristics of each provider's site (e.g., cost of living, salary, institutional overhead). (See French *et al.*, 2002 for a full description of these issues.)

### Cost-Effectiveness Analysis

Given the differences by condition in cost and the similarity of clinical outcomes, we also considered the economic efficiency with which the conditions achieve their clinical outcomes. Across trials and conditions, the average cost of CYT interventions per day of abstinence achieved over the next 12 months was $8.72 per day and the average cost per person in recovery at the end of the study was $8231.

In Trial 1, the average cost per day of abstinence over the 12 months post intake was $8.79 and varied significantly by condition (Cohen's $f = 0.48$, $p < 0.05$). Based on Tukey range tests, the primary difference was that MET/CBT5 ($4.91) and MET/CBT12 ($6.15) had significantly lower cost per day of abstinence than FSN ($15.13). The average cost per person in recovery at the end of the study was $8846 and varied significantly by condition (Cohen's $f = 0.72$, $p < 0.05$), with MET/CBT5 ($3958) costing significantly less per person in recovery than MET/CBT12 ($7377) and both of the MET/CBT models costing significantly less per person in recovery than FSN ($15,116). In short, MET/CBT5 proved to be more cost effective.

In Trial 2, the average cost per day of abstinence was $8.65 and varied significantly by condition overall (Cohen's $f = 0.22$, $p < 0.05$); while there was a trend for ACRA ($6.62) to have a lower cost per day of abstinence than MET/CBT5 ($9.00) or MDFT ($10.38), the pair-wise comparisons were not significant. When controlling for site differences, MET/CBT5 was actually less cost-effective (i.e., [condition cost − average cost]/[condition effect − average effect]) than ACRA ($26.34 versus $4.10 per additional day of abstinence over average). The average cost per person in recovery at the end of the study was $7615 and varied significantly by condition (Cohen's $f = 0.78$, $p < 0.06$), with ACRA ($4460) being lower than MET/CBT5 ($6611) and both being lower than MDFT ($11,775) in Tukey range tests. While there were still major site differences in magnitude, the above order and significance findings were replicated at Site 3 ($3123 versus $4673 versus $6490; $f = 0.61$) and Site 4 ($6029 versus $8016 versus $17,979; $f = 0.83$, $p < 0.05$). Both across and within sites, ACRA was more cost effective than MET/CBT5 and MDFT and MET/CBT5 was more cost effective than MDFT.

## Therapist's Response to Manualized Treatment

Given the controversy about the applicability of treatment manuals in real world clinical settings, we were interested in exploring therapists' reactions to using treatment manuals. Many have questioned whether manuals can address individual needs of patients, can be applied to patients with complex co-morbidities, and whether manuals will restrict therapists' necessary creative application of psychotherapy (Addis, 1997; Silverman, 1996). To explore these issues from the therapist perspective, we interviewed the 25 CYT providers at the end of the project (Godley *et al.*, 2001b). The manuals varied from highly structured psychoeducational programs (CBT group, FSN parent education) to principle driven individualized treatment (ACRA, MDFT), and so responses varied according to the different manuals.

A major concern by therapists was whether manually guided treatment could address patients' individual needs. By the end of the study, 75% of the therapists felt able to modify the treatment to meet the specific needs of individual patients. These modifications (e.g., using participants' stories as examples) were not viewed as deviations from the manual but rather as appropriate applications of the treatment approach. The CBT and psycho-education therapists felt the most restricted by the manuals, but many providers reported feeling able to easily adapt even this more structured material. Another concern was whether therapists would feel that the manuals restricted their creativity. Few therapists, however, reported feeling confined by the manuals. In fact, most staff welcomed the structure and organization and felt that the manuals provided guidance and focus. In the more structured manuals (CBT group, FSN parent education), therapists accepted the restrictions because they believed the information they were teaching was valuable. Another common misconception is that manualized treatment cannot target complex co-morbid cases. The outcome data, however, suggest that the most complex and severe cases showed similar retention rates and magnitudes of change on key outcome variables to the less complex cases (although they were often still worse off post treatment). Over all, this study suggested that the 25 therapists predominately had positive experiences with the manuals. Interestingly many of the therapists pointed to the intensive supervision that accompanied the manuals as the greatest benefit, suggesting that manuals by themselves may not have as much impact on the practice community if not accompanied by training and supervision.

## Conclusions and Recommendations

The main finding from this study, and the most important message for the field, is that brief, outpatient psychotherapy can be helpful for many adolescents with marijuana abuse or dependence. Not only did treatment work, but it had good retention rates and costs were comparable to–or lower than–estimation of current services (French *et al.*, 2002). There is also evidence to suggest that some treatments are more cost effective than other, although these findings are confounded by the location of this project and the unique context of a research study (rather than a typical clinical setting). However, the costs of these treatments differ in predictable ways associated with their intensity, but all are roughly within the bounds now commonly spent on adolescent outpatient treatment services.

Overall, these findings challenge the unfortunate fiction that treatment for this population is ineffective and undeliverable. The other good news is that these treatments are now manualized and accompanied by training and monitoring guidelines. These manuals can be downloaded for free from the CSAT web site site at http://www.samhsa.gov.csat.csat.htm. These well-designed and structured manuals should facilitate dissemination and training in these treatment approaches. Ideally, however, more efficacy studies will be conducted to garner enough support to consider these treatments empirically supported

(Chambless & Hollon, 1998) which would better position them for future effectiveness and dissemination research.

One might have expected different treatments, or at least those with higher dosage, to be associated with better outcomes. This was neither the case in CYT, nor in many other clinical trials (Luborsky *et al.*, 1975; Project MATCH Research Group, 1997). Several reasons may account for this finding. First, each treatment represents some of the best clinical thinking and modeling available in the field today. Each treatment was founded on strong clinical, if not developmental theory, had well-articulated intervention strategies, and strong empirical support. It is possible that any treatment with this kind of foundation that is brief, intensive, well structured, focused, and programmatic may produce promising results (Koss *et al.*, 1986). Second, although treatments were distinct, each had overlapping elements. In terms of modality, for instance, all three treatments in the alternative arm had individual sessions with the adolescent, and ACRA and MDFT both had meetings alone with the parents. At the level of intervention strategy, both MET/CBT and ACRA used functional analysis, and ACRA and MDFT targeted parenting practices and reducing the adolescent's involvement with deviant peers. In this regard, although these treatments are clearly distinct, the commonalities may be contributing to similar outcomes.

Third, one might have expected that treatment dosage would have contributed to differential treatment outcomes. After all, intended treatment dose ranged from 5 to 22 sessions. However, in practice, other than FSN, adolescents attended on average between four and nine sessions. Although this is long for outpatient services, the difference seems inconsequential over the course of 6–12 months. In fact, data from the adult psychotherapy literature suggest that 50% of patients are measurably improved by the eighth session (Howard *et al.*, 1986). The CYT data, and other studies (Stephens *et al.*, 2000) suggest that "very" brief treatments might be as effective as brief treatments. However, this controversial conclusion warrants more investigation. What does seem apparent is that for adolescents who meet ASAM level I or II, a good assessment and a low dose of treatment (four to eight sessions) can effectively help many adolescents make important reductions in drug use and improvement in functional status. Therefore, more research should focus on the systems of care that refer these adolescent (e.g., improving case identification and referrals success) and on early engagement strategies that can help retain adolescents in short-term treatment.

The CYT team is currently carrying out a number of analyzes to help tease apart the conundrum of no differential treatment outcomes and to better understand the active ingredients of these treatments more generally. Analysis of treatment moderators (substance use severity, delinquency, psychiatric distress, history of trauma, treatment motivation) are being examined to see if different patient characteristics interact with different treatment models. Several studies are looking at mediational factors within and across treatment that may contribute to outcomes (alliance, family functioning or participation, motivation, peer involvement, etc.). Analyzes will also compare the dosage of common treatment processes across approaches that may contribute to change. For example, did the amount of parental involvement, case management services, or an explicit focus on substance use contribute to better treatment outcome regardless of the type of treatment? Finally, the CYT research group was funded to conduct long-term follow-up evaluations (30 months) on all 600 patients. This data will allow us to look at long-term treatment effects and examine the developmental trajectory of these adolescents as they enter young adulthood.

## References

Addis, M. E. (1997). Evaluating the treatment manual as a means of disseminating empirically validated psychotherapies. *Clinical Psychology Science & Practice, 4*, 1–11.

American Society of Addiction Medicine (1996). *Patient placement criteria for the treatment of psychoactive substance disorders* (2nd ed.). Chevy Chase, MD: American Society of Addiction Medicine.

Azrin, N. H. (1976). Improvements in the community-reinforcement approach to alcoholism. *Behavioral Research and Therapy, 14*, 339–348.

Azrin, N. H., Donohue, B., Besalel, V. A., Kogan, E. S., & Acierno, R. (1994). Youth drug abuse treatment: a controlled outcome study. *Journal of Child and Adolescent Substance Abuse, 3*, 1–16.

Babor, T. F., Webb, C. P. M., Burleson, J. A., & Kaminer, Y. (2002). Subtypes for classifying adolescents with marijuana use disorders: construct validity and clinical implications. *Addiction, 97*, S58–S69.

Bukstein, O. G., Glancy, L. J., & Kaminer, Y. (1992). Patterns of affective comorbidity in a clinical population of dually diagnosed adolescent substance abusers. *Journal of the American Academy of Child and Adolescent Psychiatry, 31*, 1041–1045.

Bureau of Justice Statistics (BJS) (2000). *Sourcebook of criminal justice statistics 1999* (27th ed.). Washington, DC: U.S. Department of Justice.

Center for Substance Abuse Treatment (1993). *Guidelines for the treatment of alcohol and other drug-abusing adolescents* (DHHS Publication No. 93-2010, Treatment Improvement Protocol Series, Volume 4). Rockville, MD: U.S. Department of Health and Human Services.

Chambless, D. L., & Hollon, S. D. (1998). Defining empirically supported therapies. *Journal of Consulting and Clinical Psychology, 66*(1), 7–18.

270                                                    *Guy Diamond* et al.

Crowley, T. J., & Riggs, P. D. (1995). Adolescent substance use disorder with conduct disorder and comorbid conditions. In E. R. Rahdert, & D. Czechowicz (Eds.), *Adolescent drug abuse: clinical assessment and therapeutic intervention* (pp. 49–111). Rockville, MD: National Institute on Drug Abuse.

Dakof, G. A. (2000). Understanding gender differences in adolescent drug abuse: issues of comorbidity and family functioning. *Journal of Psychoactive Drugs, 32*, 25–32.

Dennis, M. L. (1999). *Global Appraisal of Individual Needs (GAIN): administration guide for the GAIN and related measures.* Bloomington: IL Chestnut Health Systems. Available at: www.chestnut.org/li/gain.

Dennis, M. L., Godley, S., & Titus, J. (1999). Co-occurring psychiatric problems among adolescents: variations by treatment, level of care and gender. *TIE Communiqué*, 5–8.

Dennis, M. L., Babor, T., Roebuck, C., & Donaldson, J. (2002a). Changing the focus: the case for recognizing and treating marijuana use disorders. *Addiction, 97*(Suppl. I), 4–15.

Dennis, M. L, Dawud-Noursi, S., Muck, R., & McDermeit, M. (2003). The need for developing and evaluating adolescent treatment models. In S. J. Stevens, & A. R. Morral (Eds.), *Adolescent substance abuse treatment in the United States: exemplary models from a national evaluation study* (pp. 3–56). Binghamton, NY: Haworth Press.

Dennis, M. L., Titus, J. C., Diamond, G., Donaldson, J., Godley, S. H., Tims, F., et al. (2002b). The Cannabis Youth Treatment (CYT) experiment: rationale, study design, and analysis plans. *Addiction, 97*(Suppl. I), 16–34.

Dennis, M, Godley, S. H, Diamond, G. D., Tims, F., Babor, T., Donaldson, J., Liddle, H. L., Titus, J. C., Kaminer, Y., Webb, C., Hamilton, N., & Funk, R. (2004). The Cannabis Youth Treatment (CYT) study: main findings from two randomized trials. *Journal of Substance Abuse Treatment, 27*, 197–213.

Diamond, G. S., & Liddle, H. A. (1996). Resolving a therapeutic impasse between parents and adolescents in multidimensional family therapy. *Journal of Consulting and Clinical Psychology, 64*(3), 481–488.

Diamond, G. S., & Liddle, H. A. (1999). Transforming negative parent–adolescent interactions: from impasse to dialogue. *Family Process, 38*(1), 5–26.

Diamond, G. M., Diamond, G. S., & Liddle, H. A. (2000). The therapist–parent alliance in family-based therapy for adolescents. *Journal of Clinical Psychology, 56*(8), 1037–1050.

Diamond, G. S., Godley, S. H., Liddle, H. A., Sampl, S., Webb, C., Tims, F. M., et al. (2002). Five outpatient treatment models for adolescent marijuana use: a description of the Cannabis Youth Treatment Interventions. *Addiction, 97*(Suppl. I), 70–83.

El Sholy, M. A., Ross, S. A., Mehmedic, Z., Arafat, R., Bao, Y., & Banahan, B. F. (2000). Potency trends of delta9-THC and other cannabinoids in confiscated marijuana from 1980–1997. *Journal of Forensic Science, 45*, 24–30.

Fergusson, D. M., Lynsky, M. T., & Horwood, L. J. (1996). The short-term consequences of early onset cannabis use. *Journal of Abnormal Child Psychology, 24*, 499–512.

French, M. T., Roebuck, M. C., Dennis, M. L., Diamond, G., Godley, S. H., Tims, F., *et al.* (2002). The economic cost of outpatient marijuana treatment for adolescents: findings from a multi-site field experiment. *Addiction, 97*(Suppl. I), 84–97.

Gerstein, D. R., & Johnson, R. A. (1999). *Adolescents and young adults in the National Treatment Improvement Evaluation Study.* Rockville, MD: Center for Substance Abuse Treatment.

Godley, S. H., Godley, M. D., Pratt, A., & Wallace, J. L. (1994). Case management services for adolescent substance abusers: a program description. *Journal of Substance Abuse Treatment, 11*, 309–317.

Godley, S. H., Meyers, R. J., Smith, J. E., Godley, M. D., Titus, J. M., Karvinen, T., *et al.* (2001a). *The Adolescent Community Reinforcement Approach for adolescent cannabis users* (DHHS Publication No. (SMA) 01–3489, Cannabis Youth Treatment (CYT) Series, Volume 4). Rockville, MD: Center for Substance Abuse Treatment, Substance Abuse and Mental Health Services Administration. Available online at: http://www.chestnut.org\li\cyt\findings or at www.health.org.

Godley, S. H., White, W. L., Diamond, G. S., Passeti, L., & Titus, J. C. (2001b). Therapist reactions to manual-guided therapies for the treatment of adolescent marijuana users. *Clinical Psychology: Science and Practice, 8*, 405–417.

Grella, C. E., Hser, Y. I., Joshi, V., Rounds-Bryant, J. (2001). Drug treatment outcomes for adolescents with comorbid mental and substance use disorders. *Journal of Nervous and Mental Disease, 189*(6), 384–392.

Hamilton, N., Brantley, L., Tims, F., Angelovich, N., & McDougall, B. (2001). *Family Support Network (FSN) for adolescent cannabis users* (DHHS Publication No. (SMA) 01–3488, Cannabis Youth Treatment (CYT) Manual Series, Volume 3). Rockville, MD: Center for Substance Abuse Treatment, Substance Abuse and Mental Health Services Administration. Available online at http://www.chestnut. org\li\cyt\findings or at www.health.org.

Henggeler, S. W., Borduin, C. M., Melton, G. B., Mann, B. J., Smith, L. A., Hall, J. A., *et al.* (1991). Effects of multisystemic therapy on drug use and abuse in serious juvenile offenders: a progress report from two outcomes studies. *Family Dynamics of Addiction Quarterly, 1*, 40–51.

Hofler, M., Lieb, R., Perkonigg, A., & Schuster, P. (1999). Covariates of cannabis use progress in a representative sample of adolescents: a prospective examination of vulnerability and risk factors. *Addiction, 94*, 1679–1694.

Hogue, A., Liddle, H. A., Rowe, C., Turner, R. M., Dakof, G. A., & Lapann, K. (1998). Treatment adherence and differentiation in individual versus family therapy for adolescent substance abuse. *Journal of Counseling Psychology, 45*(1), 104–114.

Howard, K. I., Kopta, S. M., Krause, M. S., & Orlinsky, D. E. (1986). The dose-effect relationship in psychotherapy. *American Psychologist, 41*, 159–164.

Hser, Y. I., Grella, C. E., Hubbard, R. L., Hsieh, S. C., Fletcher, B. W., Brown, B. S., & Anglin, M. D. (2001). An evaluation of drug treatments for adolescents in four U.S. cities. *Archives of General Psychiatry, 58*, 689–695.

Jackson-Gilfort, A., & Liddle, H. A., (1999). Using culturally syntonic themes to enhance engagement of African-American males in family therapy. *Family Psychologist*, *15*, 6–12.

Koss, M. P., Butcher, J. N., & Strupp, H. H. (1986.) Brief psychotherapy methods in clinical research. *Journal of Consulting & Clinical Psychology*, *54*, 60–67.

Liddle, H. A. (1999). Theory development in a family-based therapy for adolescent drug abuse. *Journal of Clinical Child Psychiatry*, *28*, 521–532.

Liddle, H. A. (2002). *Multidimensional Family Therapy (MDFT) for adolescent cannabis users* (DHHS Publication No. (SMA) 02–3660, Cannabis Youth Treatment (CYT) Manual Series, Volume 5). Rockville, MD: Center for Substance Abuse Treatment, Substance Abuse and Mental Health Services Administration. Available online at http://www.chestnut.org\li\cyt\findings or at www.health.org.

Liddle, H. A., & Hogue, A. (2000). A developmental, family-based, ecological preventive intervention for antisocial behavior in high-risk adolescents. *Journal of Marital and Family Therapy*, *26*, 265–279.

Liddle, H. A., Rowe, C., Diamond, G. M., Sessa, F., Schmidt, S., & Ettinger, D. (2000). Towards a developmental family therapy: The clinical utility of adolescent development research. *Journal of Marital and Family Therapy*, *26*(4), 491–505.

Liddle, H. A., Dakof, G. A., Parker, K., Diamond, G. S., Barrett, K., & Tejeda, M. (2001). Multidimensional family therapy for adolescent substance abuse: results of a randomized clinical trial. *American Journal of Drug and Alcohol Abuse*, *27*(4), 651–687.

Liddle, H. A., Rodriguez, R. A. Dakof, G. A. Kanzki, E., & Marvel, F. A. (2005). Multidimensional family therapy: a science-based treatment for adolescent drug abuse. In J. Lebow (Ed.), *Handbook of clinical family therapy* (pp. 128–163). New York: John Wiley & Sons.

Luborsky, L., Singer, B., & Luborsky, L. (1975). Comparative studies of psychotherapy: it is true that "everybody has won and all must have prizes." *Archives of General Psychiatry*, *32*, 995–1008.

McLellan, A. T., Hagan, T. A., Levine, M., Meyers, K., Gould, F., Bencivengo, M., *et al.* (1999). Does clinical case management improve outpatient addiction treatment? *Drug and Alcohol Dependence*, *55*, 91–103.

Meyers, R. J., & Smith, J. E. (1995). *Clinical guide to alcohol Treatment: the community reinforcement approach*. New York: The Guilford Press.

Meyers, R. J., Miller, W. R., Hill, D. E., & Tonigan, J. S. (1999). Community reinforcement and family training (CRAFT): engaging unmotivated drug users in treatment. *Journal of Substance Abuse*, *10*(3), 291–308.

Miller, W. R., & Rollnick, S. (1991). *Motivational interviewing: preparing people to change addictive behavior*. New York: Guilford Press.

Minuchin, S. (1974). *Families and family therapy*. Cambridge, MA: Harvard Press.

Monitoring the Future (MTF) (2000). *Percent Past-year Drug and Alcohol Use among Twelfth Graders: 1975–2000 Monitoring the Future*. Available online at: www.monitoringthefuture.org.

Monti, P. M., Abrams, D. B., Kadden, R. M., & Cooney, N. L. (1989). *Treating alcohol dependence: a coping skills training guide.* New York: Guilford Press.

National Institute of Justice (2001). *Preventing crime: what works, what doesn't, what's promising.* Washington, DC: National Institute of Justice.

Newcomb, M., & Bentler, P. (1988). *Consequences of adolescent drug use: impact on lives of young adults.* Newbury Park, CA: Sage.

Newcomb, M. D., Maddahian, E., Bentler, P. M. (1986). Risk factors for drug use among adolescents: concurrent and longitudinal analyses. *American Journal of Public Health, 76,* 525–531.

Office of Applied Studies (2000). *Year-end 1999 medical examiner data from the Drug Abuse Warning Network (DAWN).* DAWN Series, D-16. Rockville, MD: Substance Abuse and Mental Health Services Administration.

Ozechowski, T. J., & Liddle, H. A. (2000). Family-based therapy for adolescent drug abuse: knowns and unknowns. *Clinical Child and Family Psychology Review, 3,* 269–298.

Prochaska, J. O., &. DiClemente, C. C. (1984). *The transtheoretical approach: crossing traditional boundaries of therapy.* Homewood, IL: Dow Jones/Irwin.

Project MATCH Research Group (1997). Matching alcoholism treatments to client heterogeneity: project MATCH post-treatment drinking outcomes. *Journal of Studies on Alcohol, 58*(1), 7–29.

Robins, L. N., & McEvoy, L. (1990). Conduct problems as predictors of substance abuse. In L. N. Robins, & M. Rutter (Eds.), *Straight and devious pathways from childhood to adulthood* (pp. 182–204). Cambridge: Cambridge University Press.

Sampl, S., & Kadden, R. (2001). *Motivational Enhancement Therapy and Cognitive Behavioral Therapy (MET-CBT-5) for adolescent cannabis users* (DHHS Publication No. (SMA) 01–3486, Cannabis Youth Treatment (CYT) Manual Series, Volume 1). Rockville, MD: Center for Substance Abuse Treatment, Substance Abuse and Mental Health Services Administration. Available online at http://www.chestnut.org\li\cyt\findings or at www.health.org.

Schmidt, S., Liddle, H. A., & Dakof, G. (1996). Changes in parenting practices during multidimensional family therapy. *Journal of Family Psychology, 10,* 12–27.

Siegal, H. A., & Rapp, R. C. (1996). Introduction: In H. A. Siegal, & R. C. Rapp (Eds.), *Case management and substance abuse treatment.* New York: Springer Publishing.

Siemens, A. J. (1980). Effects of cannabis in combination with ethanol and other drugs. In R. C. Petersen (Ed.), *Marijuana research findings* (pp. 37–39). Rockville, MD: National Institute on Drug Abuse.

Silverman, W. H. (1996). Cookbooks, manuals, and paint-by-numbers: psychotherapies in the 90s. *Psychotherapy, 33,* 207–215.

Simpson, D. D., Savage, L. J., & Sells, S. B. (1978). *Data book on drug treatment outcomes. Follow-up study of the 1969–1977 admissions to the Drug Abuse Reporting Program.* Fort Worth, TX: Texas Christian University.

Stanton, M. D., & Todd, T. C. (1982). _The family therapy of drug abuse and addiction._ New York: Guilford Press.

Stephens, R. S., Roffman, R. A., & Curtin, L. (2000). Comparison of extended versus brief treatments for marijuana use. _Journal of Consulting and Clinical Psychology,_ _68,_ 898–908.

Webb, C. P., Burleson, J. A., & Ungemack, J. A. (2002a). Treating juvenile offenders for marijuana problems. _Addiction, 97_(Suppl. I), 35–45.

Webb, C., Scudder, M., Kaminer, Y., Kadden, R., & Tawfik, Z. (2002b). _The MET/CBT_ _5 Supplement: 7 sessions of Cognitive Behavioral Therapy (CBT 7) for adolescent_ _cannabis users_ (DHHS Publication No. (SMA) 02-3659, Cannabis Youth Treatment (CYT) Manual Series, Volume 2). Rockville, MD: Center for Substance Abuse Treatment, Substance Abuse and Mental Health Services Administration. Available online at http://www.chestnut.org\li\cyt\findings or at www.health.org.

Williams, R. C., & Chang, S. Y. (2000). A comprehensive and comparative review of adolescent substance abuse treatment outcomes. _Clinical Psychology: Science and_ _Practice, 7,_ 138–166.

World Health Organization (WHO) (1997). _Cannabis: a health perspective and research_ _agenda._ Geneva, Switzerland: World Health Organization.

# 12

# The Teen Cannabis Check-Up: Exploring Strategies for Reaching Young Cannabis Users

JAMES P. BERGHUIS, WENDY SWIFT, ROGER A. ROFFMAN, ROBERT S. STEPHENS AND JAN COPELAND

This chapter describes a motivational enhancement therapy (MET) intervention tailored to reach young people who use cannabis, motivate them to voluntarily participate in a confidential assessment and evaluation of the impact of cannabis on their lives, and offer support to those who wish to quit or reduce use. After a review of the need for brief interventions and the rationale for using a MET approach with adolescents, we provide an overview of the structure, components, and delivery of the "check-up" approach. This chapter concludes with a description of the application of this approach in two studies recently completed in the USA and Australia.

## Epidemiology of Adolescent Cannabis Use

Cannabis is so readily available and widely used that experimentation with the drug could be regarded as a normative experience among many young people. A general trend toward increased cannabis use for much of the 1990s was particularly marked among teenagers, possibly due to its ready availability and declining perceptions of risk (e.g., Johnston *et al.*, 2003; Makkai & McAllister, 1997). Despite an apparent slight decrease in use, it remains the most commonly used illicit drug among young people in the USA (Substance Abuse and Mental Health Administration, Office of Applied Studies (SAMHSA), 2003), Australia (Australian Institute of Health and Welfare (AIHW), 2002), New Zealand (Wilkins *et al.*, 2002) and the European Union (European Monitoring Centre for Drugs and Drug Addiction (EMCDDA), 2003; Ramsay & Partridge, 1999). In 2003, 8% of US 8th graders (aged 13–14 years) had used cannabis in the past month (Johnston *et al.*, 2003). In 2001, recent cannabis use was as common as tobacco use among 14–17-year-old Australians (approximately 20%) (AIHW, 2002).

While most cannabis use remains experimental and irregular, the incidence and intensity of use typically increases over the mid-to-late teens (e.g., Coffey

276                                              *James P. Berghuis* et al.

*et al.*, 2000; Perkonnig *et al.*, 1999; Poulton *et al.*, 1997), before a decline in use from the mid-20s (Bachman *et al.*, 1997; Chen & Kandel, 1995). Nevertheless, a minority of young people report use patterns that increase the likelihood of long-term use and dependence, regular use of other drugs, and exposure to cannabis-related harms (e.g., AIHW, 2002; Golub & Johnson, 2001; Johnston *et al.*, 2003; Perkonnig *et al.*, 1999; Poulton *et al.*, 1997). Thus, 6% of US high school 12th graders report daily cannabis use (Johnston *et al.*, 2003), and 19.1% and 11.6% of 14–19-year-old Australian cannabis users report at least weekly and daily use, respectively (AIHW, 2002).

Numerous factors may modify the natural history of cannabis use (e.g., Hall *et al.*, 1999). While young males typically report more frequent and heavier use, gender differences may be decreasing (Perkonnig *et al.*, 1999; Wilkins *et al.*, 2002). For example, in Australia, between 1995 and 1998, the number of 14–19-year-old females who had ever used cannabis or used it in the last year nearly doubled from 11.6% to 19.5% (Reid *et al.*, 2000). Research also indicates that an earlier age of initiation and frequent cannabis use predict the escalation and persistence of use (e.g., Coffey *et al.*, 2000; DeWit *et al.*, 2000; Perkonnig *et al.*, 1999; Poulton *et al.*, 1997). There is evidence that the age of initiation of cannabis use is decreasing among more recent birth cohorts (Degenhardt *et al.*, 2000; Hall & Swift, 2000; SAMHSA, 2003).

**Negative Consequences of Adolescent Cannabis Use**

Although experimentation is a normal part of adolescent development, young people who regularly use cannabis may risk negative effects at a time of rapid development and transitions in life roles. This may interfere with their options and choices in a range of areas in their lives, now and in the future.

In particular, earlier and/or greater involvement with cannabis is associated with an increased risk of problems such as impaired mental health, delinquency, lower-educational achievement, problematic use of other substances, risky sexual behavior and criminal offending (e.g., Arsenault *et al.*, 2002; Brook *et al.*, 1999; Fergusson & Horwood, 1997, 2000b; D. Fergusson *et al.*, 1994; D. M. Fergusson *et al.*, 2002; Lynskey *et al.*, 2003; McGee & Newcomb, 1992). There is no simple cause and effect relationship between the extent of cannabis use and other outcomes. Rather, these associations primarily arise because of common or overlapping risk factors and life pathways among young people who may be predisposed to cannabis use and those at increased risks of these other outcomes (e.g., Hall *et al.*, 1999; Lynskey & Hall, 2000).

Young people may be significantly more likely to develop cannabis dependence for a given dose than adults (Kandel *et al.*, 1997). The population prevalence of cannabis dependence and abuse increases throughout adolescence, up to levels of 10% among young adults (e.g., Coffey *et al.*, 2002; Fergusson & Horwood, 2000a; Perkonnig *et al.*, 1999; Poulton *et al.*, 1997). As spontaneous remission of cannabis use may be somewhat rare among adolescent regular cannabis users (Perkonnig *et al.*, 1999), there is a significant group who may benefit from assistance in order to overcome cannabis-related problems including abuse or dependence.

## Intervention Research with Adolescents

Currently, few young people who might benefit from professional assistance for their substance use choose to access relevant services. Fewer than 10% of adolescents reporting substance use disorder symptoms in the past year have ever received treatment (Titus & Godley, 1999) and self-referral is uncommon, with most referred by family, or the educational or juvenile justice systems (e.g., Brody & Waldron, 2000). Traditional intervention approaches for this group include: (1) 12-step (abstinence-based disease model); (2) behavioral (cognitive behavioral and other learning models); (3) family-based (therapy models in which the family system is seen as critical in the development and maintenance of substance abuse problems); and (4) therapeutic communities (intensive residential treatment for severe substance abuse problems) (Titus & Godley, 1999). Rigorous evaluations of the effectiveness of adolescent substance abuse treatments have recently been completed or are currently in progress, with greatly increased attention having been devoted to this population in recent years. Manualized therapies are now becoming available for dissemination to the field. Prior to the late 1990s, the conclusions of the few published studies had been limited by methodological problems (Deas & Thomas, 2001).

Outpatient treatments for young people have had mixed success in reducing cannabis use (see Center for Substance Abuse Research, 2000a, for review). The Treatment Outcome Prospective Study (TOPS) of 87 adolescents, for example, compared daily cannabis use in the year prior to, and the year following, treatment. It found a reduction of 42% for those receiving less than 3 months of treatment and an increase of 13% among those who received 3 or more months of treatment (Hubbard *et al.*, 1985, 1989). The Services Research Outcome Study found that cannabis use increased 2–9% among 156 adolescents in the 5 years after they received any kind of treatment (Office of Applied Studies, 1995).

However, two recent studies, the National Treatment Improvement Evaluation Study ($n = 236$) and the Drug Abuse Treatment Outcome Study – Adolescents ($n = 445$), found reductions in cannabis use of 10–18% and 21–25%, respectively, in the year following outpatient treatment (Center for Substance Abuse Treatment, 2000b; Powers *et al.*, 1999). The lack of untreated control groups in these studies makes it difficult to evaluate the outcomes. Treatment may be helpful, but relapse rates are high (20–50%), retention in treatment is problematic, and long-term outcomes are unknown (Titus & Godley, 1999).

Preliminary outcome data from the Cannabis Youth Treatment (CYT) project, a rigorous, multi-site intervention study of 600 young cannabis users aged between 12 and 18 years, compare favorably with previous studies (Center for Substance Abuse Research, 2000a; Dennis *et al.*, 1998). Participants were randomized to one of five outpatient interventions of varying type and intensity. A non-treatment control condition was not included in the design. Compared to intake, at 6 months there was an increase in reported abstinence, and decreases in symptoms of cannabis abuse or dependence and a range of other behavior problems (e.g., truancy, criminal justice involvement, school problems, family problems, and violence). There was some evidence for differential effectiveness of the five treatments by problem severity, with the briefest treatment being more effective among low-severity adolescents, and longer, more intensive interventions most effective with high-severity adolescents. Otherwise, little difference was found across the treatment conditions; 30- and 42-month follow-up assessments are also underway. While the CYT offers a menu of effective treatments, the results may apply primarily to treatment-seeking adolescents, many of whom may have been coerced into treatment in various ways. Interventions tailored to attract and enhance motivation in non-treatment-seeking adolescents have not been developed or studied systematically.

Several recent studies have shown promise utilizing brief MET approaches with adolescent substance users. MET refers to counseling that incorporates motivational interviewing, defined as "a directive, client-centered counseling style for eliciting behavior change by helping clients to explore and resolve ambivalence" (Rollnick & Miller, 1995, p. 325). In a study using MET as an adjunct to standard substance use treatment, treatment-seeking adolescents with polysubstance use problems who received MET prior to treatment attended more sessions, and had more days of abstinence and decreased drug use at follow-up than those who did not (Aubrey, 1997). Monti *et al.* (1999) used MET with adolescent drinkers in an emergency room setting and demonstrated reductions in alcohol use, drinking and driving, traffic violations, and alcohol-related injuries and problems. Colby *et al.* (1998a) compared brief advice and brief MET with adolescent tobacco smokers in an emergency room setting. While both groups reduced their days of smoking and levels of nicotine dependence, there were no significant differences between interventions. Promising results have come from a British randomized-controlled trial, in which young college students who received a single session of motivational interviewing showed reductions in cannabis and other drug use compared to those receiving their normal college education but no intervention specifically targeting drug use (McCambridge & Strang, 2004). More research is needed to examine whether MET is more efficacious than standard brief interventions in reducing cannabis and other substance use among adolescents.

**Developmental Issues in Designing Interventions for Adolescents**

Adolescence is a period of profound physical, cognitive, and social changes that need to be considered when developing interventions. Developmental tasks of adolescence include increasing psychological autonomy, expanding social roles, development of the capacity for intimacy, and the formation of value systems and life goals (Kimmel & Weiner, 1995). In addition, developmental variations occur in younger versus older adolescents in peer influence, maturation, and cognitive, affective, and social development. Peer influence, for example, tends to peak in early adolescence (11–14) years and then declines, and the ability to think abstractly and about future consequences begins to develop at age 12. Interventions directed toward adolescents need to address contextual factors that are different from those of adults. These factors include the influence of perceived peer group norms on behavior; shorter histories of cannabis use (with fewer negative health effects apparent); higher rates of binge and opportunistic use than is the case with adults (Dennis, 2002); and developmentally different affective, cognitive, decision-making, and planning processes (Irwin & Millstein, 1986). Data from treated adolescent samples indicate that when compared to adults in treatment, adolescents manifest higher rates of depression, anxiety, traumatic distress, attention deficit disorder, hyperactivity, conduct disorders, and crime and violence (Dennis, 2002). As with adults, stage of change must be considered with adolescents because use of inappropriate intervention strategies is likely to promote resistance (Werner, 1995). This may be especially important in working with adolescents for whom motivation may be even more variable and fluid a concept than with adults. Understanding these developmental and contextual factors will facilitate designing interventions that are flexible in their delivery and

280                                          *James P. Berghuis* et al.

allow for variations in developmental stage and the salient issues influencing cannabis use for different adolescents. Some adolescents are likely to benefit most from an emphasis in the intervention on peer factors and concrete, short-term consequences of cannabis use and its cessation. In contrast, adolescents who can think more abstractly, and can hypothetically plan ahead and weigh future consequences and options may benefit more from interventions that utilize these abilities to explore ambivalence and to enhance motivation for change. Interventions that take into account these individual differences and offer a somewhat flexible approach are likely to effectively reach and motivate change in a diverse range of adolescents. The check-up approach, described in the following section, is designed to meet these criteria.

**The Check-up: Tailoring an Intervention for Adolescent Cannabis Users**

The Teen Cannabis Check-Up, modeled after the Drinkers' Check-Up for problem drinkers (Miller & Sovereign, 1989), is a two-session assessment and feedback intervention developed to reach cannabis users who are neither self-initiating change nor seeking treatment. In the initial session, assessment data are collected concerning the participant's cannabis, alcohol, and other drug use in the past 90 days; recent treatment; positive and negative consequences of cannabis use; the individual's life goals; readiness for change; and other attitudinal measures of interest. This information is used to prepare a Personalized Feedback Report (PFR) that is reviewed with the participant in the feedback session conducted approximately 1 week later.

While reviewing the PFR with the participant during the feedback session, the counselor uses motivational interviewing strategies (e.g., open-ended questions, reflections, reframing, and avoidance of argumentation) to elicit the participant's active and candid involvement in the session (Lawendowski, 1998; Miller & Rollnick, 1991). The general focus is on encouraging the teen to explore the personal meaning and implications of the information in an open and balanced fashion. Expressions of motivation for change are reinforced and resistance is avoided by giving attention to motivation both favoring and opposing change. If participants clearly express a desire to change their cannabis use, the counselor supports their efficacy by discussing various change options, including self-managed change or referrals to local drug treatment providers. The counselor also facilitates a process of goal setting and strategizing, including completion of a Change Plan Worksheet and discussion of handouts describing a range of behavior change actions. An additional session may be offered for further support, as needed.

The feedback session includes a number of key elements intended to facilitate the client's candid evaluation of their experiences with cannabis:

1. *Building rapport*: The counselor assists the young person to feel safe and supported through a consistently warm, accepting, and non-judgmental interactional style.

2. *Acknowledging benefits*: The young person's positive feelings about cannabis use are explored in a balanced and non-threatening manner, without imposing any assumptions about it being a problem.

3. *Reviewing the individual's use pattern*: The participant's typical pattern of cannabis use is discussed in the context of comparative information concerning the prevalence and frequency of cannabis use by other young people. If the validity of the comparative data is questioned, the counselor doesn't argue about their accuracy, but rather reflects the participant's feelings while considering the comparisons. Subsequently, alcohol and other drug use patterns are also reviewed.

4. *Acknowledging adverse consequences*: While reviewing adverse consequences associated with cannabis, resistance is minimized by talking about "less good things" rather than "problems". Each "less good" response is inquired about and the young person is encouraged to elaborate. An integrative summary of positive and negative things about cannabis smoking for the young person is presented to highlight the decisional balance. (For example, "So, smoking cannabis helps you relax and you enjoy smoking with friends. On the other hand, you feel less motivated when you smoke and its interfering with your school work.")

5. *Anticipating consequences of reduced use*: The counselor reviews the young person's responses to an assessment item that asked what costs and benefits they anticipated *if* they were to decide to quit or reduce their cannabis use (the pros and cons of increasing their use also may be explored).

6. *Identifying supportive relationships*: Important people in the young person's life – people they feel they can count on when having a problem – are identified to get a snapshot of how cannabis use is related to those with whom the teen has key relationships. This is a useful way to find out whether key people in their life know about their cannabis use and what those individuals' opinions are about this (or their expected opinions, if they were to find out).

7. *Identifying goals and aspirations*: The counselor explores the participant's goals for the future, their confidence in being able to attain their goals, and the anticipated effects of their cannabis use on the likelihood their goals will be met.

The focus of the feedback session then shifts to a consideration of decisions concerning future cannabis use. The counselor summarizes the key information covered in the PFR and asks the young person about their current thoughts about cannabis, attempting to elicit problem recognition, concern, and intention to change statements. The decisional process includes *whether* to do something, *what* to do (goals), and *how* to go about achieving the goals (change strategies). The counselor does not rush the teen into premature decision-making, and if the participant appears unready to make a decision, additional time may be devoted to exploring ambivalence. If the young person is ready to consider changes, the counselor helps the teen think through and clearly articulate the reasons they perceive their current level of cannabis use is too high. The counselor supports their self-efficacy for change and assists in the identification of specific goals, strategies, and potential challenges to making changes. For those who want to reduce but not quit, beginning by quitting for a specified period of time (e.g., 30 days) may be recommended as an initial step so that the person can get practice saying "no" and abstaining, then revisiting the issue of finding a reduced level of smoking that works for them after this time has passed. Clinical experience suggests this method is more effective for some people with alcohol problems compared with reducing use immediately and it may be the case for cannabis as well (Sanchez-Craig, 1995). Additional skills training may occur to support the young person's efforts, and handouts (e.g., description of coping skills, meeting schedules of relevant self-help groups) also may be reviewed and distributed as appropriate. The question, "How would you know if you were using too much?" is raised with the young person who does not see their current cannabis use as problematic or is not ready to make a change in their use. The purpose is to help them consider and articulate indicators that would tell them they are smoking too much cannabis. It is important to avoid the implication that the counselor expects them to reach this point, instead emphasizing that this is a precaution to help them guard against the types of problems they have successfully avoided so far. In ending the session, the counselor affirms the young person's effort and willingness to take the time to look at their cannabis use, responds to any remaining questions, and discusses referrals as appropriate.

**US and Australian Studies in Progress**

The remainder of this chapter will describe variations of cannabis check-up interventions tailored for adolescents. Common issues in implementing the check-up approach also will be discussed. The US Teen Marijuana Check-Up was funded by National Institute on Drug Abuse (NIDA) as an exploratory study of a MET intervention with adolescent cannabis smokers. The Australian study was funded by the Australian Government's Department of Health and Ageing's Illicit Drugs Strategy.

Both interventions involve two sessions and are tailored to attract young people in the pre-contemplation (not yet considering behavior change) or contemplation (conflicted feelings about use, weighing pros and cons of use) stages of Prochaska and DiClemente's stage of change model (Prochaska & DiClemente, 1983), and promoting increased motivation to change. In both countries, the design for evaluating the interventions has involved single group, pre–post designs, with no comparison or control group. A unique feature of the Australian study is that it offers adolescents who meet diagnostic criteria for cannabis abuse or dependence the opportunity to participate in a subsequent trial involving randomization to a single skills-based strategy session or placement on a 3-month wait-list.

Both check-up programs developed a variety of informational materials for both young people and those who are concerned about them (concerned others, COs). These included a project brochure, business cards, a booklet targeted at young people, and COs describing current knowledge about the health and psychological effects of cannabis, a "communication tips" booklet on how to effectively share cannabis-related concerns with a young person, a videotape of effective and less effective communication style vignettes, and a booklet on coping strategies for young people who would like to make changes in their cannabis use.

### Recruitment Approaches

Recruitment of participants in the USA primarily involved adolescents self-referring or being referred by teachers and counselors. Project staff visited high school classrooms in order to deliver guest talks on cannabis and its effects on health and behavior. The talks included a description of the Teen Marijuana Check-Up, highlighted the confidential and no-pressure nature of this program, and made it possible for interested individuals to notify staff of their interest by writing their names on the bottom of an anonymous guest talk evaluation form collected from all students at the end of the class. Importantly, Institutional Review Board (IRB) approval was granted to waive parental consent following a review of applicable state and federal law. The researchers had argued that requiring parental consent would likely prevent voluntary enrollment by many cannabis-using adolescents.

During a 7-month recruitment period, 92 adolescents expressed interest by contacting project staff. Eighty-five percent ($n = 78$) completed a screening interview and 90% of these individuals ($n = 70$) were both eligible and interested. All of those found ineligible ($n = 8$) failed to meet the inclusion criteria of having smoked cannabis at least once in the past 30 days. Eighty-seven percent ($n = 61$) of the 70 eligible and interested adolescents attended their baseline assessment session. Seventy-seven percent ($n = 54$) completed all study components (i.e., baseline assessment, feedback session, and follow-up assessment sessions).

Recruitment of participants in Australia primarily targeted adults who were concerned about an adolescent's cannabis use. The program was designed to assist the adult in communicating their concern to the adolescent and then referring him or her to the check-up. Referred to as COs, the Australian program marketed its program through drug and alcohol agencies, community service agencies, telephone helplines, school/college counselors, as well as targeted media and advertising in newspapers, industry newsletters and magazines, and on the National Drug and Alcohol Research Centre's web site.

In a 24-month period, the Australian program was contacted by more than 300 people, 178 completed screening; 135 were eligible to participate and 109 eligible family groups, comprising 73 young people and 62 CO, were enrolled in the study. The main reasons for ineligibility of young people were: age (too young or old), heavy alcohol consumption, and severe psychiatric impairment. The majority of enrolled young people ($n = 65/73$; 87.7%) were referred by a CO, predominantly parents ($n = 50$), but also other relatives or partners ($n = 4$), and schools ($n = 10$). A small number were self-referred ($n = 9$; 12.3%). Ninety percent ($n = 66$) of the enrolled participants completed both check-up sessions.

## *Characteristics of Enrolled Teens*

Characteristics of the participants in the US and Australian programs are presented in Table 12.1. For both groups the typical participant was a white male who lived with his parents, although the Australian sample was slightly older than its US counterpart. While all US participants were currently attending secondary school, a proportion of the Australian sample was not in school and was unemployed (8.2%) or working full time (13.9%).

Cannabis use had commenced in the early teens for both groups (mean of 13 years), although on average the Australian participants reported smoking cannabis more frequently than their US peers (21.5 days versus 10.3 days out of the last 30; range: 1–30 days for both groups). One in five Australian participants (19.2%) had smoked every day in this time, compared to only one participant

Table 12.1. *Participant demographics*

| Variable | US sample ($n = 54$) | Australian sample ($n = 73$) |
|---|---|---|
| *Sex, n (%)* | | |
| Males | 39 (72.2) | 56 (76.7) |
| Females | 15 (27.8) | 17 (23.3) |
| *Age,* Mean (SD) | 15.43 (1.02) | 16.4 (1.5) |
| *Race/ethnicity,[a] n (%)* | | *Country of birth* |
| White | 36 (66.7) | Australia: 59 (80.8) |
| Hispanic | 4 (7.5) | Indigenous: 0 (0) |
| African-American | 6 (11.1) | Overseas: 14 (19.2) |
| Asian-American | 1 (1.9) | |
| Multi-racial/other | 7 (13) | |
| *Current education,[b] n (%)* | | |
| Attending school | 54 (100) | 40 (54.8) |
| Other educational | 0 (0) | 6 (8.2) |
| *Stage of change,[c] n (%)* | | |
| Pre-contemplator | 14 (25.9) | 11 (41.4) |
| Contemplator | 11 (20.4) | 21 (24.1) |
| Preparation | 8 (14.8) | 19 (13.8) |
| Action | 20 (37) | 19 (13.8) |
| Maintenance | 1 (1.9) | 3 (6.9) |
| *Age at first cannabis use* Mean (SD) | 12.56 (1.71) | 13.2 (1.7) |
| *Days of alcohol use in last 90 days* | | |
| Mean (SD) | 5.06 (5.23) | 12.8 (19.0) |
| Median | 3 | 6.5 |
| *Days of other illicit drug use in last 90 days[d]* | | |
| Mean (SD) | 1.02 (3.73) | |
| Median | 0 | <Weekly $n = 73$ (100%) |

[a] This variable was measured differently in the two studies.
[b] In the US study this was ascertained from study records as there was no specific question on educational status.
[c] Assessed how they felt about their cannabis use "right now". Those in the action and maintenance stages had made changes to their use in the past 6 months.
[d] Other illicit drug use was measured in days of use in the last 90 days for the US study, but in the Australian study it was measured as "at least weekly or more" or "less than weekly" in the past 90 days.

(1.9%) in the US sample. Over half the participants in both studies reported at least one occasion on which they had voluntarily reduced (US: 56%; AUS: 64.3%), and the great majority reported at least one occasion on which they had ceased their cannabis use (US: 80%; AUS: 79.5%). Slightly more of the US sample appeared interested in change, with more than half of in the preparation to maintenance stages of change, compared to a third of the Australian sample. Alcohol use was much less common than cannabis use in both samples, but the frequency of alcohol use among Australian participants was more than twice that of the US participants. Illicit drug use other than cannabis use was only infrequently reported over the past 90 days.

### *Outcomes*

Reductions in cannabis use were found in both groups at the 3-month follow-up (see Table 12.2). Firstly, more than three quarters of both follow-up samples

Table 12.2. *Use outcomes*

| Variable | US sample ($n = 54$) | Australian sample ($n = 54$ unless specified)[a] |
|---|---|---|
| *Voluntarily stopped/reduced use in last 90 days, N (%)* | 45 (83) | 42 (77.7) |
| *Complete abstinence in past 30 days (%)* | | |
| Baseline | 0 | 0 |
| 3 months[b] | 14.8 | 16.7 |
| *Days of cannabis use in past 30 days* | | ($n = 52$) |
| Baseline mean (SD) | 10.30 (8.20) | 18.98 (10.8) |
| Median | 8.00 | 23.5 |
| 3-month mean (SD) | 8.39 (9.03) | 14.0 (11.7) |
| Median | 5.00 | 11.5 |
| Wilcoxin test (*p*-value) | $z = -2.04, p = 0.04$ | $z = -2.63, p = 0.009$ |

[a] Of these followed at 3 months, 17 had received the additional single session of cognitive-behavioral therapy (CBT) as part of the randomized trial component prior to the follow-up interview. Another 15 had been randomized to the wait-list condition and were offered this session at the follow-up interview.
[b] For the US study, the 3-month follow-up occurred 3 months after their baseline assessment, while for the Australian study it occurred 3 months after their final participation in the study.

reported having made voluntary reductions (stopping or reducing use) in their cannabis use in the previous 90 days. This is supported by data showing that, compared to the frequency of cannabis consumption in the 30 days prior to baseline, there were substantial decreases in consumption in the 30 days prior to the 3-month follow-up. Further, 15% (*n* = 8) of the US sample and 17% (*n* = 9) of the Australian sample reported complete abstinence from cannabis in the 30 days prior to their follow-up session. In fact, all of those in the Australian sample who reported 30-day abstinence had been abstinent for the entire 3-month follow-up period. The consistency of the outcome data is surprising given the higher levels of cannabis use among the Australian sample, although 17 of the Australian participants received the additional skills-based session.

*Perceptions of the Intervention*

Program evaluation measures completed after the feedback session typically indicated a positive response from both samples. Nearly all participants felt their counselor listened to them (US: 98%; AUS: 100%), was helpful (US: 98%; AUS: 97%), and was non-judgmental of them and their attitudes about their cannabis use (US: 91%; AUS: 83%). Seventy-seven percent of US participants and 87% of Australian participants also reported that receiving feedback about their cannabis use was moderately to extremely helpful. At least a half of the participants (US: 50%; AUS: 75%) reported they would be interested in attending additional sessions to discuss their cannabis use, if offered.

## Issues in Implementing a Check-up Intervention

*Working with Persons Concerned About an Adolescent*

COs may include family members, friends, and school staff (e.g., teachers, counselors), as well as staff members at drug and alcohol agencies, community service agencies, and telephone helplines. For COs who choose to attend a session with the counselor, the focus is on: providing accurate information on cannabis, clarifying and assessing the nature of their specific concerns, enhancing their skills in effectively communicating concerns to the young person, providing a clear understanding of the nature and purpose of the check-up, and helping them to consider and practice ways of encouraging the young person to participate in the check-up.

The COs recruited to the Australian study typically expressed substantial, and often long-standing, concerns about their young person's cannabis use. Concerns largely focused on the teen's level of use and its perceived impact on mental health and behavior; family and social peer issues; physical health; school and work performance and general interests. Most COs believed the young person had a cannabis problem or needed treatment and typically wanted the check-up to allow the young person a chance to recognize they had a problem or to be better informed about their use. They also hoped the check-up could effect a decrease in the young person's levels of cannabis use and improvements in areas such as mental health and behavior (e.g., improved self-esteem, less aggression/hostility) and family relationships.

It is important to spend time listening to and legitimizing the concerns of COs, without passing judgment. They may feel isolated, and in some cases this will be the first time they have spoken to an objective person about their experiences, so a lot of time may be spent listening. However, this session also provides a valuable opportunity for education about the effects of cannabis and a sounding board for approaches to communicating with the young person. The exact content of the session will depend to some extent on the interests and situation of the CO, so the amount of coverage of each area will be flexible.

One issue, which should be clarified, is the extent to which the check-up is a "treatment" program. As there are relatively few services for COs, some may be disappointed if their expectations (e.g., of the young person ceasing their use or the provision of long-term counseling and support) are not met. As described earlier, the check-up targets those who may not be committed to change, so even if there is an improvement in the motivation of the young person to change, this may be less perceptible than the changes desired by a parent (e.g., in behavior). It is likely that the expected outcomes of the check-up will differ for the CO and the young person. Particularly in cases where the young person (and/or the family) have other long-standing issues such as serious co-morbid disorders or behavioral problems, or family problems, referral to other services providing longer-term support will be necessary.

### Marketing Strategies

Recruitment is a significant issue among young people who often have low motivation to change, so marketing and recruitment methods need to be flexible and target a variety of sources. Adequate time, money, and effort are necessary to plan and develop effective recruitment strategies, particularly in fostering liaisons with schools, drug and alcohol agencies, community service agencies, telephone helplines, and school/college counselors. Tailored approaches and messages are necessary to attract persons who are concerned about a young person (and may refer an adolescent to the project) versus those for young cannabis users themselves (who may initiate contact with the project on their own). In marketing to persons who are in frequent contact with young people and may be a referral source (e.g., alcohol and drug services, school counselors, helpline staff), the marketing message may focus more on a straightforward description of the project and contact information. Marketing messages geared to persons who are concerned about a young person and are not sure what to do (e.g., parents or other family members), may additionally focus on addressing and legitimizing their concerns, and offering an opportunity for an educational session regarding cannabis and communication.

## *Confidentiality and Consent*

In the context of research studies, informed consent is obtained from all participants. The assurance of confidentiality is an important factor in successfully recruiting and encouraging an open, honest dialog with adolescents. Research suggests that parents are often unaware of cannabis use by their teenaged children (Colby *et al.*, 1998b). Some adolescents may forego health care because of concerns that their parents might find out, but giving assurances of confidentiality may increase their willingness to disclose sensitive information (Ford *et al.*, 1997). To allow for young people who may not want their parents to be aware of their smoking status, or in situations where there is no relevant or interested CO, ethics approval was granted for a waiver of parental consent. Secondly, unless requested by the young person, the check-up sessions are conducted without the attendance of the CO, to foster an open discussion and maximize the benefits of the program. In clinical practice, states or localities may have laws governing whether teens may obtain treatment services without parental consent and these issues should be discussed upfront with teens, noting any limitations to confidentiality. The general principle is to create an environment in which the young person feels able to talk candidly about drug use.

## *Coercion*

CO attempts to engage a young person who may not be motivated or interested in change raise the issue of coercion (see Brody & Waldron, 2000). This may range from promises of reward for attendance to more direct threats of punishment for non-attendance, such as grounding, suspension or expulsion from school, or some legal consequence. While the anxiety of COs for the young person to address what they perceive to be problematic cannabis use is understandable, the check-up approach is particularly careful not to make the young person feel forced into

290                                         *James P. Berghuis* et al.

making unwanted change. While COs can play a powerful role in facilitating treatment entry (e.g., Landau *et al.*, 2000; Szapocznik *et al.*, 1988), undue external pressure may increase the resistance of young people to participate. The CO's session actively discourages coercion, stressing the importance of allowing the young person to make the decision to participate, and ultimately, they must provide informed consent. However, even if a young person attends the check-up unwillingly, this does not necessarily mean they won't become engaged in the process and actually benefit from it. The main issue is to ensure they are fully informed of what the check-up entails so they can make an informed choice about participation. This process should allow for developmental differences in adolescents' cognitive and decision-making abilities and processes.

*Counselor Training and Quality Assurance*

Good clinical skills, experience working with young people, and an understanding of adolescent/family issues are desirable attributes for the MET approach. In particular, the ability to be non-judgmental when discussing substance use is critical and will facilitate a good rapport and an open exploration of substance use issues by the young person. Good rapport is especially important in order to encourage young people who are not motivated to return for further sessions.

Training in the delivery of the check-up focused on addressing issues such as counselors' lack of confidence, knowledge, and skills in this area, and stressed the need to be non-judgmental of illicit drug use. It included readings and discussion to provide a thorough grounding in current knowledge of substance use (e.g., reasons for use, pharmacology and withdrawal). The counselors need to be prepared to provide education and answer at least basic questions about cannabis, or to be able to know where to obtain the relevant information. Training also included reading materials and discussion of MET principles and technique, watching videotaped examples of motivational interviewing, didactic presentation of MET components, role plays of motivational interviewing with young people, and practice deliveries of the intervention which were audio- or videotaped and reviewed. We also audiotaped our sessions, had them audited, and provided clinical supervision to maximize understanding of the techniques and an opportunity to debrief sessions.

**Summary and Discussion**

The check-up approach makes developmental sense as a potentially effective way of working with, and assisting, adolescent cannabis smokers. It contrasts with traditional treatment approaches in several ways. First, it can be tailored for a voluntary, non-treatment-seeking population recruited from schools and the community at large as well as for a treatment-seeking population. Schools, in particular, are an effective way to reach young people and recommendations for conducting school-based research are available in the literature (Gans & Brindis, 1995; Harrington *et al.*, 1997; Lytle *et al.*, 1994; O'Hara *et al.*, 1991; Olds & Symons, 1990; Petosa & Goodman, 1991). Most drug and alcohol interventions with young people, however, have primarily dealt with "captive" populations of young people in drug and alcohol treatment facilities, the juvenile justice system, or various aftercare programs. Second, the brevity of the check-up (two to three sessions), and its low barriers to access (i.e., an opportunity for a confidential and in-depth "no-pressure" evaluation as contrasted with a treatment intervention with accompanying expectations for change), encourage participation with minimal effort. This is important because the check-up is seeking to reach a population whose members may not be committed to making changes in their use. In other words, the level of motivation for change is not presumed; rather it is explored as part of the intervention. Third, the check-up approach views ambivalence as normal, does not label young people as having a problem with cannabis, and treats them as the experts and decision-makers regarding their cannabis use. This approach is intended to enhance the likelihood that the young person will feel engaged and empowered in the interaction. Traditional treatments emphasize behavior change (i.e., abstinence) rather than motivation, and place pressure on the young person to make changes.

Two promising applications of this intervention in the USA and Australia have been described. The results of the US and Australian check-ups indicate that this approach was able to effectively recruit and retain voluntary, non-treatment-seeking adolescent cannabis smokers, almost half of whom were in the pre-contemplation or contemplation stages of change. The programs attracted samples reporting a wide range of cannabis use patterns. In comparison with the Australian study, recruitment through schools was much more successful for the US study than efforts to recruit through family members or others who might be concerned about an adolescent's cannabis use. The heavier use patterns evident in the Australian study may reflect the fact that most participants were recruited as a result of someone else's often serious concerns. Nevertheless, the interventions were well received by those who participated and at least half of the participants were interested in additional sessions. Each of these findings supports the feasibility of this type of intervention with a broad voluntary sample of adolescent cannabis smokers not seeking other services for their cannabis use. However, long-term outcomes are unknown and more research is needed.

Randomized-controlled trials of the check-up are currently underway in the USA (with funding from the National Institute on Drug Abuse) and Australia (funded by the National Health and Medical Research Council) that will provide important additional data on the efficacy this approach.

## References

Arsenault, L., Cannon, M., Poulton, R., Murray, R., Caspi, A., & Moffitt, T. E. (2002). Cannabis use in adolescence and risk for adult psychosis: longitudinal prospective study. *British Medical Journal, 325*, 1212–1213.

Aubrey, L. (1997). Motivational interviewing with adolescent poly-substance users. Paper presented at the *31st Annual Meeting of the Association for Advancement of Behavior Therapy*, New York, USA.

Australian Institute of Health and Welfare (2002). *2001 National Drug Strategy Household Survey: detailed findings* (Drug Statistics Series No. 11). Canberra, Australian Capital Territory: Australian Institute of Health and Welfare.

Bachman, J. G., Wadsworth, K. N., O'Malley, P. M., Johnston, L. D., & Schulenberg, J. E. (1997). *Smoking, drinking, and drug use in young adulthood: the impacts of new freedoms and new responsibilities.* Mahwah, NJ: Lawrence Erlbaum Associates.

Brody, J. L., & Waldron, H. B. (2000). Ethical issues in research on the treatment of adolescent substance use disorders. *Addictive Behaviors, 25*, 217–228.

Brook, J. S., Balka, E. B. & Whiteman, M. (1999). The risks for late adolescence of early adolescent marijuana use. *American Journal of Public Health, 89*, 1549–1554.

Center for Substance Abuse Research (2000a). Substance Abuse and Mental Health Services Administration. The Cannabis Youth Treatment (CYT) Experiment: Preliminary Findings. *Report to H.W. Clark, Director.*

Center for Substance Abuse Treatment (2000b). The National Treatment Improvement Evaluation Study: Adolescents and young adults in treatment [online]. Available: http://www.health.org/nties/young/yungall.htm

Chen, K., & Kandel, D. B. (1995). The natural history of drug use from adolescence to the mid-thirties in a general population sample. *American Journal of Public Health, 85*, 41–47.

Coffey, C., Wolfe, R., & Patton, G. C. (2000). Initiation and progression of cannabis use in a population-based Australian adolescent longitudinal study. *Addiction, 95*, 1679–1690.

Coffey, C., Carlin, J. B., Degenhardt, L., Lynskey, M., Sanci, L., & Patton, G. C. (2002). Cannabis dependence in young adults: an Australian population study. *Addiction, 97*, 187–194.

Colby, S. M., Monti, P. M., Barnett, N. P., Rohsenow, D. J., Weissman, K., Spirito, A., et al. (1998a). Brief motivational interviewing in a hospital setting for adolescent smoking: a preliminary study. *Journal of Consulting and Clinical Psychology*, *66*(3), 574–578.

Colby, S. M., Wood, M., Chung, T., Spirito, A., Rohsenow, D., & Monti, P. (1998b). Diagnostic issues related to marijuana use disorders among adolescents. Paper presented at the *Annual Meeting of the Association for the Advancement of Behavior Therapy*, Washington, DC.

Deas, D., & Thomas, S. E. (2001). An overview of controlled studies of adolescent substance abuse treatment. *The American Journal on Addictions*, *10*, 178–189.

Degenhardt, L., Lynskey, M., & Hall, W. (2000). Cohort trends in the age of initiation of drug use in Australia. *Australian and New Zealand Journal of Public Health*, *24*, 421–426.

Dennis, M. (2002). Treatment research on adolescent drug and alcohol abuse: despite progress, many challenges remain. *Connection*, *May*, pp. 1, 2, 7.

Dennis, M., Babor, T., Diamond, G., Donaldson, J., Godley, S., & Tims, F. (1998). *The Cannabis Youth Treatment (CYT) Cooperative Agreement Study* (SAMHSA/CSAT Grant TI11320). Bloomington, IL: Chestnut Health Systems.

DeWit, D. J., Hance, J., Offord, D. R., & Ogborne, A. (2000). The influence of early and frequent use of marijuana on the risk of desistance and progression to marijuana-related harm. *Preventive Medicine*, *31*, 455–464.

European Monitoring Centre for Drugs and Drug Addiction (2003). *Annual Report 2003: The State of the Drugs Problem in the European Union and Norway*. Luxembourg: Office for Official Publications of the European Communities.

Fergusson, D., Horwood, L., & Lynskey, M. (1994). Parental separation, adolescent psychopathology and problem behaviors. *Journal of the American Academy of Child and Adolescent Psychiatry*, *33*, 1122–1131.

Fergusson, D. M., & Horwood, L. J. (1997). Early onset cannabis use and psychosocial adjustment in young adults. *Addiction*, *92*, 279–296.

Fergusson, D. M., & Horwood, L. J. (2000a). Cannabis use and dependence in a New Zealand birth cohort. *New Zealand Medical Journal*, *113*, 156–158.

Fergusson, D. M., & Horwood, L. J. (2000b). Does cannabis use encourage other forms of illicit drug use? *Addiction*, *95*, 505–520.

Fergusson, D. M., Horwood, L. J., & Swain-Campbell, N. (2002). Cannabis use and psychosocial adjustment in adolescence and young adulthood. *Addiction*, *97*, 1123–1135.

Ford, C. A., Millstein, S. G., Halpern-Felsher, B. L., & Irwin, C. E. J. (1997). Influence of physician confidentiality assurances on adolescents' willingness to disclose information and seek future health care: a randomized trial. *Journal of the American Medical Association*, *278*(12), 1029–1034.

Gans, J. E., & Brindis, C. D. (1995). Choice of research setting in understanding adolescent health problems. *Journal of Adolescent Health*, *17*(5), 306–313.

Golub, A., & Johnson, B. A. (2001). The rise of marijuana as the drug of choice among youthful adult arrestees. *National Institute of Justice Research in Brief*, *June*, 1–19.

Hall, W., & Swift, W. (2000). The THC content of cannabis in Australia: evidence and implications. *Australian and New Zealand Journal of Public Health*, 24, 503–508.

Hall, W., Johnston, L., & Donnelly, N. (1999). The epidemiology of cannabis use and its consequences. In H. Kalant, W. Corrigall, W. Hall, & R. Smart (Eds.), *The health effects of cannabis* (pp. 71–125). Toronto, Canada: Centre for Addiction and Mental Health.

Harrington, K. F., Brinkley, D., Reynolds, K. D., Duvall, R. C., Copeland, J. R., Franklin, F., *et al.* (1997). Recruitment issues in school based research: lessons learned from the High 5 Alabama Project. *Journal of School Health*, 67(10), 415–421.

Hubbard, R. L., Cavanaugh, E. R., Craddock, S. G., & Rachel, J. V. (1985). *Characteristics, behaviors, and outcomes for youth in the TOPS: treatment services for adolescent substance abusers* (DHHS Publication No. ADM 85-1342). Washington, DC: National Institute on Drug Abuse.

Hubbard, R. L., Marsden, M. E., Rachal, J. V., Harwood, H. J., Cavanaugh, E. R., & Ginzburg, H. M. (1989). *Drug abuse treatment: a national study of effectiveness*. Chapel Hill, NC: University of North Carolina Press.

Irwin, C., & Millstein, S. (1986). Biopsychosocial correlates of risk taking behaviors during adolescence: can a physician intervene? *Journal of Adolescent Health Care*, 7(Suppl. 6), 82–96.

Johnston, L. D., O'Malley, P. M., & Bachman, J. G. (2003). *Monitoring the future: National results on adolescent drug use: overview of key findings 2003*. Bethesda, MD: National Institute on Drug Abuse.

Kandel, D., Chen, K., Warner, L. A., Kessler, R. C., & Grant, B. (1997). Prevalence and demographic correlates of symptoms of last year dependence on alcohol, nicotine, marijuana and cocaine in the US population. *Drug and Alcohol Dependence*, 44, 11–29.

Kimmel, D. C., & Weiner, I. B. (1995). *Adolescence: a developmental transition*. New York: John Wiley and Sons, Inc.

Landau, J., Garrett, J., Shea, R., Stanton, M. D., Brinkman-Sull, D., & Baciewicz, G. (2000). Strength in numbers: the ARISE method for mobilizing family and network to engage substance abusers in treatment. *American Journal of Drug and Alcohol Abuse*, 26, 379–398.

Lawendowski, L. A. (1998). A motivational intervention for adolescent smokers. *Preventive Medicine*, 27, A39–A46.

Lynskey, M., & Hall, W. (2000). The effects of adolescent cannabis use on educational attainment: a review. *Addiction*, 95, 1621–1630.

Lynskey, M. T., Heath, A. C., Bucholz, K. K., Slutske, W. S., Madden, P. A. F., Nelson, E. C., Statham, D. J., & Martin, N. G. (2003). Escalation of drug use in early-onset cannabis users vs. co-twin controls. *Journal of the American Medical Association*, 289, 427–433.

Lytle, L. A., Johnson, C. C., Bachman, K., Wambsgans, K., Perry, C. L., Stone, E. J., *et al.* (1994). Successful recruitment strategies for school-based health promotion: experiences from CATCH. *Journal of School Health, 64*(10), 405–409.

Makkai, T., & McAllister, I. (1997). *Marijuana in Australia: patterns and attitudes* (Monograph No. 31). Canberra, Australian Capital Terriotory: Australian Government Publishing Service.

McCambridge, J., & Strang, J. (2004). The efficacy of single-session motivational interviewing in reducing drug consumption and perceptions of drug-related risk and harm among young people: results from a multi-site cluster randomized trial. *Addiction, 99*, 39–52.

McGee, L., & Newcomb, M. D. (1992). General deviance syndrome: expanded hierarchical evaluations at four ages from early adolescence to adulthood. *Journal of Consulting and Clinical Psychology, 60*, 766–776.

Miller, W. R., & Rollnick, S. (1991). *Motivational interviewing: preparing people to change addictive behavior*. New York: The Guilford Press.

Miller, W. R., & Sovereign, R. G. (1989). The check-up: a model for early intervention in addictive behaviors. In T. Loberg, W. R. Miller, P. E. Nathan, & G. A. Marlatt (Eds.), *Addictive behaviors: prevention and early intervention* (pp. 219–231). Amsterdam: Swets and Zeitlinger.

Monti, P. M., Colby, S. M., Barnett, N. P., Spirito, A., Rohsenow, D. J., Myers, M., *et al.* (1999). Brief intervention for harm reduction with alcohol-positive older adolescents in a hospital emergency department. *Journal of Consulting and Clinical Psychology, 67*(6), 989–994.

Office of Applied Studies (OAS) (1995). *Services Research Outcome Study (SROS).* Rockville, MD: SAMHSA [online]. Available: http://www.samhsa.gov/oas/sros/httoc.htm

O'Hara, N. M., Brink, S., Harvey, C., Harrist, R., Green, B., & Parcel, G. (1991). Recruitment strategies for school health promotion research. *Health Education Research, 6*(3), 363–371.

Olds, R. S., & Symons, C. W. (1990). Recommendations for obtaining cooperation to conduct school-based research. *Journal of School Health, 60*(3), 96–98.

Perkonnig, A., Lieb, R., Höffler, M., Schuster, P., Sonntag, H., & Wittchen, H.-U. (1999). Patterns of cannabis use, abuse and dependence over time: incidence, progression and stability in a sample of 1228 adolescents. *Addiction, 94*, 1663–1678.

Petosa, R., & Goodman, R. M. (1991). Recruitment and retention of schools participating in school health research. *Journal of School Health, 61*(10), 426–429.

Poulton, R. G., Brooke, M., Moffitt, T. E., Stanton, W. R., & Silva, P. A. (1997). Prevalence and correlates of cannabis use and dependence in young New Zealanders. *New Zealand Medical Journal, 110*, 68–70.

Powers, K., Grella, C., Hser, Y., & Anglin, M. (1999). *Differential assessment of treatment effectiveness on property crime and drug dealing among adolescents.* Collage on problems of drug dependence, Acapulco, June 1999. Available: http://www.datos.org/posters/CPDD_99_Powers/sld001.htm

Prochaska, J. O., & DiClemente, C. C. (1983). Stages and processes of self-change of smoking: toward an integrative model of change. *Journal of Consulting and Clinical Psychology*, *51*(3), 390–395.

Ramsay, M., & Partridge, S. (1999). *Drug misuse declared in 1998: results from the British Crime Survey*. London: Home Office.

Reid, A., Lynskey, M., & Copeland, J. (2000). Cannabis use among Australian adolescents: findings of the 1998 National Drug Strategy Household Survey. *Australian and New Zealand Journal of Public Health*, *24*, 596–602.

Rollnick, S., & Miller, W. R. (1995). What is motivational interviewing? *Behavioural and Cognitive Psychotherapy*, *23*, 325–334.

Sanchez-Craig, M. (1995). *Drinkwise: how to quite drinking or cut down* (2nd ed., revised). Toronto: Addiction Research Foundation.

Substance Abuse and Mental Health Administration, Office of Applied Studies (2003). *Results from the 2002 National Survey on Drug Use and Health: National findings* (NHSDA Series H-22, DHHS Publication No. SMA 03-3836). Rockville, MD: Department of Health and Human Services, Substance Abuse and Mental Health Services Administration, Office of Applied Studies.

Szapocznik, J., Perez-Vidal, A., Brickman, A. L., Foote, F. F., Santisteban, D., Hervis, O., et al. (1988). Engaging adolescent drug abusers and their families in treatment: a strategic structural systems approach. *Journal of Consulting and Clinical Psychology*, *56*, 552–557.

Titus, J. C., & Godley, M. D. (1999). What research tells us about the treatment of adolescent substance use disorders. Paper prepared for the *Governor's Conference on Substance Abuse Prevention, Intervention, and Treatment for Youth*, Bloomington, IL.

Werner, M. J. (1995). Principles of brief intervention for adolescent alcohol, tobacco, and other drug use. *Pediatric Clinics of North America*, *42*(2), 335–349.

Wilkins, C., Casswell, S., Bhatta, K., & Pledger, M. (2002). *Drug use in New Zealand: National Surveys Comparison 1998 and 2001*. Auckland: Alcohol and Public Health Research Unit.

# 13

# Engaging Young Probation-Referred Marijuana-Abusing Individuals in Treatment

KATHLEEN M. CARROLL, RAJITA SINHA AND CAROLINE EASTON

For the past several years, our group has been working on developing effective treatments for young adults who are referred for treatment of marijuana abuse and dependence through the legal system, as well as other criminal justice populations. This chapter provides a brief overview of the rationale for the treatments we have developed, summarizes the initial small trial we conducted to evaluate these approaches (Sinha *et al.*, 2003), and describes how results from that study are informing our ongoing work in this area.

## Why Target Young Adult Marijuana Users?

Marijuana is the most commonly used illicit substance in the USA, with approximately 5.5 million regular weekly users (see Anthony *et al.*, 1994; and Anthony's chapter in this volume). Moreover, marijuana use among adolescents and young adults has increased dramatically in recent years (Johnson *et al.*, 1996). This is significant because longitudinal epidemiological studies have consistently identified marijuana as a gateway drug for progression to use of other illicit substances among young adults (Kandel & Yamaguchi, 1993; Kandel *et al.*, 1992). The segment with the highest prevalence of marijuana use is the 18–25 age range, where 48% report lifetime use, 23% report use in the last year, and 11% report marijuana use in the last month, with higher rates among males than females (Kandel *et al.*, 1997).

Frequent marijuana use during young adulthood significantly increases the risk of lifetime experiences with other illicit drugs, greater involvement in drugs, earlier onset of cocaine and opioid use, health problems, depression, and involvement with the legal system (Kandel & Davies, 1996; Kandel *et al.*, 1992). As (a) marijuana use peaks between the ages of 18 and 25, (b) frequent marijuana use is the best predictor of persistent use, and (c) initiation of drug use after age 29 is rare, an important strategy may be targeting individuals

297

at risk during early adulthood (Chen & Kandel, 1995) as a means of preventing progression to more severe problems.

## Why Target Marijuana Users Referred by the Legal System?

Frequent marijuana use in young adults is associated with greater delinquency and involvement with the legal system (Kandel & Davies, 1996), and early involvement with the legal system is a predictor of further problematic substance use and legal involvement. Moreover, young adult marijuana users are unlikely to present for treatment by themselves; many individuals seeking treatment for marijuana dependence do not do so until their mid-30s (Stephens et al., 1994). This reduces opportunities to identify and intervene with individuals whose marijuana use puts them at risk for the development of heavier drug use. Thus, their involvement with the legal system presents a unique opportunity for intervention.

This approach is consistent with other efforts to identify and intervene with individuals at risk for more severe substance abuse, typically in primary care, legal, and occupational settings where affected individuals would not be seeking treatment for a substance use disorder (Babor, 1994; Institute of Medicine, 1990; Saunders et al., 1995). This approach is exemplified by the World Health Organization (WHO) Brief Intervention Project (WHO Brief Intervention Study Group, 1996), which was conducted in 10 countries, and focused on brief interventions for problem drinkers recruited from primary care centers, hospitals, and work settings. Six-month follow-up evaluations indicated that brief interventions exerted significant durable effects on substance use and related problems (WHO Brief Intervention Study Group, 1996).

The point at which drug abusers confront legal consequences of their substance use may be a particularly effective means and time at which to intervene. Most drug abusers do not seek formal treatment (Regier et al., 1993); moreover, more drug users are involved with the legal system than the drug abuse treatment system (Weisner & Schmidt, 1995). Legal pressures can exert substantial pressure to change drug use (Leukefeld & Tims, 1988). For example, Cornish et al. (1997) reported reduced substance use, lower re-arrest rates, and lower rates of revocation of probation status for a group of federal probationers offered a 6-month naltrexone program versus those who received probation without drug treatment.

## Why Evaluate a Motivational Enhancement Approach?

Program evaluation data from our community-based outpatient substance abuse treatment facility in New Haven suggested that over 80% of 218 individuals referred to treatment for marijuana use over the period of 1 year were young

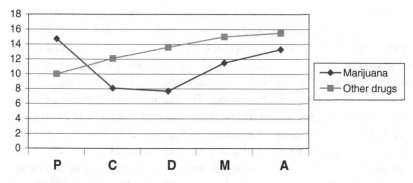

Figure 13.1  SOCRATES scores for SATU probation referrals, marijuana versus
other drug users, N 5 1064 (P: Precontemplation; C: Contemplation; D: Determination;
M: Maintenance; A: Action).

adults (in the 18–25 age group) and referred by the legal system. Furthermore,
compared with probation-referred individuals using other substances (e.g.,
cocaine, opioids, or alcohol), the marijuana-using group were significantly less
likely to engage in treatment (i.e., return for second appointment after the initial
intake session) compared with other probation-referred clients (43% versus
57%; $X^2 = 4.73$; $p < 0.03$). This group also had significantly lower motivation
for change compared with probation referees who were using other drugs, as
assessed by the Stages of Change Readiness and Treatment Eagerness Scale
(SOCRATES) (Miller & Tonigan, 1996a), with the majority of marijuana-
abusing individuals providing precontemplation profiles. As shown in Figure 13.1,
precontemplation (poorly motivated) scores were significantly ($p = 0.01$) higher
for the marijuana group as compared to probation-referred patients using cocaine,
alcohol, or opioids; moreover, scores on the contemplation, determination, and
maintenance subscales were significantly lower ($p < 0.05$) for the marijuana
users compared to the other groups.

The low rate of retention in the targeted population, coupled with our data
implying particularly low readiness to change in this group, suggested the importance of addressing issues of motivation in this group. Brief motivational
approaches that focus on mobilizing the individual's own resources to change
have very high levels of empirical support in the cigarette and alcohol treatment
literature (Babor, 1994; Bien *et al.*, 1993; Miller *et al.*, 1995; Wilk *et al.*, 1997).
However, with the exception of the work of Roffman and colleagues (Stephens
*et al.*, 1994, 2000), only a handful of studies have been done evaluating the effectiveness of motivational enhancement therapy (MET) or motivational interviewing (MI) among drug users (Carroll *et al.*, 2001; Martino *et al.*, 2000; Saunders
*et al.*, 1995; Swanson *et al.*, 1999).

One factor that may be related to the paucity of efficacy data on MET with drug abusers is the complexity of the issues around implementing this approach with comparatively severe, treatment-seeking drug users. For example, the bulk of studies of brief motivational approaches have targeted less severe problem drinkers who have not necessarily met Diagnostic and Statistical Manual (DSM) criteria for alcohol abuse or dependence. This had led to questions as to whether MET will be sufficient as sole treatment for treatment-seeking drug users, given the severity and the range of problems seen among drug-dependent patients. However, an apt role for motivational approaches may be as a means of bolstering drug users' motivation to change as preparation for treatment or as a means of enhancing treatment engagement or compliance. Moreover, motivational approaches may also be particularly appropriate for marijuana users and specifically the population targeted here, given their low level of readiness for change.

**Why Evaluate a Contingency Management Approach?**

A notable recent finding in the drug abuse field is the effectiveness of the contingency management (CM) approaches developed by Steve Higgins and colleagues at the University of Vermont (Higgins *et al.*, 1991, 1993, 1994, 2000). This elegant series of studies has demonstrated that the provision of incentives for desired behaviors (i.e., abstinence) in the form of vouchers redeemable for items consistent with a drug-free lifestyle, has been associated with high rates of retention and abstinence in several samples and settings (Petry *et al.*, 2000; Silverman *et al.*, 1996). An intriguing finding from this literature is that this approach can be used to target specific desired behaviors. For example, when abstinence is reinforced through the voucher system, rates of abstinence increase. On the other hand, when attendance in treatment is targeted, attendance increases but drug use does not change appreciably (Iguchi *et al.*, 1996). Thus, contingent reinforcement of abstinence from marijuana is a potentially promising approach for the targeted population, but only one trial on the effectiveness of this approach with a marijuana-dependent sample has been conducted (see Budney 2001; and Budney's chapter in this volume).

**Description of the Interventions**

*MET*

We adapted a manual specifically for the needs of this population, drawing from the MET manuals used in Project MATCH (Project MATCH Research Group,

1997) and the Center for Substance Abuse Treatment (CSAT) Multi-Site Marijuana Treatment Project (MTP Research Group, 2004). In MET, the therapeutic stance is one in which empathy is expressed, resistance and argumentation are avoided, and self-efficacy is supported. In the trial described below, we evaluated a three-session treatment, in which the first session focused on building rapport and providing information and feedback to the participants regarding the effects of marijuana use on their day-to-day functioning. Therapists sought to increase the participant's willingness to participate in treatment and reduce their marijuana use by heightening their awareness of the personal consequences resulting from marijuana use. Preparation of a "quit contract," where participants would commit to a date for stopping marijuana use, was encouraged. The second session focused on assessing the participant's current level of motivation, formulating a change plan, and discussing strategies to avoid high-risk situations. The final session focused on reviewing the change plan, assessing high-risk situations that had occurred in the past week, and providing strategies for coping with high-risk situations, cravings and slips. A recommendation for continued treatment at the outpatient facility was made to facilitate further reduction in marijuana use.

## MET and CM

To evaluate whether providing incentives for session participation enhanced retention, we also evaluated the value of adding vouchers to the MET sessions. Thus, in addition to the MET sessions described above, a second group of participants received vouchers redeemable for items selected by the participant contingent on prompt session attendance. Vouchers worth $25 were provided for attending the first session, $35 for the second session, and $45 for the third and final session. Missing or rescheduling a session reset the voucher value to $25. In our initial piloting of the study with a few participants, we noted that they tended to be late for session. Thus, we added an additional incentive where, if the participant was prompt for the therapy appointment (i.e., within 5 min of the scheduled appointment time), an additional $5 bonus was provided. Thus, participants who attended all three sessions and were on time for each session received vouchers worth $120.

In the first session, the therapist described the voucher system and reviewed a voucher catalogue that contained descriptions of items and services supporting a drug-free lifestyle. Sporting goods, clothing, music items, entertainment (i.e., tickets to museums, amusement parks, and gift certificates for local restaurants), payment for General Educational Development (GED) courses and other technical courses are examples of items listed in the catalogue. Early in treatment, participants were encouraged to identify specific items that they were interested in working to earn through attending treatment as a strategy to enhance goal setting.

## Therapists and Training

In our clinical trial, the MET and MET + CM interventions were delivered by comparatively experienced clinicians (three Ph.D. level and four masters level) who had an average of 6 years of experience in treating substance abusers. The following therapist selection criteria were used:

1. demonstration of an interest and commitment to this therapeutic approach;
2. willingness to take an active stance in treatment;
3. an ability to balance empathy and validation of the client's current state with problem solving; and
4. a change orientation and the ability to generate hope and confidence in the patient's ability to achieve success.

Therapists attended a didactic training seminar that included:

(i) a didactic seminar on MET principles and strategies including review of the treatment manual, videotaped examples of MET techniques, and role-play exercises;
(ii) review of additional procedures for managing the CM component of the MET + CM condition; and
(iii) successful completion of at least two closely supervised MET cases.

The didactic seminar on MET principles and strategies began with a discussion of the basic principles of MET. The major principles included expressing empathy, developing discrepancies, rolling with resistance, avoiding argumentation/confrontation, and supporting self-efficacy. This discussion was followed by a specific description of the process of implementing MI. We placed special emphasis on techniques such as asking open-ended questions, affirming, using reflective listening techniques, and providing summaries. Each of these skills involved specific strategies to accomplish them. The discussion of the overall MET procedures and content was followed by watching the MI professional training videotape series developed by Miller *et al.* (1998). The tapes were used to demonstrate the style in which MET sessions are typically delivered. After a thorough discussion and demonstration of these styles occurred, the therapists' role played various case examples and were given feedback.

The ultimate goal of the MET portion of this seminar was to train therapists to achieve the following aims:

(i) create an accepting and non-judgmental therapeutic alliance with the patient;
(ii) begin the process of developing motivation for change;
(iii) reduce resistance; and
(iv) develop discrepancy between the patient's self-assessment, the personal feedback and his/her stated goals.

This discussion also focused on strategies for integrating teaching of basic coping skills while using an MET style (consistent emphasis on empathy, rolling with resistance, avoiding confrontation).

This training seminar also included discussion on how and when to integrate the CM component (vouchers) into therapy sessions. This was illustrated through discussion and role plays. The discussion focused on the importance of supporting the CM system wherever possible. This included strategies such as:

(i) Discussing how the CM system might help the patient reach his/her personal goals (spending their vouchers on joining the gym to achieve their goal of increasing exercise and obtaining a healthier lifestyle).
(ii) Discussing what items and services the patient might like to earn with the vouchers (i.e., items supporting a drug-free lifestyle, that is, no illegal or drug-related items).
(iii) Checking back with the patient to find out how he or she "spent" their vouchers.
(iv) Talking with the patient about whether he/she is finding the voucher program helpful.

This training also involved illustrating basic guidelines for incorporating CM into the MET condition. This included encouraging patients to use vouchers to redeem low-value gifts fairly early in treatment so that patients could receive fairly rapid and concrete reinforcement for behavior change. Additionally, therapists used judgment regarding the timing of discussions around the vouchers and goals. For example, discussion of vouchers and goals were reserved for later sessions for patients who were precontemplators. Lastly, discussions about vouchers and the CM system were typically of short duration and only take up a very small part of the therapy session (e.g., no more than 5–10 minutes in any session). For patients who questioned or resisted the CM system, therapists were instructed to maintain the MET approach and roll with resistance and highlight the general principles of CM (i.e., rewards or incentives are used for "positive changes").

304                                                                  *Kathleen M. Carroll* et al.

All treatment sessions were videotaped and regularly reviewed for adherence and competence to manual guidelines. Furthermore, the therapists were also rated on their ability to successfully integrate the CM component into the MET + CM condition. All the therapists received ongoing supervision based on supervision procedures used in previous psychotherapy projects (Carroll *et al.*, 1994b). The supervision focused on (1) questions of implementation, (2) problems with adherence to treatment protocols, and (3) preparation for the next group treatment session. Supervision was provided on a weekly basis to the therapists and the supervisory group met quarterly to review tapes and discuss supervisory issues.

**Review of Study**

Sixty-five marijuana-using individuals (aged 18–25) were recruited from clients entering treatment at the Substance Abuse Treatment Unit of the Connecticut Mental Health Center, a publicly-funded outpatient substance abuse treatment facility. All participants were referred to the treatment facility for substance abuse evaluation and treatment by the adult probation departments in the greater New Haven area. In addition to the referral from adult probation, all clients met current DSM-IV criteria for marijuana abuse (25%) or dependence (75%) as assessed via Structured Clinical Interview for DSM (SCID) interviews (25). All subjects were positive for marijuana on the urine toxicology specimen at intake. Individuals were excluded who

(i)  were currently abusing opiates or cocaine, or whose principal substance of abuse was not marijuana,
(ii)  were currently receiving treatment for substance use, or
(iii)  had severe psychiatric or medical problems that would interfere with participation in outpatient treatment.

Seventy individuals were screened for the study; five did not meet inclusion/exclusion criteria or refused to participate.

Participants were interviewed before treatment, weekly during the treatment period, at a post-treatment (28-day) interview and at the 1-month follow-up. Marijuana use over the 28-day treatment period was assessed via self-report (using a weekly substance use calendar) and validated via weekly urine toxicology screens, which were also collected at follow-up. It is of note that participants appear to provide valid self-reports: Of 225 urine specimens collected, 211 (93.7%) were consistent with self-report and 6.3% indicated marijuana use in cases where the participant had denied use. The Addiction Severity Index (ASI) (McLellan *et al.*, 1992) was used to assess severity of drug use, psychosocial problems and legal problems. Readiness to change substance abuse behaviors was also assessed at pre and post-treatment and follow-up using the brief 20-item SOCRATES (Miller & Tonigan, 1996b), with specific attention to the precontemplation subscale.

## Results

Pretreatment characteristics of the 65 participants randomized to treatment are presented in Table 13.1. The sample was composed predominantly of young (mean age 20.4) males (93%) who were members of ethnic minority groups (76% were African-American). Participants were largely unemployed (74%), almost all were single and about two-thirds had not completed high school. The sample, while quite young, reported a high number of previous arrests (mean of 5.0) and had spent an average of 10 months in jail or prison. Participants reported using marijuana an average of 14 days of the past 28 and had been using marijuana regularly for an average of 7 years. The baseline ASI composite scores indicate that this group of young adults reported problems in a number of areas other than substance use, particularly in the areas of employment and legal problems.

Effects on retention, the outcome that was targeted by the CM intervention, are presented in Table 13.2. A significantly higher number of participants in the MET + CM condition completed treatment in 28 days as compared to participants in the MET alone condition (64% versus 39%, $X^2 = 3.85$, $p < 0.05$). Similarly, participants in the MET + CM condition attended a higher number of treatment sessions in 28 days as compared to the MET alone condition (2.3 versus 1.8 sessions), although this difference fell just short of statistical significance ($p < .07$). While more participants in the MET + CM condition continued in treatment at the clinic compared with those receiving MET alone (14 versus 8), this difference was not statistically significant. Regarding effects on marijuana use, there was a significant decrease in frequency of marijuana use, ASI drug use composite scores, ASI legal composite scores, and SOCRATES precontemplation scores for the group as a whole. Across time, however, there were no main effects for group or group by time effects.

## Conclusions and Future Directions

Our work has focused on developing and evaluating strategies to engage a poorly motivated, treatment resistant sample of young, probation-referred marijuana users in treatment and improve treatment outcomes as a strategy to prevent escalation into more severe forms of drug use and further legal and social

Table 13.1. *Pretreatment characteristics of all randomized participants*
*(N = 65)*

| Characteristic | MET alone (*N* = 28) | | MET + CM (*N* = 37) | |
|---|---|---|---|---|
| *Demographic* | | | | |
| Age mean (SD) | 20.25 | (2.38) | 20.86 | (2.29) |
| Female % (*N*) | 3.6 | (1) | 11 | (4) |
| Minority % (*N*) | 78.6 | (22) | 75.7 | (28) |
| Unemployed % (*N*) | 78.6 | (22) | 70.3 | (26) |
| Single/unmarried % (*N*) | 100 | | 97.3 | (36) |
| Education % (*N*) | | | | |
|   Completed HS | 35.7 | (10) | 45.9 | (17) |
|   Less than HS | 64.3 | (18) | 54.1 | (20) |
| *Marijuana use* mean (SD) | | | | |
| Days of use/month* | 10.25 | (9.51) | 16 | (12.45) |
| Years of regular use | 7.93 | (8.13) | 5.38 | (2.88) |
| Previous treatment | 0.79 | (1.2) | 0.49 | (.8) |
| Age of first marijuana use | 14.57 | (2.81) | 14.68 | (1.96) |
| *Legal involvement* mean (SD) | | | | |
| Lifetime # of arrests | 5.11 | (5.3) | 5.08 | (5.4) |
| Lifetime months of incarceration | 10.11 | (13.23) | 9.3 | (16.94) |
| *Other drug use disorder* % (*N*) | | | | |
| Alcohol abuse/dependence | 37 | (10) | 21.6 | (8) |
| Cocaine abuse/dependence | 3.6 | (1) | 10.8 | (4) |
| *ASI composite scores* mean (SD)** | | | | |
| Medical | 0.09 | (0.2) | 0.13 | (0.25) |
| Employment | 0.85 | (0.2) | 0.8 | (0.26) |
| Marijuana use | 0.28 | (0.22) | 0.33 | (0.26) |
| Alcohol use | 0.11 | (0.13) | 0.1 | (0.12) |
| Drug use | 0.01 | (0.02) | 0.02 | (0.04) |
| Legal | 0.27 | (0.21) | 0.26 | (0.23) |
| Family/social | 0.12 | (0.13) | 0.1 | (0.13) |
| Psychological | 0.11 | (0.13) | 0.09 | (0.15) |

*Note*: *denotes $p < 0.05$. MET alone denotes Motivation Enhancement Therapy
alone; MET + CM denotes Motivational Enhancement Therapy + Contingency
Management; SD = standard deviation.
**ASI Composite scores range from 0 to 1, higher scores (HS) indicate greater severity.

Table 13.2. *Treatment engagement variables for all participants randomized*
*(N = 65)*

| Measure | Treatment condition | | | |
|---|---|---|---|---|
| | MET alone (*N* = 28) | MET + CM (*N* = 37) | *F* or $X^2$ | *p* |
| Number of sessions attended, mean (SD) | 1.82 (1.19) | 2.32 (1.06) | *F* = 3.25 | 0.07 |
| Percent attending three sessions/28 days, % (*N*) | 39.3 (11) | 64.8 (24) | $X^2$ = 3.85 | 0.05 |
| Percent entering treatment after study, % (*N*) | 29.6 (8) | 39 (14) | $X^2$ = 0.6 | NS |

problems. This population was targeted because of their low motivation for changing drug use behaviors and poor treatment engagement rate compared with other drug-abusing probationers seeking treatment in our clinic. In this initial study, we found that a treatment that combined CM and MET was associated with a significantly higher rate of treatment completion and more session attendance compared with an MET alone condition. Moreover, the rate of treatment engagement (defined as remaining in treatment for more than 1 month after the end of the study) in the combined MET + CM condition (69%) was much higher than that historically found for this population in our outpatient program (43%).

Although the sample size was small, our findings suggest that the addition of CM to MET in this sample had an effect on treatment retention but not on marijuana use. Previous controlled trials of CM have suggested that that treatment effects are usually specific to the behavior being reinforced (Higgins *et al.*, 1994; Iguchi *et al.*, 1996; Petry, 2000). Thus, our findings are consistent with this literature and extend these findings to a marijuana-dependent population.

Analysis of secondary outcomes indicated substantial improvements in marijuana use, severity of legal problems, and readiness for change (as evidenced by reduction in precontemplation scores) over time for participants as a whole, although no main effects were seen by treatment condition. The lack of significant treatment differences on the marijuana use outcomes also suggest that direct reinforcement of abstinence may be needed to produce further reductions in marijuana use in this population. It is of note that urine toxicology screen results were not shared with probation officers while participants were in the study (the only information that was shared with the referring probation officers is whether participants were still enrolled in the treatment program).

308

*Kathleen M. Carroll* et al.

Thus, although this may have been a factor in the high rate of correspondence between self-reports and urine toxicology reports, the substantial pressure that could be exerted by probation officers generally did not appear to be a major factor in the findings.

Also, because we did not include a no-treatment comparison group, we can draw no conclusions regarding the efficacy of MET in this population. Nevertheless, these findings suggest that scientifically validated treatments such as MET and CM were well accepted by this population and seem to be of benefit to them in several important areas.

The success of our initial work in this area suggests that MET is compatible with the voucher approach. That is, both treatments target substance user's motivation to change their behavior in highly complementary ways: MET through enhancing the individuals' internal change resources for change, CM through providing incentives for change. Our experience in combining MET and CM within the study was that the participants experienced this as "we think abstinence is the best idea and we will offer you some incentives to talk with us and give abstinence a try while you are here, but ultimately you are free to decide what you want to do about your marijuana use". One patient said, "it showed you guys cared about what happens with me; you actually put something behind it".

It should be noted that this small study did not permit an extended follow-up of the participants, and thus it is not clear whether the study treatments had durable effects on the participants' marijuana use, criminal behavior, and other outcomes. Nevertheless, our hope is that this type of early intervention targeted to this important, understudied population may be associated with important long-term benefits. This group had several risk factors known to increase the likelihood of continued involvement in drug abuse, crime and deviant behavior (DuRant *et al.*, 1999; Kandel *et al.*, 1997). These included an early age of onset of drug use, a high rate of school dropout, minimal previous treatment and an average of over five arrests in this comparatively young sample, with a lifetime average of 10 months in prison. Furthermore, the arrests were not only limited to drug-related charges (mean of 1.5), but also included violent crimes (1.5) and charges associated with property-related crimes (2.0), underscoring their involvement in multiple deviant behaviors.

**Summary**

In this chapter we described the rationale for and results from a preliminary study of the efficacy of strategies to engage probation-referred marijuana-abusing young adults in substance abuse treatment. It is a population that is frequently referred to substance abuse treatment by the criminal justice system, that is at high risk for progression to more severe problems and for which few empirically validated treatments have been described. It should be noted that the present study was limited by a small sample size, the use of brief interventions that targeted a limited range of outcomes, and lack of a control condition which permitted evaluation of the efficacy of MET itself. Moreover, the CM intervention targeted only retention and not abstinence; thus we are currently conducting a larger randomized trial evaluating the effects of providing reinforcement for both retention as well as abstinence. Future research on the development of effective treatment interventions for this population is needed on the extent to which these and other behavioral strategies can be used to achieve marijuana abstinence, to assess whether improvements in marijuana use can be sustained over time and whether targeting marijuana use in the population is an effective strategy for reducing the risk of progression to more severe drug use and legal involvement in this highly vulnerable population.

## References

Anthony, J. C., Warner, L. A., & Kessler, R. C. (1994). Comparative epidemiology of dependence on tobacco, alcohol, controlled substances and inhalants. Basic findings from the National Comorbidity Study. *Experimental and Clinical Psychopharmacology*, 2, 244–268.

Babor, T. F. (1994). Avoiding the horrid and beastly sin of drunkenness: Does dissuasion make a difference? *Journal of Consulting and Clinical Psychology*, 62, 1127–1140.

Bien, T. H., Miller, W. R., & Tonigan, J. S. (1993). Brief interventions for alcohol problems: a review. *Addiction*, 88, 315–335.

Carroll, K. M., Libby, B., Sheehan, J., & Hyland, N. (2001). Motivational interviewing to enhance treatment initiation in substance abusers: an effectiveness study. *American Journal on Addictions*, 10, 335–339.

Chen, K., & Kandel, D. B. (1995). The natural history of drug use from adolescence to the mid-thirties in a general population sample. *American Journal of Public Health*, 85, 41–47.

Cornish, J. W., Metzger, D., Woody, G. E., Wilson, D., McLellan, A. T., Vandergrift, B., *et al.* (1997). Naltrexone pharmacotherapy for opioid dependent federal probationers. *Journal of Substance Abuse Treatment*, 14, 529–534.

DuRant, R. H., Smith, J. A., Kreiter, S. R., & Krowchuk, D. P. (1999). The relationship between early age onset of initial substance use and engaging in multiple health risk behaviors among young adolescents. *Archives of Pediatric & Adolescent Medicine*, 153, 286–291.

Higgins, S. T., Delany, D. D., Budney, A. J., Bickel, W. K., Hughes, J. R., Foerg, F., *et al.* (1991). A behavioral approach to achieving initial cocaine abstinence. *American Journal of Psychiatry*, 148, 1218–1224.

Higgins, S. T., Budney, A. J., Bickel, W. K., & Hughes, J. R. (1993). Achieving cocaine abstinence with a behavioral approach. *American Journal of Psychiatry, 150,* 763–769.

Higgins, S. T., Budney, A. J., Bickel, W. K., Foerg, F. E., Donham, R., & Badger, G. J. (1994). Incentives improve outcome in outpatient behavioral treatment of cocaine dependence. *Archives of General Psychiatry, 51,* 568–576.

Higgins, S. T., Wong, C. J., Badger, G. J., Haug-Ogden, D. E., & Dantona, R. L. (2000). Contingent reinforcement increases cocaine abstinence during outpatient treatment and one year follow-up. *Journal of Consulting and Clinical Psychology, 68,* 64–72.

Iguchi, M. Y., Lamb, R. J., Belding, M. A., Platt, J. J., Husband, S. D., & Morral, A. R. (1996). Contingent reinforcement of group participation versus abstinence in a methadone maintenance program. *Experimental and Clinical Psychopharmacology, 4,* 1–7.

Institute of Medicine (1990). *Broadening the base of treatment for alcohol problems.* Washington, DC: National Academy Press.

Johnson, L. D., O'Malley, P. M., & Bachman, J. G. (1996). *National survey results on drug use from monitoring the future study, 1975–1995.* Rockville, MD: NIDA.

Kandel, D. B., & Davies, M. (1996). High school students who use crack and other drugs. *Archives of General Psychiatry, 53,* 71–80.

Kandel, D., & Yamaguchi, K. (1993). From beer to crack: developmental patterns of drug involvement. *American Journal of Public Health, 83,* 851–855.

Kandel, D. B., Yamaguchi, K., & Chen, K. (1992). Stages of progression in drug involvement from adolescence to adulthood. *Journal of Studies on Alcohol, 53,* 447–457.

Kandel, D. B., Chen, K., Warner, L. A., Kessler, R. C., & Grant, B. (1997). Prevalence and demographic correlates of symptoms of last year dependence on alcohol, nicotine, marijuana, and cocaine in the U.S. population. *Drug and Alcohol Dependence, 44,* 11–29.

Leukefeld, C. G., & Tims, F. M. (1988). Compulsory treatment: a review of findings. In C. G. Leukefeld, & F. M. Tims (Eds.), *Compulsory treatment of drug abuse: research and clinical practice* (pp. 236–249). Rockville, MD: NIDA.

Martino, S., Carroll, K. M., O'Malley, S. S., & Rounsaville, B. J. (2000). Motivational interviewing with psychiatrically ill substance abusing patients. *American Journal on Addictions, 9,* 88–91.

McLellan, A. T., Kushner, H., Metzger, D., Peters, R., Smith, I., Grissom, G., *et al.* (1992). The fifth edition of the addiction severity index. *Journal of Substance Abuse Treatment, 9,* 199–213.

Miller, W. R., & Tonigan, J. S. (1996a). Assessing drinker's motivation for change: the stages of change readiness and treatment eagerness scale (SOCRATES). *Psychology of Addictive Behaviors, 10,* 81–89.

Miller, W. R., & Tonigan, J. S. (1996b). Assessing drinker's motivation for change: the stages of change readiness and treatment eagerness scale (SOCRATES). *Psychology of Addictive Behaviors, 10,* 81–89.

Miller, W. R., Brown, J. M., Simpson, T. L., Handmaker, N. S., Bien, T. H., Luckie, L. F., *et al.* (1995). What works? A methodological analysis of the alcohol treatment literature. In R. K. Hester, & W. R. Miller (Eds.), *Handbook of alcoholism treatment approaches: effective alternatives* (pp. 12–44). Boston, MA: Allyn & Bacon.

Miller, W. R., Rollnick, S., & Moyers, T. B. (1998). *Motivation an interviewing: professional videotape series, 1998.* Washington, DC: American Psychological Association.

MTP Research Group (Babor, T. F., Carroll, K. M., Christiansen, K., Kadden, R., Litt, M. McRee, B., Miller, M. Roffman, R., Solowij, N., Steinberg, K., Stephens, R. Vendetti, J., Donaldson, J., & Herrell, J.) (2004). Brief treatments for cannabis dependence. Findings from a randomized multisite trial. *Journal of Consulting and Clinical Psychology, 72,* 455–466.

Petry, N. M. (2000). A comprehensive guide to the application of contingency management procedures in clinical settings. *Drug and Alcohol Dependence, 58,* 9–25.

Petry, N. M., Martin, B., Cooney, J. L., & Kranzler, H. R. (2000). Give them prizes and they will come: contingency management treatment of alcohol dependence. *Journal of Consulting and Clinical Psychology, 68,* 250–257.

Project MATCH Research Group (1997). Matching alcohol treatments to client heterogeneity: project MATCH post-treatment drinking outcomes. *Journal of Studies on Alcohol, 58,* 7–29.

Regier, D. A., Narrow, W. E., Rae, D. S., Manderscheid, R. W., Locke, B. Z., & Goodwin, F. K. (1993). The defacto US mental health and addictive disorders service system: epidemiological catchment area prospective one-year prevalence rates of disorders and services. *Archives of General Psychiatry, 50,* 85–91.

Saunders, B., Wilkinson, C., & Philips, M. (1995). The impact of a brief motivational intervention with opiate users attending a methadone programme. *Addiction, 90,* 415–424.

Silverman, K., Higgins, S. T., Brooner, R. K., Montoya, I. D., Cone, E. J., Schuster, C. R., *et al.* (1996). Sustained cocaine abstinence in methadone maintenance patients through voucher-based reinforcement therapy. *Archives of General Psychiatry, 53,* 409–415.

Sinha, R., Easton, C., Renee-Aubin, L., & Carroll, K. M. (2003). Engaging young probation-referred marijuana-abusing individuals in treatment: a pilot trial. *American Journal on Addictions, 12,* 314–323.

Stephens, R., Roffman, R. A., & Simpson, E. E. (1994). Treating adult marijuana dependence: a test of the relapse prevention model. *Journal of Consulting and Clinical Psychology, 62,* 92–99.

Stephens, R., Roffman, R. A., & Curtin, L. (2000). Comparison of extended versus brief treatments for marijuana use. *Journal of Consulting and Clinical Psychology, 68*, 898–908.

Swanson, A. J., Pantalon, M. V., & Cohen, K. R. (1999). Motivational interviewing and treatment adherence among psychiatric and dually diagnosed patients. *Journal of Nervous and Mental Disease, 187*, 630–635.

Weisner, C., & Schmidt, L. A. (1995). Expanding the frame of health services research in the drug abuse field. *Health Services Research, 30*, 707–726.

WHO Brief Intervention Study Group (1996). A randomized cross-national clinical trial of brief interventions with heavy drinkers. *American Journal of Public Health, 86*, 948–955.

Wilk, A. I., Jensen, N. M., & Havighurst, T. C. (1997). Meta-analysis of randomized controlled trials addressing brief interventions in heavy alcohol drinkers. *Journal of General Internal Medicine, 12*, 274–283.

# Part IV
Policy

# 14

# The Policy Implications of Cannabis Dependence

WAYNE HALL AND WENDY SWIFT

## Introduction

In this chapter, we discuss the potential policy implications of the observation that some cannabis users become dependent on the drug in the sense that they lose control of their use, and find themselves unable to cut down or stop using cannabis despite health and personal problems caused by its use. We begin by summarizing the key features of cannabis dependence, and briefly discussing why dependence requires a policy response. The various ways in which the public health system may respond to cannabis dependence are then explored. These options are not limited to specialist interventions for people who request assistance to stop using cannabis. We place specialist interventions in a spectrum of interventions ranging from education about the risks of developing dependence, to screening, early intervention, and specialist treatment. The appropriateness of these interventions will vary with the severity of cannabis dependence. Within specialist treatment programs, we discuss the need for management of withdrawal, comorbid substance disorders (e.g., alcohol and opioid use disorders), comorbid mental disorders (e.g., depression and schizophrenia), and the special problems of cannabis-dependent adolescents. In the absence of evidence on many of these issues, these sections pose questions rather than provide definitive answers.

The final section of the chapter discusses the role that cannabis dependence may play in policy debates about medical cannabis use and the legal status of recreational cannabis use. This section is necessarily speculative given the dearth of evidence. We consider the most probable effects that changing legal sanctions for recreational cannabis use would have on the prevalence and severity of cannabis dependence in the community. This is done in light of the limited evidence on the impact of two popular policy options: "decriminalization" (i.e., removing criminal penalties for personal possession and use of cannabis); and "legalization" (i.e., making the use and sale of cannabis legal in much the same way as alcohol and tobacco).

## Key Features of the Epidemiology of Cannabis Use and Dependence

Cannabis use in Western societies typically begins in the mid to late teens and is most prevalent in the early 20s (Bachman *et al.*, 1997). Use steadily declines from the early and mid 20s to the early 30s. This is similar to patterns of alcohol use, but quite different from tobacco use which is much more persistent. Major role transitions (e.g., entering tertiary education, entering full-time employment, marrying, and having children) explain a substantial part of these changes (see Chapter 4). There is an increase in cannabis use among those who enter college, but their rates of use only catch up with those among students who did not enter college. The largest decreases are seen in cannabis use among males and females after marriage, and especially during pregnancy and after childbirth in women (Bachman *et al.*, 1997; Chen & Kandel, 1995, 1998).

Community mental health surveys (reviewed in Chapter 4) indicate that after alcohol and tobacco dependence, cannabis dependence is one of the most prevalent forms of drug dependence in many developed societies (Anthony & Helzer, 1991; Hall *et al.*, 1999; Kessler *et al.*, 1994). The prevalence of cannabis dependence is around 2% of the adult population per annum (Swift *et al.*, 2001a), with an estimated lifetime risk of 9% among persons who have ever used cannabis (Anthony *et al.*, 1994).

Among general population samples, most people who meet criteria for cannabis dependence do not seek professional help (Degenhardt *et al.*, 2001b; Regier *et al.*, 1993). In the Australian National Survey of Mental Health and Well-being (NSMHWB), for example, 36% of persons who met criteria for any type of drug dependence in the past year (of which cannabis was the most common) sought treatment for that problem. Cannabis-dependent females were more likely to seek treatment than males (45% versus 25%). In 74% of these cases, treatment-seeking was confined to a consultation with a family medical practitioner. Very few sought assistance from mental health or addiction professionals (Degenhardt *et al.*, 2000). Help-seeking is also uncommon among population based (Sas & Cohen, 1997) and convenience (Copeland *et al.*, 1999; Swift *et al.*, 1998a, b) samples of regular, long-term cannabis users.

## Does Cannabis Dependence Require a Policy Response?

The title of our chapter presupposes that cannabis dependence requires a policy response. There are two types of skeptical responses to this assumption: the first questions whether there is a cannabis dependence syndrome; the second concedes that there are people who fit the diagnostic criteria for the syndrome, but argues that cannabis dependence is a trivial problem that has, at worst, minor adverse health or other consequences for affected users. Both objections need to be discussed before we consider how we should respond to cannabis dependence.

Whether there is, indeed, a cannabis dependence syndrome is one of the most contested claims in the cannabis policy debate. Some proponents of prohibition argue that the existence of cannabis dependence is a strong reason to continue this policy, citing animal evidence of tolerance to the effects of tetrahydro-cannabinol (THC) and reports of withdrawal symptoms in heavy users (e.g., Nahas & Latour, 1992). Some critics of current policy contend that cannabis is not a drug of dependence because it does not have a clearly defined withdrawal syndrome (e.g., Zimmer & Morgan, 1997). Both arguments assume that with-drawal and tolerance are defining characteristics of cannabis dependence.

Modern concepts of dependence emphasize impaired control over use and continued use despite problems caused or exacerbated by drug use. In this sense, there is no doubt that some cannabis users want to stop or cut down, and find it very difficult to do so without assistance and support (Hall *et al.*, 2001). For example, the Australian NSMHWB found that approximately one third (36.6%) of recent cannabis users reported these difficulties in controlling their use – this was particularly prevalent among dependent users (86.9% versus 23.2% of non-dependent users) (Swift *et al.*, 2001b). More importantly, an increasing number of individuals are seeking help from drug treatment services in the USA, Europe, and Australia to cut down or stop using cannabis (AIHW, 2003; Dennis *et al.*, 2002; EMCDDA, 2003; SAMHSA, 2004; Shand & Mattick, 2001).

Some skeptics have argued that this increase is an artifact of workplace drug testing, the promotional activities of the "cannabis treatment industry" and increased diversion of cannabis users into treatment by the courts in the USA (Zimmer & Morgan, 1997). In Australia, however, cannabis is widely used, workplace-based drug testing is uncommon, and there is no large private cannabis (or any other drug) treatment industry. Yet treatment services that have tradi-tionally catered for people with alcohol and opiate problems have seen the pro-portion of persons seeking help to stop using cannabis increase from 4% in 1990 (Webster *et al.*, 1991) to 21% in 2001 (AIHW, 2003). This increase has paralleled increases in rates of regular cannabis use among young Australians (Hall *et al.*, 2001). There have also been increases in numbers seeking treat-ment in the Netherlands between 1994 and 2001 in a country in which personal use of cannabis and small scale retail sales have been decriminalized (Dutch National Alcohol and Drug Information System, 2004).

The second type of skeptic argues that if there is a "cannabis dependence syndrome," its health and social consequences are minimal. The most skeptical contest the claim that cannabis use has any major adverse health effects (Grinspoon & Bakalar, 1993; Zimmer & Morgan, 1997). Others could conceivably argue that the adverse health effects identified in recent reviews (e.g., Hall *et al.*, 2001; Hall & Pacula, 2003) are uncommon except among very heavy users, and even then they are not very severe (e.g., chronic bronchitis and other respiratory disease, possibly an increased risk of accidental injury, subtle forms of cognitive impairment, impaired psychosocial development in adolescents, and exacerbation of schizophrenia).

The second form of skepticism seems more defensible but for two reasons we believe that it does not mean that cannabis dependence is an issue of no policy importance. First, these are the health effects so far identified from a minimal amount of epidemiological research. We should avoid the fallacy of inferring that the absence of evidence of harm is equivalent to evidence that cannabis is harmless (Hall & Babor, 2000). We can be sure that cannabis-dependent persons are at the highest risk of experiencing any of the harms that future research may reveal are caused by regular cannabis use.

Second, the loss of control over one's drug use, which is a cardinal feature of dependence, can be a problem in and of itself, regardless of the severity of its adverse health and psychological consequences. Indeed, it is this loss of control, as reflected in repeated failed efforts to stop or cut down, that prompts many dependent cannabis users to seek help (Budney *et al.*, 1998; Copeland *et al.*, 2001b; Stephens *et al.*, 2000, 2002). If the fact that individuals seek help to cut down or stop provides sufficient reason for providing services for problem drinkers and gamblers, then there is the same warrant to respond to cannabis dependence.

**Public Health System Responses to Cannabis Dependence**

The low rate of specialist treatment-seeking among persons with cannabis use disorders in population surveys does not necessarily mean that treatment services should actively seek out all community members with cannabis use disorders. Since a substantial proportion of these disorders will remit in the absence of professional help, it would be inefficient to use scarce clinical resources to deal with time-limited and minimally-disabling disorders. Also, a substantial proportion of persons with less severe cannabis use disorders may not be interested in treatment, as is the case for alcohol use disorders (Grant, 1997). The attempt to identify and treat persons with these disorders may also medicalize behavior that is better dealt with in other ways.

In considering how to address cannabis dependence in the population, we have used as our point of departure a similar analysis of a public health approach to addressing alcohol use disorders (Hall & Teesson, 2000). In the absence of similarly rich outcome data on the treatment of cannabis dependence, the following analysis should be seen as identifying opportunities for intervention that need to be evaluated, rather than as a set of specific recommendations about what should be done.

## Public Health Policies for Cannabis

A major development in responding to alcohol dependence and alcohol-related health problems has been the adoption of a public health perspective on alcohol use (Edwards *et al.*, 1994). This approach considers the spectrum of health problems caused by alcohol, for example, road traffic accidents, dependence, lost productivity, violence, and diseases such as cancer, liver cirrhosis, brain damage, and heart disease (Edwards *et al.*, 1994). A similar perspective could usefully inform our thinking about responding to cannabis-related problems, including cannabis dependence.

A public health approach examines the characteristics of the physical and social environment that encourage heavy drinking, as well as the characteristics that predispose some drinkers to develop alcohol use disorders. This includes the role of advertising and promotion of alcohol, and the ready availability of alcohol at low prices (Edwards *et al.*, 1994; Walsh & Hingson, 1987). Among the measures proposed for decreasing hazardous alcohol consumption are: laws and regulations which aim to reduce the availability of alcohol (e.g., licensing regulations which restrict trading hours for liquor outlets, and the enforcement of laws on underage drinking); measures which increase the price of alcohol to reduce consumption (e.g., increased taxes levied on the alcohol content of beverages); and regulations to control the promotion of alcohol (Edwards *et al.*, 1994; Walsh & Hingson, 1987).

The prohibition on the recreational use, cultivation, and sale of cannabis is primarily aimed at preventing young people from using cannabis. Enforcement of the prohibitions on cultivation and sales are intended to reduce the availability of cannabis, and criminal penalties for use are intended to deter young people from using. Prohibition also maintains a high price for cannabis which may discourage adolescents from initiating cannabis use, and may shorten the duration of use among young adults who do use it (Hall & Pacula, 2003). The policy options of regulation and price (such as, age restrictions on purchase, restrictions on hours of sale, and taxation based on THC content) cannot be used for cannabis while its use remains prohibited. It has proven difficult to assess the impact that cannabis prohibition has on cannabis use (see Hall & Pacula, 2003, Chapter 14).

**Public Education about Cannabis Dependence**

Public education campaigns can be used to inform drinkers about the risks of alcohol use. In Australia, for example, guidelines about the maximum number of standard drinks that can be legally consumed before driving, in combination with random breath testing, have reduced overall road fatalities and the proportion in which drivers have a blood alcohol level above the prescribed level of 0.05% (Homel, 1990). These campaigns enjoy widespread public support, and may have reduced alcohol consumption by providing an excuse to moderate consumption (Homel, 1990; Peek-Asa, 1999). Alcohol campaigns have primarily addressed the risks of intoxication, but there is no reason why more attention could not be paid to patterns of alcohol consumption that pose a risk of developing dependence.

In countries that prohibit the use of cannabis, it is difficult to implement public health education about ways to use cannabis that reduce the risks of dependence because the advocacy of "safe" levels of use is seen as condoning its use. This is especially true in countries that advocate a "drug-free society" or pursue a policy of "zero tolerance" towards cannabis use, such as Sweden and the USA (Hall & Pacula, 2003). More limited information on dependence risks can be given by explaining that the risks of cannabis dependence increase with regular use. Such information can be included in health education about cannabis, usually along with a clear message that cannabis use is illegal. An important question for health education is whether including messages about the illegality of cannabis use compromises the credibility of information about its adverse health effects, including dependence.

A sensible strategy in communicating the risks of cannabis dependence may be to capitalize on knowledge about the dependence potential of alcohol and tobacco. In most developed societies, it is reasonably well appreciated that alcohol and tobacco are drugs of dependence, although the public could be better educated about the dependence risks of alcohol. Any health education about these risks for alcohol and other drug dependence could also include information on the risks of cannabis dependence. This should avoid exaggerating the prevalence and the adverse effects of cannabis dependence by emphasizing that the risk increases when cannabis is used daily for weeks or months, as is true for alcohol and tobacco dependence. This approach is currently being included in the drug education curriculum in some Australian schools (e.g., *Cannabis: Know the Risks*) (New South Wales Department of Education and Training, 2003).

## Screening and Brief Intervention for Hazardous Cannabis Use

Persons who present for medical treatment can be screened for hazardous alcohol use and alcohol-related problems. Screening and brief advice for excessive alcohol consumption in general practice and hospital settings reduces consumption and the problems caused by alcohol (Chick *et al.*, 1985; Elvy *et al.*, 1988; Kristenson *et al.*, 1983; Shand *et al.*, 2003; Wallace *et al.*, 1988). There is a good economic argument for such interventions (Shand *et al.*, 2003). They usually involve 1–3 h in screening and brief advice which can potentially reach a far greater number of persons whose drinking is hazardous or harmful than can specialist alcohol treatment services.

The same approach could conceivably be adopted for cannabis use disorders in primary care settings where there is likely to be a reasonable prevalence of cannabis use among young adults. For example, young adults with respiratory problems could be routinely screened about their cannabis use, along with their use of tobacco. Similarly, young adults with symptoms of anxiety and depression may be screened because of evidence that there are high rates of these disorders among cannabis-dependent persons who seek help from family physicians (Degenhardt *et al.*, 2001b). Training and support of primary health workers is vital to maximize screening and intervention. Such health workers may not be very knowledgeable about the effects of cannabis use; they may not be confident about raising the issue, engaging clients or having an effect on their behavior; and they may also be unsure of the legal implications of discussing illegal behavior (Penrose-Wall *et al.*, 2000; Roche & Freeman, 2004).

A "Check-up" approach modeled on the Brief Drinker Check-up (Miller & Sovereign, 1989) provides a promising model for raising the health risks of cannabis use in a non-confrontational way (see Chapters 8 and 12). This approach combines an assessment of cannabis use and health with personalized feedback of information. The screening could include symptoms of cannabis dependence and patterns of cannabis use that place the user at increased risk of developing dependence. Simple advice and self-help material can be provided. If more time is available, a brief session containing guided materials could be provided (e.g., a single session of motivational enhancement therapy and/or skills training). If a brief session is insufficient or inappropriate, the person can be referred to specialist treatment. While clinical lore suggests that dependent users would not benefit from such brief interventions, recent trials of severely dependent cannabis users have found that even one or two sessions of counseling can improve outcomes up to 6 months later, compared to a wait-list control group (Copeland *et al.*, 2001b; Stephens *et al.*, 2000) (see Chapter 6).

Cannabis-dependent persons who do not want to stop using cannabis could be given advice on how to minimize some of the potential adverse health effects of their cannabis use (Hall, 1995c; Swift *et al.*, 2000). An obvious way of reducing the respiratory risks of cannabis use is to change the route of administration from smoking to swallowing. This is unlikely to be a popular suggestion given the pharmacology of smoked and swallowed cannabis (Hall *et al.*, 2001). The next best options may be to advise against smoking tobacco and cannabis together, and to discourage the use of waterpipes, deep inhalation, and breath holding. A recent trial of vaporization suggests this method may deliver levels of THC comparable to that of cannabis cigarettes with substantial decreases in several pyrolytic smoke compounds (Gieringer *et al.*, 2004). We should also advise cannabis users against driving or operating machinery after using cannabis or feeling its effects. Such advice may help dependent cannabis users to reduce some of the risks of their use.

**Specialist Treatment for Cannabis Dependence**

There will be a role for specialist treatment for cannabis dependence, as there is for alcohol use disorders, because self-help and brief interventions are not sufficient to produce cessation or moderation of use for all dependent users. A number of trials have now established that cannabis dependence can be successfully treated on an outpatient basis in the sense that rates of cannabis use and cannabis-related problems are substantially reduced after treatment (Babor *et al.*, 2004; Budney *et al.*, 1998, 2000; Copeland *et al.*, 2001b; Stephens *et al.*, 1994, 2000). Abstinence rates have been modest in many of these trials (e.g., around 15% reporting continuous abstinence at 6-month follow-ups according to Copeland, *et al.* (2001b), and 12-month follow-ups according to Stephens *et al.* (1994)). These low rates of abstinence may tempt some to advocate residential or inpatient treatment for the more severely cannabis-dependent. Experience with the treatment of alcohol dependence suggests that we should be wary of pursuing this path.

Controlled evaluations of treatment for alcohol dependence suggest that treatment should not be *routinely* provided in an inpatient or residential setting

(Shand *et al.*, 2003). Reviews of the alcohol research literature (Finney *et al.*, 1996; Heather & Tebbutt, 1989; Shand *et al.*, 2003), large scale follow-up studies of treatment (Armor *et al.*, 1978), and well-controlled studies comparing brief advice with more intensive treatment (Orford & Edwards, 1977), indicate that there is, at most, a small benefit from inpatient treatment rather than outpatient assessment and advice to stop drinking.

Given that cannabis use disorders are likely to be less disabling and life threatening than alcohol disorders, the onus of proof should be on those who advocate residential treatment programs for cannabis dependence to demonstrate that this is more effective and cost-effective than outpatient treatment programs. Until this has been done, inpatient and residential treatment for cannabis should be confined to research programs rather than becoming routine forms of care. In the interim it would be better to provide outpatient treatment programs based upon approaches that have been trialed to date.

*Withdrawal Management*

Cannabis withdrawal symptoms are much less severe than withdrawal symptoms of alcohol dependence (Budney *et al.*, 2001; Hall & Zador, 1997). Nonetheless, a substantial proportion of persons seeking help with cannabis problems do report withdrawal symptoms (Budney *et al.*, 1999; Copeland *et al.*, 2001a; Stephens *et al.*, 2002). If failure to complete withdrawal proves to be a barrier to achieving controlled use or abstinence from cannabis, then we may need to improve our management of cannabis withdrawal symptoms, perhaps by using pharmacological assistance to complete withdrawal. It is unlikely, however, that many cannabis users will require an inpatient program to manage withdrawal symptoms.

*Dealing with Comorbid Substance Disorders*

The most common types of comorbidity among cannabis-dependent persons are with other substance use disorders, such as, alcohol, sedative, and opiate disorders (e.g. Degenhardt *et al.*, 2001a; Swift *et al.*, 2001a). Community surveys show that people with cannabis use disorders are more likely to have alcohol and other illicit substance use disorders than those without (Degenhardt *et al.*, 2001a; Swift *et al.*, 2001a). Treatment programs for cannabis dependence that exclude persons with other substance use disorders are therefore excluding an important part of the target population. Accordingly, they will need to incorporate program elements to address alcohol and other drug use disorders among patients affected by them.

Treatment programs for other types of substance dependence may also need to address cannabis disorders. For example, among opioid-dependent people in methadone maintenance treatment cannabis dependence is a common diagnosis (Darke & Ross, 1997; Kidorf *et al.*, 1996). As cannabis dependence does not present such serious consequences as alcohol and opioid dependence, it is often low on the list of clinical priorities. It may deserve more research attention. Some evidence suggests that cannabis dependence predicts a poorer prognosis among opioid-dependent methadone clients (e.g., Bell *et al.*, 1995), whereas other evidence suggests that addressing cannabis dependence makes no difference to the outcome of treatment for opioid dependence (Budney *et al.*, 1998).

### Dealing with Comorbid Mental Disorders

There is no prospective research on the impact of comorbid mental disorders on the treatment of cannabis dependence. Research suggests, however, that alcohol dependence complicated by other comorbid mental disorders, such as anxiety and depression, has a poorer prognosis and is more difficult to treat (Drake *et al.*, 1993; McLellan *et al.*, 1983) than alcohol disorders without comorbid disorders. Persons with comorbid disorders are more likely to have chronic and disabling conditions and to use more health services (Kessler, 1995).

In community surveys, persons with cannabis use disorders report higher rates of anxiety and affective disorders than persons who do not have this diagnosis, and comorbid anxiety and affective disorders predict treatment-seeking (Degenhardt *et al.*, 2001b; Grant, 1995; Regier *et al.*, 1990). In treating cannabis dependence, we may therefore need to improve our recognition and treatment of comorbid anxiety and affective disorders (Hall & Farrell, 1997). There are brief, valid, and reliable screening tests that can be used to detect anxiety and depressive disorders among cannabis-dependent persons (Dawes & Mattick, 1997).

A special difficulty for specialist mental health services is responding to cannabis dependence among young adults with schizophrenia (Hall, 1998). In Australia and the USA, around a third of persons with schizophrenia and other psychoses are daily users of cannabis (Jablensky *et al.*, 2000), a much higher rate than the 2% reported in the general population (Hall *et al.*, 1999). A number of retrospective and prospective studies have shown that cannabis use *exacerbates* the symptoms of schizophrenia (Hall & Degenhardt, 2000).

The treatment of schizophrenic patients is complicated by the presence of cognitive deficits, poor motivation and compliance, impaired social functioning, limited support networks, and the use of neuroleptic medication (Bellack & Gearon,

1998; Mueser *et al.*, 1992). Specific interventions have been developed, including modified 12 step, relapse prevention, motivational enhancement therapy, contingency management approaches, and assertive community treatment (Bellack & Gearon, 1998; Bennett *et al.*, 2001; Kavanagh, 1995; Ziedonis & Brady, 1997). Pharmacotherapeutic approaches have also been proposed (Krystal *et al.*, 1999), but there are few controlled evaluations of their efficacy. The evidence suggests that comprehensive programs that integrate psychiatric and substance use interventions are effective, but their cost is a barrier to their widespread use (Bellack & Gearon, 1998; Drake *et al.*, 1993; Ziedonis & Brady, 1997).

## Responding to Adolescent Cannabis Dependence

Adolescents are a priority group for research into treatment of cannabis dependence. Cannabis use is at its highest during late adolescence, and early initiators are at increased risk of developing dependence (Chen & Kandel, 1995; DeWit *et al.*, 2000), perhaps because adolescents are at greater risk of developing cannabis dependence than adults when using at the same level (Chen *et al.*, 1997). Earlier onset of cannabis use also increases the risk of problems at school (Lynskey & Hall, 2000), later substance-related problems (Anthony & Petronis, 1995; Fergusson *et al.*, 1996; Lynskey *et al.*, 2003; Robins *et al.*, 1970), and involvement in crime (Fergusson *et al.*, 1994).

Anthony (2000) makes a persuasive argument for focusing intervention efforts at the early stages of drug involvement in adolescence, before drug dependence is diagnosed. He contends that "epidemics" of drug use largely spread by "altruistic sharing among non-dependent users," with users typically making a rapid transition from first use to more regular use. Early intervention may prevent spread to others and reduce the transition to dependent use. It also provides an opportunity for primary prevention or improved treatment of psychological disorders such as anxiety, depression or schizophrenia, if prodromal symptoms are recognized and appropriate interventions are provided (see also Häfner & Maurer, 2000).

Cannabis use and dependence may be only one of several behaviors during adolescence that have overlapping risk or protective factors and compromise health and well-being. Gender and developmental issues and adolescents' burgeoning autonomy and changing social relationships indicate the need for a unique approach with this group. In addition, many young cannabis users may not be motivated to change because they neither consider their use a problem, nor see the need to change, despite the concerns of parents and difficulties at school and with the law. Promising research using motivational approaches (e.g., McCambridge & Strang, 2004), which include the "Check-up" approach to enhance motivation with this group (Chapter 6), suggest that further investment in early intervention efforts is warranted. This research is making it clear that families have an important role to play in engaging and supporting substance-using adolescents in help-seeking (see Chapter 11).

A range of approaches is needed for adolescents, from preventive measures to tertiary interventions. There remain large gaps in the provision of services to this group, particularly for adolescents in the criminal justice system and among ethnic minorities. Policy responses to cannabis dependence in adolescents need to be evaluated and the results used to improve the design of more effective services.

## Cannabis Dependence and the Cannabis Policy Debate

The existence of cannabis dependence is a contested issued in the cannabis policy debate in the USA, as has been discussed above. Proponents of cannabis law reform are understandably skeptical about the existence of a cannabis dependence syndrome because it increases the difficulty of making a case for changing legal sanctions against cannabis use. Cannabis law reformers already face a difficult political task; a much stronger case needs to be made to remove the prohibition of cannabis than is required to continue the current policy of cannabis prohibition (MacCoun & Reuter, 2001).

Nonetheless, advocates of cannabis law reform can acknowledge that some cannabis users will become dependent on the drug, but still argue for a change in the legal sanctions for cannabis use. Developed societies allow the use, sale, and promotion of alcohol and tobacco, substances which have more serious health consequences for dependent users than cannabis (Hall, 1995a). The governments of many developed societies also derive substantial taxation revenue from gambling, an activity that can share many of the compulsive features of cannabis dependence (Elster, 1999). In the cases of alcohol, tobacco, and gambling, the societal judgment has been that the social costs of prohibition do not justify any health gains that it may bring by reducing use (MacCoun & Reuter, 2001). The same type of argument can be made for changing current cannabis policy (Hall, 2000; Hall & Pacula, 2003).

## Dependence and Therapeutic Cannabinoid Use

It is not clear how relevant the risk of cannabis dependence in recreational users is to patients who use cannabinoids for therapeutic reasons (Institute of Medicine, 1999). A review of several indicators of the abuse potential of dronabinol (synthetic THC) found little evidence of dependence on THC when it was used therapeutically (Calhoun *et al.*, 1998; Neff *et al.*, 2002), but the risks and severity of dependence from therapeutic cannabinoid use is a research priority.

Until further research is undertaken the following generalizations can be made (Swift & Hall, 2002). First, the risk of dependence is likely to be low if THC or cannabis is used for a limited period, as in a short course of treatment to reduce nausea and vomiting during chemotherapy or radiotherapy. Given the benefits of increased compliance with potentially life-saving treatment (e.g., cancer chemotherapy), the small risk of dependence may be judged by patients and doctors to be worth taking.

Second, there is a greater risk of dependence if cannabinoids are used to treat chronic disorders, such as glaucoma, multiple sclerosis, and neurological disorders. Tolerance is likely to develop, even though many patients seem able to achieve a therapeutic benefit at a stable dose (Beal *et al.*, 1997; Grinspoon & Bakalar, 1993; Maurer *et al.*, 1990). However, even if the risk of dependence is as high as it is among daily recreational cannabis users, patients may judge this to be a reasonable price for the relief of distressing symptoms that disable and interfere with their lives. In the case of terminal illnesses, such as cancers and AIDS, dependence may be a minor concern (Gurley *et al.*, 1998).

The major ethical issue in the chronic therapeutic use of cannabinoids is ensuring that there is informed patient consent to their use. Patients need to be informed about the risk of dependence so they can weigh it among the costs and benefits of therapeutic cannabinoid use. Patients need to be told about the type of dependence symptoms that they may experience, the possible side effects of daily cannabinoid use (e.g., on memory and concentration), the severity of withdrawal symptoms they may experience if they choose to stop, and where to seek assistance if it is required.

## Possible Effects of Changes in the Legal Status of Cannabis Use

No studies have directly examined the effects of changes in the legal status of cannabis on the prevalence of cannabis dependence. An argument by analogy to our experience with alcohol would suggest that an increase in the availability of cannabis would increase the rates and frequency of cannabis use, and, all else being equal, this would increase rates of cannabis dependence (Edwards *et al.*, 1994). The available evidence on the effects of changes in cannabis policy assesses the effect that changes in penalties for the use of cannabis have on the prevalence of its use. These changes are often described as cannabis decriminalization and *de facto* cannabis legalization.

## Decriminalization of Cannabis Use

The decriminalization of cannabis use involves replacing penal sanctions (i.e., a period of imprisonment) with civil penalties (e.g., a fine, probation or education). It has a number of appeals: it is a modest and easily reversed policy option that promises to reduce some of the harms caused by cannabis prohibition, namely, the harms to users of having a criminal record, the discriminatory enforcement of the law, and the inappropriate use of scarce police and criminal justice system resources (Criminal Justice Commission, 1994; Hall & Pacula, 2003; Single *et al.*, 1999).

Decriminalization was a popular policy option among proponents of cannabis law reform in the USA in the 1970s (Himmelstein, 1983; Maloff, 1981; Single, 1989) and in Australia in the 1980s (Bowman & Sanson-Fisher, 1994; Criminal Justice Commission, 1994). A form of this policy has been implemented in 11 US states (Single, 1989) and in the Australian states of South Australia (1987), the Australian Capital Territory (1992), and the Northern Territory (1997) (Ali *et al.*, 1999).

Assessments of the effects of decriminalization in the USA (Single, 1989), South Australia (Donnelly *et al.*, 1995, 1999), and the Netherlands (MacCoun & Reuter, 1997) have found that decriminalization had little or no effect on rates of cannabis use in surveys of school children and adults. While these studies have their limitations (Maloff, 1981; Single, 1989) they have reasonably and consistently found that the substitution of civil for criminal penalties does not substantially increase rates of cannabis use in the lifetime or the past year (MacCoun & Reuter, 2000). None of these studies, however, has had sufficient statistical precision to examine the impact of decriminalization on rates of monthly or more frequent cannabis use, and none has estimated its effects on the prevalence of cannabis dependence (Hall & Pacula, 2003).

## De Facto Legalization of Cannabis Use

Since 1983, The Netherlands has had a *de facto* legal market in cannabis in its largest cities. In 1976, the Netherlands introduced a policy of not enforcing the criminal penalties for the possession and use of small quantities of cannabis. Since 1983, it has also tolerated the sale of cannabis in coffee shops in Amsterdam and other large cities. Cannabis sales are allowed in these shops if there are no sales to minors, no alcohol or hard drugs are sold, and there are limits on the quantity of cannabis that coffee shops can hold and that users can purchase.

There have been conflicting evaluations of the impact of the Netherlands policies on rates of cannabis use (Cohen & Sas, 1998; MacCoun & Reuter, 1997). Cohen and Sas have argued, using Dutch survey data, that cannabis use has increased at the same rate in the Netherlands as elsewhere in Europe, thereby reflecting shared trends in youth culture rather than the effects of Dutch policy. MacCoun and Reuter (1997, 2001) have drawn a different conclusion from comparisons of trends in cannabis use in surveys in the Netherlands, the USA, Norway, and Sweden. They argued that the policy of not enforcing criminal penalties against cannabis use had no discernible effect on rates of cannabis use in the Netherlands between 1976 and the early 1980s. However, they also argued that the policy of tolerating a legal cannabis market since 1983, in combination with the promotional activities of youth and popular culture, have led to a greater increase in cannabis use in the Netherlands than in comparable European countries (MacCoun & Reuter, 2001). It is not known whether any such increase in rates of use has led to increased rates of cannabis dependence. There are reports of increased numbers of persons presenting to treatment services in the Netherlands for cannabis dependence (Dutch National Alcohol and Drug Information System, 2004) but it is not clear that this has been at a faster rate than elsewhere in Europe.

### De Jure Legalization of Cannabis

The legalization of cannabis would make it legal for any adult to use cannabis and produce and sell it, in much the same way that it is legal to use, manufacture and sell alcohol and tobacco in developed societies. The major roles for government under cannabis legalization would be to control the quality of cannabis products, regulate the behavior of manufacturers and distributors, tax cannabis sales, and restrict sales to minors (Hall & Pacula, 2003). No developed country has a policy of cannabis legalization because most are signatories to the Single Convention on Narcotic Drugs, which rules out this policy option. There is consequently no evidence on the effects of this policy on rates of cannabis use or cannabis dependence (Hall & Pacula, 2003).

Since no country has enacted *de jure* cannabis legalization, we can only speculate about the likely effects of this policy (Hall & Pacula, 2003). It is a reasonable prediction, given our experience with alcohol (Edwards *et al.*, 1994), that legalizing cannabis sales would lead to more people using cannabis regularly because availability would increase and price would fall (Hall & Pacula, 2003). If cannabis were legal, more cannabis users may also use cannabis for a much longer part of their adult lives than is the case under prohibition when most users discontinue in their mid to late 20s (Bachman *et al.*, 1997; Chen & Kandel, 1995). More regular cannabis use would probably also mean more cannabis-related health and psychological problems, such as dependence, impaired school performance among adolescents, and exacerbation of psychoses in the population (Hall, 1995b). Some increase in cannabis use and dependence seems likely after legalization but it is difficult to predict how large an increase might occur or to what extent increased use may be offset by countervailing measures, such as taxation policies (Hall & Pacula, 2003; MacCoun & Reuter, 2001).

A legal cannabis market would allow the taxation of cannabis sales to regulate use but, since cannabis is already effectively taxed at a high rate by the illicit market, taxation could not increase its price above existing black market prices because an incentive would remain for a cannabis black market (Courtwright, 2001). In order to undercut the black market it is much more likely that the cannabis price under a legal market will be considerably less than the current black market price (Hall & Pacula, 2003).

A legal cannabis market would make it easier to adopt other measures that may limit the increase in cannabis use or reduce rates of harmful cannabis use. It would be much easier, for example, to teach users ways of using cannabis that reduce the risks of developing dependence (e.g., by limiting use to less than weekly) and other adverse health effects (e.g., eating rather than smoking cannabis). A legal regime may also allow the development of social norms that stigmatize, and thereby discourage, regular cannabis intoxication and compulsive cannabis use, although it is uncertain how effective such norms may be. It is difficult to predict what the net effects of legalization would be because no one knows how the effects of increased availability and reduced price would be offset by the type of efforts to reduce harmful use that would become available under a legal cannabis regime. Our experience with alcohol suggests that such educational initiatives would have at most a modest effect.

## Conclusions

Cannabis use disorders are among the most common forms of drug dependence after alcohol and nicotine in community surveys, but very few persons with these disorders seek or receive treatment. This does not necessarily mean that cannabis dependence is under-treated, because many cases identified in population surveys will remit without professional help. Public education about the risks of cannabis use may be the best way of preventing and ameliorating the public health impact of the more common and less severe forms of cannabis use disorders. Good advice on self-help strategies for quitting or cutting down may obviate the need for further professional assistance in these cases. For individuals whose problems resist self-help, treatment needs to be provided on an outpatient basis. Special issues that need to be addressed are: comorbidity between cannabis dependence, other drug dependence, and other mental disorders; and the special needs of adolescents with cannabis dependence.

The existence of cannabis dependence complicates the political task of those who want to decriminalize or legalize cannabis use. This has led some cannabis law reformers to attempt to debunk the idea of cannabis dependence. Our experience with alcohol, tobacco, and gambling indicates that having a potential for dependence is not sufficient to justify prohibition. The existence of cannabis dependence does not preclude the medical uses of cannabis and cannabinoids, provided that patients are informed about the risks.

There is limited evidence on the impact of proposed changes to the legal status of cannabis on the prevalence of cannabis dependence. The available evidence suggests that cannabis decriminalization is likely to have, at most, a modest impact on rates of cannabis use, and, by implication, on rates of cannabis dependence. It is much less certain what the effects would be of legalizing cannabis, but experience with alcohol would suggest that a legal cannabis market would increase the availability and reduce the price of cannabis and permit more promotion of its use, all of which would probably increase rates of regular cannabis use and hence the prevalence of cannabis dependence. It is unclear how large an increase there would be and to what extent it might be offset by measures designed to reduce hazardous patterns of cannabis use.

## References

Ali, R., Christie, P., Lenton, S., Hawks, D., Sutton, A., *et al.* (1999). *The Social Impacts of the Cannabis Expiation Notice Scheme in South Australia: Summary Report Presented to the Ministerial Council on Drug Strategy* (National Drug Strategy Monograph, Vol. 34). Canberra, Australian Capital Territory: Commonwealth Department of Health and Aged Care.

Anthony, J. C. (2000). Putting epidemiology and public health in needs assessment: drug dependence and beyond. In G. Andrews, & S. Henderson (Eds.), *Unmet need in psychiatry: problems, resources, responses* (pp. 302–308). Cambridge, MA: Cambridge University Press.

Anthony, J. C., & Helzer, J. E. (1991). Syndromes of drug abuse and dependence. In L. N. Robins, & D. A. Regier (Eds.), *Psychiatric disorders in America: the epidemiologic catchment area* (pp. 116–154). New York: Free Press.

Anthony, J. C., & Petronis, K. R. (1995). Early-onset drug use and risk of later drug problems. *Drug and Alcohol Dependence, 40*(1), 9–15.

Anthony, J. C., Warner, L., & Kessler, R. (1994). Comparative epidemiology of dependence on tobacco, alcohol, controlled substances and inhalants: basic findings from the National Comorbidity Survey. *Experimental and Clinical Psychopharmacology*, 2(3), 244–268.

Armor, D., Polich, J. M., & Stambul, H. (1978). *Alcoholism and treatment*. New York: John Wiley and Sons.

Australian Institute of Health and Welfare (AIHW) (2003). *Alcohol and Other Drug Treatment Services in Australia 2001–2002: Report on the National Minimum Data Set*. Canberra, Australian Capital Territory: AIHW.

Babor, T. F., Carroll, K. M., Christiansen, K., Kadden, R., Litt, M., *et al.* (2004). Brief treatments for cannabis dependence: findings from a randomized multisite trial. *Journal of Consulting and Clinical Psychology*, 72(3), 455–466.

Bachman, J. G., Wadsworth, K. N., O'Malley, P. M., Johnston, L. D., & Schulenberg, J. (1997). *Smoking, drinking, and drug use in young adulthood: the impacts of new freedoms and new responsibilities*. Mahwah, NJ: Lawrence Erlbaum.

Beal, J., Olson, R., Lefkowitz, L., Laubenstein, L., Bellman, P., *et al.* (1997). Long-term efficacy and safety of dronabinol for acquired immunodeficiency syndrome-associated anorexia. *Journal of Pain and Symptom Management*, 14, 7–14.

Bell, J., Ward, J., Mattick, R. P., Hay, A., Chan, J., & Hall, W. (1995). *An Evaluation of Private Methadone Clinics* (National Drug Strategy Research Report Series, Report No. 4). Canberra, Australian Capital Territory: Australian Government Publishing Service (AGPS).

Bellack, A. S., & Gearon, J. S. (1998). Substance abuse treatment for people with schizophrenia. *Addictive Behaviors*, 23(6), 749–766.

Bennett, M. E., Bellack, A. S., & Gearon, J. S. (2001). Treating substance abuse in schizophrenia: an initial report. *Journal of Substance Abuse Treatment*, 20(2), 163–175.

Bowman, J., & Sanson-Fisher, R. (1994). *Public Perceptions of Cannabis Legalization*, (National Drug Strategy Monograph, Vol. 28). Canberra: Australian Government Publishing Service (AGPS).

Budney, A. J., Radonovich, K. J., Higgins, S. T., & Wong, C. J. (1998). Adults seeking treatment for marijuana dependence: a comparison with cocaine-dependent treatment seekers. *Experimental and Clinical Psychopharmacology*, 6(4), 419–426.

Budney, A. J., Novy, P. L., & Hughes, J. R. (1999). Marijuana withdrawal among adults seeking treatment for marijuana dependence. *Addiction*, 94(9), 1311–1322.

Budney, A. J., Higgins, S. T., Radonovich, K. J., & Novy, P. L. (2000). Adding voucher-based incentives to coping skills and motivational enhancement improves outcomes during treatment for marijuana dependence. *Journal of Consulting and Clinical Psychology*, 68(6), 1051–1061.

Budney, A. J., Hughes, J. R., Moore, B. A., & Novy, P. L. (2001). Marijuana abstinence effects in marijuana smokers maintained in their home environment. *Archives of General Psychiatry*, 58(10), 917–924.

Calhoun, S. R., Galloway, G. P., & Smith, D. E. (1998). Abuse potential of dronabinol (Marinol). *Journal of Psychoactive Drugs, 30*(2), 187–196.

Chen, K., & Kandel, D. B. (1995). The natural history of drug use from adolescence to the mid-thirties in a general population sample. *American Journal of Public Health, 85*(1), 41–47.

Chen, K., & Kandel, D. B. (1998). Predictors of cessation of marijuana use: an event history analysis. *Drug and Alcohol Dependence, 50*(2), 109–121.

Chen, K., Kandel, D. B., & Davies, M. (1997). Relationships between frequency and quantity of marijuana use and last year proxy dependence among adolescents and adults in the United States. *Drug and Alcohol Dependence, 46*(1–2), 53–67.

Chick, J., Lloyd, G., & Crombie, E. (1985). Counselling problem drinkers in medical wards: a controlled study. *British Medical Journal, 290*(6473), 965–967.

Cohen, P., & Sas, A. (1998). *Cannabis use, a stepping stone to other drugs? The case of Amsterdam.* Amsterdam: Centre for Drug Research, University of Amsterdam.

Copeland, J., Rees, V., & Swift, W. (1999). Health concerns and help-seeking among a sample entering treatment for cannabis dependence. *Australian Family Physician, 28*, 540–541.

Copeland, J., Swift, W., & Rees, V. (2001a). Clinical profile of participants in a brief intervention program for cannabis use disorder. *Journal of Substance Abuse Treatment, 20*(1), 45–52.

Copeland, J., Swift, W., Roffman, R., & Stephens, R. (2001b). A randomized controlled trial of brief cognitive-behavioral interventions for cannabis use disorder. *Journal of Substance Abuse Treatment, 21*(2), 55–64.

Courtwright, D. T. (2001). *Forces of habit: drugs and the making of the modern world.* Cambridge, MA: Harvard University Press.

Criminal Justice Commission (1994). *Report on Cannabis and the Law in Queensland,* Brisbane: Criminal Justice Commission, Queensland.

Darke, S., & Ross, J. (1997). Polydrug dependence and psychiatric comorbidity among heroin injectors. *Drug and Alcohol Dependence, 48*(2), 135–141.

Dawes, S., & Mattick, R. (1997). *Review of Diagnostic and Screening Instruments for Alcohol and Other Psychiatric Disorders* (2nd ed., Monograph Series No. 48). Canberra, Australian Capital Territory: Australian Government Publishing Service (AGPS).

Degenhardt, L., Hall, W. D., & Lynskey, M. (2000). *Cannabis Use and Mental Health among Australian Adults: Findings from the National Survey of Mental Health and Well-being* (NDARC Technical Report, Vol. 98). Sydney, Australia: National Drug and Alcohol Research Centre, University of New South Wales.

Degenhardt, L., Hall, W., & Lynskey, M. (2001a). The relationship between cannabis use and other substance use in the general population. *Drug and Alcohol Dependence, 64*(3), 319–327.

Degenhardt, L., Hall, W., & Lynskey, M. (2001b). The relationship between cannabis use, depression and anxiety among Australian adults: findings from the National

Survey of Mental Health and Well-being. *Social Psychiatry and Psychiatric Epidemiology, 36*(5), 219–227.

Dennis, M., Babor, T. F., Roebuck, M. C., & Donaldson, J. (2002). Changing the focus: the case for recognizing and treating cannabis use disorders. *Addiction, 97*, 4–15.

DeWit, D. J., Hance, J., Offord, D. R., & Ogborne, A. (2000). The influence of early and frequent use of marijuana on the risk of desistance and of progression to marijuana-related harm. *Preventive Medicine, 31*(5), 455–464.

Donnelly, N., Hall, W. D., & Christie, P. (1995). The effects of partial decriminalisation on cannabis use in South Australia, 1985 to 1993. *Australian Journal of Public Health, 19*(3), 281–287.

Donnelly, N., Hall, W. D., & Christie, P. (1999). *Effects of the Cannabis Expiation Notice Scheme on Levels and Patterns of Cannabis Use in South Australia: Evidence from the National Drug Strategy Household Surveys 1985–1995* (National Drug Strategy Monograph, Vol. 37). Canberra, Australian Capital Territory: Australian Government Publishing Service (AGPS).

Drake, R. E., Bartels, S. J., Teague, G. B., Noordsy, D. L., & Clark, R. E. (1993). Treatment of substance abuse in severely mentally ill patients. *Journal of Nervous and Mental Disease, 181*(10), 606–611.

Dutch National Alcohol and Drug Information System (2004). Treatment demand of cannabis clients in outpatient addiction care in the Netherlands (1994–2002). *LADIS Bulletin, April.*

Edwards, G., Anderson, P., Babor, T. F., Casswell, S., Ferrence, R., et al. (1994). *Alcohol policy and the public good.* Oxford: Oxford University Press.

Elster, J. (1999). Gambling and addiction. In J. Elster, & O. Skog (Eds.), *Rationality and addiction* (pp. 208–234). Cambridge, MA: Cambridge University Press.

Elvy, G. A., Wells, J. E., & Baird, K. A. (1988). Attempted referral as intervention for problem drinking in the general hospital. *British Journal of Addiction, 83*(1), 83–89.

European Monitoring Centre for Drugs and Drug Addiction (EMCDDA) (2003). *Annual Report 2003: The State of the Drugs Problem in the European Union and Norway.* Luxembourg: Office for Official Publications of the European Communities.

Fergusson, D. M., Horwood, L. J., & Lynskey, M. T. (1994). Parental separation, adolescent psychopathology, and problem behaviors. *Journal of the American Academy of Child and Adolescent Psychiatry, 33*(8), 1122–1131; discussion 31–33.

Fergusson, D. M., Lynskey, M. T., & Horwood, L. J. (1996). The short-term consequences of early onset cannabis use. *Journal of Abnormal Child Psychology, 24*(4), 499–512.

Finney, J. W., Hahn, A. C., & Moos, R. H. (1996). The effectiveness of inpatient and outpatient treatment for alcohol abuse: the need to focus on mediators and moderators of setting effects. *Addiction, 91*(12), 1773–1796; discussion 803–820.

Gieringer, D., St. Laurent, J., & Goodrich, S. (2004). Cannabis vaporizer combines efficient delivery of THC with effective suppression of pyrolytic compounds. *Journal of Cannabis Therapeutics, 4*, 7–27.

Grant, B. F. (1995). Comorbidity between DSM-IV drug use disorders and major depression: results of a national survey of adults. *Journal of Substance Abuse, 7*(4), 481–497.

Grant, B. F. (1997). Prevalence and correlates of alcohol use and DSM-IV alcohol dependence in the United States: results of the National Longitudinal Alcohol Epidemiologic Survey. *Journal of Studies on Alcohol, 58*(5), 464–473.

Grinspoon, L., & Bakalar, J. (1993). *Marihuana, the forbidden medicine.* New Haven, CT: Yale University Press.

Gurley, R. J., Aranow, R., & Katz, M. (1998). Medicinal marijuana: a comprehensive review. *Journal of Psychoactive Drugs, 30*(2), 137–147.

Häfner, H., & Maurer, K. (2000). The early course of schizophrenia: new concepts for early intervention. In G. Andrews, & S. Henderson (Eds.), *Unmet need in psychiatry: problems, resources, responses* (pp. 318–332). Cambridge, MA: Cambridge University Press.

Hall, W. D. (1995a). The public health significance of cannabis use in Australia. *Australian Journal of Public Health, 19*(3), 235–242.

Hall, W. D. (1995b). The public health implications of cannabis use. *Australian Journal of Public Health, 19,* 235–242.

Hall, W. D. (1995c). What advice should family physicians give their patients about the health effects of cannabis? *Australian Family Physician, 24,* 1237–1242.

Hall, W. D. (1998). Cannabis use and psychosis. *Drug and Alcohol Review, 17*(4), 433–444.

Hall, W. D. (2000). The cannabis policy debate: finding a way forward. *Canadian Medical Association Journal, 162*(12), 1690–1692.

Hall, W. D., & Babor, T.F. (2000). Cannabis use and public health: assessing the burden. *Addiction, 95*(4), 485–490.

Hall, W. D., & Degenhardt, L. (2000). Cannabis use and psychosis: a review of clinical and epidemiological evidence. *Australian and New Zealand Journal of Psychiatry, 34*(1), 26–34.

Hall, W., & Farrell, M. (1997). Comorbidity of mental disorders with substance misuse. *British Journal of Psychiatry, 171,* 4–5.

Hall, W. D., & Pacula, R.L. (2003). *Cannabis use and dependence: public health and public policy.* Cambridge, MA: Cambridge University Press.

Hall, W. D., & Teesson, M. (2000). Alcohol use disorders: who should be treated and how? In G. Andrews, & S. Henderson (Eds.), *Unmet need in psychiatry: problems, resources, responses* (pp. 291–301). Cambridge, MA: Cambridge University Press.

Hall, W. D., & Zador, D. (1997). The alcohol withdrawal syndrome. *Lancet, 349*(9069), 1897–1900.

Hall, W. D., Teesson, M., Lynskey, M.T., & Degenhardt, L. (1999). The 12-month prevalence of substance use and ICD-10 substance use disorders in Australian adults: findings from the National Survey of Mental Health and Well-being. *Addiction, 94*(10), 1541–1550.

Hall, W. D., Degenhardt, L., & Lynskey, M.T. (2001). *The health and psychological effects of cannabis use* (National Drug Strategy Monograph, Vol. 44). Canberra, Australian Capital Territory: Commonwealth Department of Health and Aged Care.

Heather, N., & Tebbutt, J. (1989). *An overview of the effectiveness of treatment for drug and alcohol problems.* (NCADA Monograph, Vol. 11). Canberra, Australian Capital Territory: Australian Government Publishing Service (AGPS).

Himmelstein, J. L. (1983). *The strange career of marihuana: politics and ideology of drug control in America.* Westport, CT: Greenwood Press.

Homel, R. (1990). Crime on the roads: drinking and driving. In J. Veron (Ed.), *Alcohol and crime.* Canberra, Australian Capital Territory: Australian Institute of Criminology.

Institute of Medicine (1999). *Marijuana and medicine: assessing the science base.* Washington, DC: National Academy Press.

Jablensky, A., McGrath, J., Herrman, H., Castle, D., Gureje, O., *et al.* (2000). Psychotic disorders in urban areas: an overview of the Study on Low Prevalence Disorders. *Australian and New Zealand Journal of Psychiatry, 34*(2), 221–236.

Kavanagh, D. J. (1995). An intervention for substance abuse in schizophrenia. *Behaviour Change, 12*(1), 20–30.

Kessler, R. C. (1995). Epidemiology of psychiatric comorbidity. In M. T. Tsuang, M. Tohen, & G. E. P. Zahner (Eds.), *Textbook in psychiatric epidemiology* (pp. 179–197). New York: Wiley and Sons.

Kessler, R. C., McGonagle, K. A., Zhao, S., Nelson, C. B., Hughes, M., *et al.* (1994). Lifetime and 12-month prevalence of DSM-III-R psychiatric disorders in the United States: results from the National Comorbidity Survey. *Archives of General Psychiatry, 51*(1), 8–19.

Kidorf, M., Brooner, R. K., King, V. L., Chutuape, M. A., & Stitzer, M. L. (1996). Concurrent validity of cocaine and sedative dependence diagnoses in opioid-dependent outpatients. *Drug and Alcohol Dependence, 42*(2), 117–123.

Kristenson, H., Ohlin, H., Hulten-Nosslin, M. B., Trell, E., & Hood, B. (1983). Identification and intervention of heavy drinking in middle-aged men: results and follow-up of 24–60 months of long-term study with randomized controls. *Alcoholism, Clinical and Experimental Research, 7*(2), 203–209.

Krystal, J. H., D'Souza, D. C., Madonick, S., & Petrakis, I. L. (1999). Toward a rational pharmacotherapy of comorbid substance abuse in schizophrenic patients. *Schizophrenia Research, 35* (Suppl.), S35–S49.

Lynskey, M., & Hall, W. (2000). *Educational outcomes and adolescent cannabis use.* Sydney: New South Wales Department of Education and Training.

Lynskey, M. T., Heath, A. C., Bucholz, K. K., & Slutske, W. S. (2003). Escalation of drug use in early-onset cannabis users vs. co-twin controls. *Journal of the American Medical Association, 289*(4), 427–433.

MacCoun, R., & Reuter, P. (1997). Interpreting Dutch cannabis policy: reasoning by analogy in the legalization debate. *Science, 278*(5335), 47–52.

MacCoun, R., & Reuter, P. (2000). *Beyond the drug war: Learning from other vices, other time.* Cambridge, MA: Cambridge University Press.

MacCoun, R., & Reuter, P. (2001). *Drugwar heresies: learning from other vices, times and places.* Cambridge, MA: Cambridge University Press.

Maloff, D. (1981). A review of the effects of the decriminalization of marijuana. *Contemporary Drug Problems, 10,* 307–322.

Maurer, M., Henn, V., Dittrich, A., & Hofmann, A. (1990). Delta-9-tetrahydrocannabinol shows antispastic and analgesic effects in a single case double-blind trial. *European Archives of Psychiatry and Clinical Neuroscience, 240*(1), 1–4.

McCambridge, J., & Strang, J. (2004). The efficacy of single-session motivational interviewing in reducing drug consumption and perceptions of drug-related risk and harm among young people: results from a multi-site cluster randomized trial. *Addiction, 99*(1), 39–52.

McLellan, A. T., Luborsky, L., Woody, G. E., O'Brien, C. P., & Druley, K. A. (1983). Predicting response to alcohol and drug abuse treatments: role of psychiatric severity. *Archives of General Psychiatry, 40*(6), 620–625.

Miller, W. R., & Sovereign, R. G. (1989). The check-up: a model for early intervention in addictive behaviors. In T. Leberg, W. Miller, G. Nathan, & G. Marlatt (Eds.), *Addictive behaviors: prevention and early intervention* (pp. 219–231). Amsterdam: Swets and Zeitlinger.

Mueser, K. T., Bellack, A. S., & Blanchard, J. J. (1992). Comorbidity of schizophrenia and substance abuse: implications for treatment. *Journal of Consulting and Clinical Psychology, 60*(6), 845–856.

Nahas, G., & Latour, C. (1992). The human toxicity of marijuana. *Medical Journal of Australia, 156*(7), 495–497.

Neff, G. W., O'Brien, C. B., Reddy, K. R., Bergasa, N. V., Regev, A., et al. (2002). Preliminary observation with dronabinol in patients with intractable pruritus secondary to cholestatic liver disease. *American Journal of Gastroenterology, 97*(8), 2117–2119.

New South Wales Department of Education and Training (2003). *Cannabis: Know the Risks* (interactive educational material). Sydney: New South Wales (NSW) Department of Education and Training.

Orford, J., & Edwards, G. (1977). *Alcoholism: a comparison of treatment and advice, with a study of the influence of marriage.* Oxford: Oxford University Press.

Peek-Asa, C. (1999). The effect of random alcohol screening in reducing motor vehicle crash injuries. *American Journal of Preventive Medicine, 16*(Suppl. 1), 57–67.

Penrose-Wall, J., Copeland, J., & Harris, M. (2000). *Shared Care of Illicit Drug Problems by General Practitioners and Primary Health Care Providers: A Literature Review.* Sydney: Centre for General Practice Integration Studies, University of New South Wales.

Regier, D. A., Farmer, M. E., Rae, D. S., Locke, B. Z., Keith, S. J., et al. (1990). Comorbidity of mental disorders with alcohol and other drug abuse. Results from the Epidemiologic Catchment Area (ECA) Study. *Journal of the American Medical Association, 264*(19), 2511–2518.

Regier, D. A., Narrow, W. E., Rae, D. S., Manderscheid, R. W., Locke, B. Z., *et al.* (1993). The *de facto* US mental and addictive disorders service system. Epidemiologic catchment area prospective 1-year prevalence rates of disorders and services. *Archives of General Psychiatry, 50*(2), 85–94.

Robins, L., Darvish, H. S., & Murphy, G. E. (1970). The long-term outcome for adolescent drug users: a follow-up study of 76 users and 146 nonusers. In J. Zubin and A. M. Freedman (Eds.), *The psychopathology of adolescence.* New York: Grune and Stratton.

Roche, A.M., & Freeman, T. (2004). Brief interventions: good in theory but weak in practice. *Drug and Alcohol Review, 23*(1), 11–18.

Sas, A., & Cohen, P. (1997). *Patterns of Cannabis Use in Amsterdam Among Experienced Cannabis Users: some Preliminary Data from the 1995 Amsterdam Cannabis Survey.* Amsterdam: Centrum voor Drugsonderzoek, Universiteit van Amsterdam.

Shand, F., & Mattick, R. (2001). *Clients of Treatment Service Agencies: May 2001 Census Findings* (National Drug Strategy Monograph, Vol. 47). Canberra, Australian Capital Territory: Commonwealth Department of Health and Ageing.

Shand, F., Gates, J., Fawcett, J., & Mattick, R. (2003). *The treatment of alcohol problems: a review of the evidence.* Canberra, Australian Capital Territory: Commonwealth Department of Health and Ageing.

Single, E., Christie, P., & Ali, R. (1999). *The Impact of Cannabis Decriminalization in Australia and the United States.* Adelaide, Australia: Drug and Alcohol Services Council.

Single, E.W. (1989). The impact of marijuana decriminalization: an update. *Journal of Public Health Policy, 9*(4), 456–466.

Stephens, R. S., Roffman, R. A., & Simpson, E. E. (1994). Treating adult marijuana dependence – a test of the relapse prevention model. *Journal of Consulting and Clinical Psychology, 62*(1), 92–99.

Stephens, R. S., Roffman, R. A., & Curtin, L. (2000). Comparison of extended versus brief treatments for marijuana use. *Journal of Consulting and Clinical Psychology, 68*(5), 898–908.

Stephens, R. S., Babor, T. F., Kadden, R., & Miller, M. (2002). The Marijuana Treatment Project: rationale, design and participant characteristics. *Addiction*, 97, 109–124.

Substance Abuse and Mental Health Services Administration (SAMHSA), Office of Applied Studies (2004). *Treatment Episode Data Set (TEDS). Highlights – 2002. National Admissions to Substance Abuse Treatment Services*, DAIS Series: S-22, DHHS Publication No. (SMA) 04-3946, Rockville, MD: Office of Applied Studies.

Swift, W., & Hall, W. (2002). Dependence. In F. Grotenhermen (Ed.), *Cannabis and cannabinoids: pharmacology, toxicology and therapeutic potential* (pp. 257–268). New York: Springer-Verlag.

Swift, W., Hall, W. D., & Copeland, J. (1998a). Characteristics of long-term cannabis users in Sydney, Australia. *European Addiction Research*, *4*(4), 190–197.

Swift, W., Hall, W. D., Didcott, P., & Reilly, D. (1998b). Patterns and correlates of cannabis dependence among long-term users in an Australian rural area. *Addiction*, *93*(8), 1149–1160.

Swift, W., Copeland, J., & Lenton, S. (2000). Cannabis harm reduction. *Drug and Alcohol Review*, *19*(1), 101–112.

Swift, W., Hall, W., & Teesson, M. (2001a). Cannabis use and dependence among Australian adults: results from the National Survey of Mental Health and Well-being. *Addiction*, *96*(5), 737–748.

Swift, W., Hall, W. D., & Teesson, C. (2001b). Characteristics of DSM-IV and ICD-10 cannabis dependence among Australian adults: results from the National Survey of Mental Health and Well-being. *Drug and Alcohol Dependence*, *63*(2), 147–153.

Wallace, P., Cutler, S., & Haines, A. (1988). Randomised controlled trial of general practitioner intervention in patients with excessive alcohol consumption. *British Medical Journal*, *297*(6649), 663–668.

Walsh, D., & Hingson, R. (1987). Epidemiology and alcohol policy. In S. Levine, & A. Lilienfeld (Eds.), *Epidemiology and public policy* (pp. 265–291). New York: Tavistock.

Webster, P., Mattick, R., & Baillie, A. (1991). *Clients of Treatment Service Agencies: March 1990 Census Findings*. Canberra, Australian Capital Territory: Australian Government Publishing Service Government Publishing Service (AGPS).

Ziedonis, D., & Brady, K. (1997). Dual diagnosis in primary care. Detecting and treating both the addiction and mental illness. *Medical Clinics of North America*, *81*(4), 1017–1036.

Zimmer, L., & Morgan, J. P. (1997). *Marijuana myths, marijuana facts: a review of the scientific evidence*. New York: The Lindesmith Center.

# Part V
Conclusion

# 15

# The Nature, Consequences and Treatment of Cannabis Dependence: Implications for Future Research and Policy

ROBERT S. STEPHENS AND ROGER A. ROFFMAN

The phenomenon of cannabis dependence has been a topic of interest and vary-ing levels of concern for well over 100 years. As Roffman and colleagues recount in the first chapter of this book, our conceptions and understanding of it have been shaped by many social and political forces over time, but it is only in the last 20–25 years that science has directly been brought to bear on its nature, con-sequences, and treatment. It is this concentrated growth in knowledge that serves as the impetus for this book. We would be naïve to believe that social and political forces no longer affect the current cannabis Zeitgeist. Yet the research reviewed in this volume offers a starting point for a rational consensus regard-ing a condition that some still argue does not exist and others would say is a major problem plaguing our societies. In this chapter we attempt some integra-tion of the research findings, reach some tentative conclusions, and revisit direc-tions for future research. Although the book is organized into sections that loosely correspond to what we know about the nature, consequences, and treat-ment of cannabis dependence, there is great potential for cross-fertilization of ideas across these different research areas and levels of analysis. Its nature and consequences ought to shape its treatment and results from treatment trials tell us something more about its nature. Hopefully, research in all areas will inform policy in a logical fashion.

## What is the Nature of Cannabis Dependence?

By nature we mean the description of the condition or disorder, its etiology and development, the underlying processes that maintain it, and its course if left untreated. As Tom Babor reviews in the second chapter, the description of drug dependence today is heavily influenced by the dependence syndrome concept. Signs of impaired control, preoccupation with using, and neurological adaptation define the syndrome and have been codified in the most widely used diagnostic systems. A number of psychometric studies support the applicability of this syndrome to cannabis and some subset of users displays enough of the syndrome elements to qualify as dependent. Thus, cannabis dependence appears to resemble dependence on a variety of other drugs of abuse when these common criteria are used.

These findings support the existence of cannabis dependence but we must be careful in assuming that they provide an adequate description. Each of the diagnostic criteria associated with the dependence syndrome occurs in cannabis users and other drug users but their meanings may be somewhat different. Recent evidence also questions the utility of these symptoms in distinguishing milder versus more severe forms of drug use disorders and the current distinction between dependence and abuse (Langenbucher *et al.*, 2004). The dependence syndrome concept separates the definition of dependence from an appraisal of the negative consequences that ensue, but complete separation may not capture different levels of severity. For instance, the concepts of loss of control and preoccupation with use are likely relative rather than absolute phenomena. The consequences associated with drug use likely affect the effort one puts into controlling that drug use. If the negative consequences of drug use are not very severe the need to exert control and the effort expended may be lessened. One may still meet the diagnostic criterion but the degree of loss of control may be judged quite differently than for another drug with more debilitating consequences. Similarly, preoccupation with use, as indexed by spending large amounts of time using or giving up other activities, is also relative to the impairment created by the use and the extent to which it interferes with other activities. In the next section we discuss further the implications of cannabis dependence consequences for our understanding of its nature.

Signs of tolerance and withdrawal associated with chronic drug use have long been the sin qua non of drug dependence criteria. In fact, the belief that these symptoms did not occur with cannabis use fueled the debate over the existence of cannabis dependence. In the absence of such signs of neurological adaptation to the drug, preoccupation with cannabis use was at most considered "psychological dependence" and of an entirely different nature than for drugs that could produce true "physical dependence." Lichtman and Martin's review of the animal and human literatures in Chapter 3 provides strong evidence that cannabis tolerance and withdrawal can and do occur. The identification of an endocannabinoid system that mediates the acute effects of cannabis and is affected by chronic dosing of cannabinoids provides the biological underpinnings of both the positive and negative reinforcement processes that may help explain the etiology and maintenance of cannabis dependence.

Once again we have findings suggesting that cannabis dependence is not as different from other drug dependencies as was once thought. And again we must be careful in the emphasis we place on these findings. The advent of the dependence syndrome concept occurred in part because the signs of physical dependence (tolerance and withdrawal) were neither necessary nor sufficient in accounting for cases of compulsive drug taking that fit what most people think of as drug dependence. While many cannabis-dependent users report tolerance and withdrawal symptoms upon cessation, a sizable subgroup of the heaviest users do not (e.g., Stephens *et al.*, 2002). Many of those who do report withdrawal may actually be noticing offset effects or the reemergence of pre-existing negative psychological/somatic states that were suppressed by chronic marijuana use. Recent controlled laboratory and natural environment studies document the existence of true withdrawal effects in a subset of cannabis-dependent users and it has been suggested that the severity of cannabis withdrawal may be similar to that of nicotine withdrawal (Budney *et al.*, 2004). Nevertheless, research is needed linking withdrawal severity to an increased probability of relapse following abstinence before emphasis is placed on this aspect of cannabis dependence.

Regardless of the importance of withdrawal phenomena in understanding cannabis dependence, our increasing understanding of the neurobiological mediators of cannabis effects is important. Positive reinforcement from the drug likely serves as a primary incentive for initiating and maintaining use over time. This positive reinforcement has been linked to the effect of cannabinoids on the endogenous opioid system and the dopaminergic system. Greater understanding of relationships with these reward pathways may explain genetically increased risk for developing cannabis dependence. It may also lead to pharmacological interventions for cannabis dependence. While one type of potential pharmacological intervention could make use of agonists to curb withdrawal symptoms (e.g., Haney *et al.*, 2004) others may be based in antagonists that block the effects of cannabinoids and hence lessen the reinforcement value (e.g., Haney *et al.*, 2003). Research in this area is escalating rapidly but there are no controlled pharmacological treatment trials as of yet.

Jim Anthony used data from a variety of epidemiological studies in Chapter 4 to estimate that approximately 2–3% of users in the US progress to cannabis dependence within the first 2 years after initiation to cannabis use. Multiple studies also converge on a lifetime risk of users developing dependence at around 10% with rates increasing as the frequency of marijuana use increases. Preliminary studies in other cultures are largely consistent with these risk estimates.

One study indicates that the risk of developing cannabis dependence peaks around 3–4 years after initiation and then drops sharply. Apparently most users will develop dependence within a few years or not at all. Although based on the retrospective recall of symptom development, and in need of prospective longitudinal confirmation, these data raise questions about the processes involved. For instance, in contrast to the time course for cannabis, cocaine users show a much higher probability of developing dependence in the first year after initiation with a rapid drop in risk thereafter. Although the data are subject to alternate interpretations, they characterize the onset of dependence to cannabis as a gradual process more similar to alcohol. The relatively protracted risk period for both drugs may be related to the relatively mild levels of euphoria provided by the drugs and the ability to use them moderately without immediate negative consequences or loss of control. On the other hand, the finding that risk for cannabis dependence decreases rapidly after several years while remaining moderately high for alcohol for many years, suggests the influence of social forces. In contrast to alcohol, the illicit nature of cannabis leads to lower acceptability with age and increasing social responsibilities.

Anthony also addresses the limited research on etiological factors. Behavior genetic research shows cannabis dependence to be moderately heritable, but we are cautioned that gene-environment covariation is not addressed well in the studies to date. What is inherited may be a dispositional tendency to put oneself into situations that foster drug use, rather than a specific propensity to become addicted to marijuana. The common genetic vulnerability for dependence on multiple drugs suggests that some people may be more attracted to a variety drugs. Indeed, Anthony notes that the presence of an alcohol use disorder increases the probability of being cannabis dependent. There are also promising lines of research concerning the importance of parents and parenting and socialization processes more generally. While our understanding of these social–environmental influences on drug initiation is solid, we are still limited in our knowledge of their direction and degree of influence in the development of dependence. More research addressing risk factors for the transition from use to dependence is needed.

Assessment of the risks for developing cannabis dependence is limited by our ability to accurately measure the amount of cannabis consumed. If we assume that neurochemical processes underlie the development of dependence it makes sense that there would be some dose–response relationship with those using higher doses of the active ingredient more likely to develop dependence. In fact, some researchers have suggested that the small but statistically significant increase in cannabis use disorders over the past 10 years is due to an increase in the potency of cannabis available (Compton *et al.*, 2004). Others have challenged this interpretation. The resolution of the debate may rest on better assessment of cannabis potency in future research. All too often our measure of cannabis exposure is almost exclusively a crude recall of relative frequency of use across days in a specific time period or the lifetime number of uses with little attention given to the definition of a single use or the effects of multiple uses per day. Creative ways of assessing the consumption of differential doses are needed (see Stephens & Roffman, 2005 for a review).

We know little about the long-term course of cannabis dependence. While most recreational users cease use without intervention in early adulthood, longitudinal studies have yet to track those who develop cannabis dependence for prolonged periods. A small retrospective study of natural recovery from cannabis dependence provides a glimpse of how some dependent users recall overcoming dependence in the absence of treatment (see Chapter 9). Decrements in the expected positive effects of cannabis use, increased involvement in activities unrelated to cannabis use, actively avoiding other users, and changing lifestyles were some of the most commonly reported factors associated with the cessation of use. The waning of drug induced reinforcements and the growth of environments reinforcing drug abstinence may be common processes that permit some dependent users to regain control. Given the expense of longitudinal studies, larger well-designed retrospective studies may provide further insight into factors that maintain cannabis dependence or promote change. Comparing those who have recovered with continuing users matched on demographic and drug use history variables would increase confidence in conclusions about the causal role of specific environmental or developmental factors associated with change.

We end this section with some speculation on the nature of cannabis dependence gleaned from treatment studies. Treatment studies typically include participants at the extreme end of severity and we must be cautious in generalizing to the full range of users who may be dependent. Nevertheless, treatment studies inform us of the course drug dependence after an intervention designed to end it. What we know from the studies reviewed in this book is that of cannabis dependence can be as tenacious as any other drug dependency. While there is consistent evidence that treatment works better than no treatment, the majority of those treated either never achieves abstinence or returns to use within a short time after treatment ends. On the one hand these treatment outcomes are not surprising in the context of a drug treatment literature that has repeatedly found relapse to be common. However, the fact that such treatment outcomes occur for a drug that produces relatively mild euphoria and withdrawal reminds us that there may be multiple paths to the same outcome. Cannabis dependence may persist in a subset of users, not so much because of the physiological changes in endocannabinoid systems, but because motivation to achieve and remain abstinent may be limited at the start and may dwindle quickly. Low motivation is likely linked, in part, to the limited negative consequences associated with continued use. We look at those consequences more closely in the next section.

## What are the Consequences of Cannabis Dependence?

Hall and Solowij provide a comprehensive review of how cannabis can affect health and human functioning. They note at the outset that research rarely directly addresses the consequences produced by dependence. Rather, dependent users are likely at higher risk for many of the consequences believed to stem from the cumulative effects of cannabis use because of their high rate of use. The single greatest health concern arises not from the psychoactive ingredients in cannabis, but from the effects of smoking on the lungs and respiratory system more generally. There appears to be good evidence that smoking cannabis impairs lung functioning in a manner similar to tobacco. The carcinogenic nature of the smoke may increase the likelihood of respiratory cancers but no convincing evidence has been found yet. Larger cohort studies and good case control studies are needed to inform this important issue.

Chronic cannabis use does not produce gross changes in cognitive functioning but may impair learning and memory on more sensitive neuropsychological tests. Some research suggests even these deficits recover with short periods of abstinence while other studies suggest more durable but still subtle deficits. A major problem in this research is ruling out pre-existing differences in cognitive functioning and ancillary behaviors (e.g., alcohol abuse) that may account for the apparent deficiencies in performance relative to non-user controls. Cross-sectional studies must be careful in selecting well matched controls. Some recent studies suggest that the risk for enduring impairment may be greater in those who begin smoking at younger ages, perhaps because the brain is still developing. It is also possible that the negative effects on brain functioning are more substantial in a subset of users whose premorbid attentional and memory functioning is compromised. The debate on the practical significance of these effects as well as their recovery with abstinence is far from resolved. More prospective studies with large samples and sensitive measures of cognitive functioning are needed, but one recent meta-analysis concludes that "the 'real life' impact of such a small and selective effect is questionable" (Grant *et al.*, 2003, p. 686). It is also interesting to note that the acute effects of cannabis use in regular heavy users may not further compromise complex cognitive performance, presumably because behavioral tolerance develops (Hart *et al.*, 2001).

Although the severity of marijuana use on cognitive functioning is not resolved, there is some evidence that adolescent users are at risk for lower educational attainment and greater likelihood of involvement with other illicit drugs. The causal link between cannabis use and these outcomes is not certain. Better controlled studies continue to show relationships between cannabis use and these outcomes after statistically controlling for alternative explanations, but even these remaining direct effects may be mediated by social forces rather than the pharmacological effects of the drug. While it seems prudent to recommend against excessive cannabis use during adolescent development we are not yet sure what the target of our prevention efforts should be.

Cannabis's acute effects on attention, reaction time, and motor coordination predict impairment of driving and increased risk for accidents. The frequent coincidence of cannabis and alcohol use, a known contributor to motor vehicle accidents, has made it difficult to directly identify a causal link for cannabis. More recent research has found cannabis to independently increase risk for accidents. However, it is not clear to what extent these effects are related to cannabis dependence. History of use is rarely assessed in these studies and it is possible that dependent users are actually at lower risk than other cannabis users because tolerance develops too many psychomotor effects.

Other behavior genetic and epidemiological studies reviewed by Anthony have failed to find long-term economic or psychosocial consequences in heavy marijuana users once alternative vulnerabilities to these outcomes are taken into account. Other health concerns primarily affect subgroups of users with pre-existing health problems (e.g., those with heart disease or those at risk for psychoses) and therefore do not constitute a widespread concern related to cannabis dependence.

Thus, other than the threats to respiratory health, the consequences of continued cannabis use may not appear all that serious to the cannabis-dependent user. Examination of the types of problems that bring some users to treatment suggests that the primary concerns of those who seek treatment for dependence may be personal and relatively subtle (Stephens *et al.*, 2002). Issues of self-control and self-image along with beliefs that cannabis use may be interfering with productivity seem to be the primary motivators for change. The relative absence of more concrete negative consequences may undermine motivation for quitting or reducing use and consequently must be considered in our understanding of the nature of cannabis dependence. Motivation for stopping or reducing drug use is often thought to reflect the weighing of the costs and benefits of making that change versus the costs and benefits of continuing to use. If the costs for continuing and the benefits of stopping are small, as may be perceived by many cannabis users, then there is little reason to exert more effort to gain control. The issue of motivation for change has great relevance for the treatment of marijuana dependence and is discussed in the next section.

**Is the Treatment of Cannabis Dependence Effective?**

When we began conducting our first treatment study with cannabis-dependent users in 1987, there were no controlled trials in the literature. Almost 20 years later there are now at least 10 published studies and more on the way. A variety of therapeutic approaches used to treat alcohol and other drug dependencies have been shown to be efficacious with cannabis-dependent adults. Cognitive-behavioral (Chapters 6, 7, and 9), motivational enhancement (Chapters 6, 8, and 9), contingency management (CM) (Chapter 7), and supportive–expressive therapies (Chapter 10) show promise in helping adults achieve abstinence or reductions in use. Adaptations of these same approaches, as well as family systems, community reinforcement, and multi-component therapies, are beginning to be evaluated with adolescents and young adults with encouraging results (Chapters 11–13). The reductions in cannabis use resulting from treatment were often substantial and accompanied by equally large decrements in self-reported problems. Long-term abstinence, however, is rare, occurring in about 20% or less of participants in these trials. As noted earlier, the types of outcomes seen in these studies are generally similar to those for the treatment of alcohol and other drug disorders.

Few of these studies have directly compared different therapeutic approaches and, when they have, differences in treatment modality and intensity confounded clear interpretations. Thus, we can say little about which approach shows the most promise for helping dependent cannabis users achieve abstinence or meaningful sustained reductions in use. At least two studies found clear superiority for longer versus shorter durations of treatment (Chapter 10; Marijuana Treatment Project Research Group, 2004), but other studies did not (Budney et al., 2000; Copeland et al., 2001; Stephens et al., 2000). So the optimal treatment dose is uncertain as well. On the one hand it is good that there are a variety of relatively effective approaches for treating cannabis users. Clinicians can choose familiar approaches, increasing the likelihood that therapy will be conducted with a high degree of skill. On the other hand, the fact that different approaches and durations of treatment yield similar results tells us little about how or why the treatments work. Without knowledge of the processes through which treatments work it is difficult to improve on them.

It may be that non-specific factors common to most therapies (e.g., support, encouragement) are the primary active ingredients, but it seems premature to discount specific processes proposed by underlying theoretical models. For instance, evidence was provided that supportive–expressive therapy may work by increasing self-assertion and interpersonal awareness, thus improving inter-personal relations and reducing one motive for continued cannabis use (Chapter 10). Although this study lacked a control condition to rule out the possibility that these changes were the result of reduced cannabis use, rather than the cause, it illustrates the type of questions that must be asked. In contrast, use of coping strategies and self-efficacy for resisting cannabis use are primary mediating con-structs in cognitive-behavioral treatment (CBT) but have not yet been shown to be differentially affected by CBT versus non-CBT treatments (e.g., Stephens *et al.*, 1995). Future studies will profit from more attention to the measurement of pro-posed mediating processes and the use of designs that disentangle the effects of modality (i.e., group versus individual), duration or length, and type of treatment.

The notion that motivation for change may be a particular issue for cannabis-dependent users was given further credence in one treatment study by observa-tions that cannabis users were less likely to attend treatment and more likely to relapse than other drug users receiving the same intervention (Chapter 9). Comparisons of cannabis and cocaine users entering treatment in another study also identified lower levels of initial readiness for change (Budney *et al.*, 1998). Thus, therapies designed to increase motivation would be expected to demon-strate particularly good outcomes. Motivational enhancement treatment (MET) directly targets motivation by attempting to increase users' intrinsic motivation for change through problem recognition and self-efficacy enhancement. MET was effective with cannabis-dependent users relative to no treatment even in very small doses (Copeland *et al.*, 2001; Marijuana Treatment Project Research Group, 2004; Stephens *et al.*, 2000). However, no studies have convincingly demonstrated that its effects on reduced cannabis use were mediated by increased motivation for change.

Nevertheless, these promising findings with brief MET led to attempts to use this strategy with non-treatment-seeking populations recruited to a marijuana check-up (Chapter 8). The most noteworthy aspect of this study may be the success in reaching dependent cannabis users who were not interested in treat-ment. Although those exposed to the MET intervention reduced marijuana use more than those in the control conditions, the magnitude of change was modest.

The much larger impact of MET in treatment-seeking populations underscores the importance of the motivation for change that treatment seekers bring to the behavior change effort. Even though this initial level of motivation may be less in cannabis users than many other treatment-seeking drug users, it is greater than found in similar cannabis users who are not approaching treatment and it likely interacts with the intervention to create much larger change than can be accomplished in non-treatment-seeking populations. Still, the brevity of the approach and promising findings with a non-treatment-seeking population warrant further investigation in a variety of settings to learn more about the parameters of its efficacy.

CM also directly targets motivation for change by providing extrinsic incentives. CM added to the effectiveness of MET and CBT in cannabis-dependent users during the treatment period (Budney *et al.*, 2000; Chapter 7). CM's mechanism of action (i.e., contingent reinforcement of negative urine specimens) has been established in research with other drug using populations. Studies with longer-term follow-ups of treated cannabis users are now needed to address the durability of change once the contingent reinforcement is discontinued. Interestingly, this initial study with cannabis-dependent users suggested that the incremental effects of CM beyond those of MET and CBT may be fairly specific to abstinence outcomes. Treatment groups did not differ on their self-reported frequency of cannabis use or problems associated with use at the end of treatment. It may be that making reinforcement contingent solely on abstinence creates an all or none effect such that once the person has used there is little incentive to control use. In another study (Chapter 13), CM was effective in increasing treatment attendance, but had no effect on drug use when monetary incentives were contingent solely on treatment attendance. These findings raise questions regarding the ideal behavioral targets for CM and the generalizability of effects to related behaviors and outcomes.

CM also faces challenges in dissemination to treatment agencies because of its frequent reliance on monetary payments for drug abstinence. Alternative reinforcers have been suggested and are beginning to be studied. Extensions and adaptations of CM interventions with special populations and polydrug users show promise and support the continued testing of these interventions (Chapter 7). The effectiveness of CM further informs our understanding of the nature of cannabis dependence. By demonstrating that increased incentives for drug abstinence motivate change, it highlights how the lack of such incentives may maintain drug use and explain dependence.

Most treatment studies with cannabis-dependent adults have explicitly or implicitly imposed the goal of abstinence on participants. This is not surprising given the illicit status of the drug and political concerns about condoning its use. However, abstinence is a relatively rare outcome across studies and Sobell and colleagues (Chapter 9) remind us that there is little evidence that assigned goal makes a difference in the outcome of treatment with alcohol users. Therefore, their Guided Self-Change (GSC) approach allows users to decide on their own goals, in part to increase the appeal of treatment to less motivated participants who may not accept the goal of abstinence. Two-thirds of the cannabis users in their study chose a non-abstinent goal. Although the small sample size in this initial study of GSC with cannabis-dependent users probably precluded sub-analyses for users with abstinent versus moderate use goals, future research could be designed to explore the effects of different types of goals, both self-selected and imposed, on both treatment retention and cannabis use outcomes.

Systematic evaluation of treatment for adolescent cannabis users is in its early stages. Results from the landmark CYT study (Chapter 11) in many ways parallel the findings with adults in showing that a variety of therapeutic approaches and intensities of treatment appear to yield equivalent, but modest, reductions in cannabis use. However, adolescents in drug treatment differ from their adult counterparts in several potentially important ways. Adolescents rarely initiate drug treatment on their own and instead are generally coerced into treatment by legal, parental, or other social forces. They tend to feel relatively invulnerable to negative outcomes and thus have even less intrinsic motivation for change than the adults who seek treatment. Further, adolescents have less control over their immediate environment, are heavily influenced by peers, and have less power to enact changes in the environment that would support drug abstinence. These obstacles predict less treatment success and call for multi-component interventions that involve parents, teachers, and peer networks. Given these obstacles to successful treatment outcomes, it is particularly surprising that the CYT study did not find the substantially more intensive multi-component and family-based interventions to be superior to a brief MET/CBT intervention. Although future analyses of the data in this large study may yield clues as to what was more or less effective with different sub-populations, the overall findings are humbling. They suggest once again that the support and reinforcement for change common to all treatment approaches may be the primary active ingredients.

One avenue for exploration is to try and reach adolescent cannabis users on a more voluntary basis. Coercion to treatment likely engages reactance and defensive processes that are counterproductive to treatment. Although some users will always come to treatment in this manner, reducing help-seeking barriers for adolescents may increase the proportion who approach treatment with a more open mind and willingness to consider the pros and cons of drug use. The TMCU (Chapter 12) showed promise in attracting adolescents, many of whom were not considering change, to a brief MET intervention. Although the lack of control groups in these initial studies make it impossible to know the efficacy of the MET intervention, the substantial reductions in cannabis use following participation calls for further examination. Studies with control groups are needed to examine whether the reductions in use are related to pre-existing motivation for change, the assessment process, or the feedback. It will also be interesting to explore whether subgroups of less motivated adolescents profit more from participation.

Finally, as noted earlier, the explosion in research on the neurobiological substrate that mediates both acute and chronic effects of cannabis is likely to lead to a number of pharmacological approaches to the treatment of cannabis dependence. Preclinical studies are starting to appear (e.g., Haney *et al.*, 2003, 2004) and the best candidate agents will eventually be tested in randomized controlled trials in clinical populations. As with pharmacological treatments for other drugs of abuse, these trials will likely explore the efficacy of drug treatments in combination with some of the behavioral treatment approaches reviewed in this volume. The question of whether pharmacological treatments can augment the impact of behavioral interventions awaits these studies.

**What Should the Policy on Cannabis Dependence Be?**

Hall and Swift (Chapter 14) address the implications of research on cannabis dependence for public policy. While acknowledging that the full public health burden of cannabis dependence is difficult to estimate, they argue that the number of users seeking treatment demands a policy response. They rightly caution against a premature conclusion that the negative consequences associated with prolonged cannabis use are trivial given the relatively young state of the literature. And they note that the loss of control reported by dependent users is sufficient to justify a focus on treatment program development regardless of the severity of consequences associated with use.

Education about the risks of cannabis dependence should be part of any policy because it may deter initiation or escalation of use that could lead to dependence. But messages need to be honest in presenting that the risks of dependence increase with increasing frequency of use. Exaggerated messages about the likelihood of becoming dependent may elicit outright rejection among recreational users. Such messages may be hard to incorporate in prohibitionist societies that fear sending a message of tolerance for moderate levels of use. On the other hand, prohibition likely serves to decrease the number of users and thus reduces the number who will become dependent. Hall and Swift conclude that there is too little data to adequately address the effect of relaxing penalties for cannabis use on the prevalence of cannabis dependence.

Hall and Swift suggest roles for a full spectrum of programs that include prevention efforts targeted at adolescents, screening, and identification of at-risk users in a variety of settings, brief treatments and interventions as initial low cost means of promoting change, and more intensive specialist treatments for those who do not respond to briefer interventions. They acknowledge that attention to issues of comorbidity and withdrawal management may be needed in the development of comprehensive treatment policy.

## Conclusion

The recommendations for policy are largely consistent with the conclusions reached in the chapters of this book. We know cannabis dependence exists, we know it comes with a potential for increased negative consequences that affect millions of users, and we know that many of those users want help in overcoming dependence. The consequences of cannabis dependence may not be as severe as other drug dependencies. Indeed, we have argued that the relative lack of negative consequences may fuel low motivation for change and undermine the effectiveness of treatment interventions. But this is a reason to develop better treatments that capitalize on and build motivation, rather than an argument that treatment is not needed.

## References

Budney, A. J., Radonovich, K. J., Higgins, S. T., & Wong, C. J. (1998). Adults seeking treatment for marijuana dependence: a comparison to cocaine-dependent treatment seekers. *Experimental and Clinical Psychopharmacology, 6*, 1–8.

Budney, A. J., Higgins, S. T., Radonovich, K. J., & Novy, P. L. (2000). Adding voucher-based incentives to coping skills and motivational enhancement improves outcomes during treatment for marijuana dependence. *Journal of Consulting and Clinical Psychology, 68*, 1051–1061.

Budney, A. J., Hughes, J. R., Moore, B. A., & Vandrey, R. (2004). Review of the validity and significance of cannabis withdrawal syndrome. *American Journal of Psychiatry, 161*, 1967–1977.

Compton, W. M., Grant, B. F., Colliver, J. D., Glantz, M. D., & Stinson, F. S. (2004). Prevalence of marijuana use disorders in the United States: 1991–1992 and 2001–2002. *Journal of the American Medical Association, 291*, 2114–2121.

Copeland, J., Swift, W., Roffman, R., & Stephens, R. (2001). A randomized controlled trial of brief cognitive-behavioral interventions for cannabis use disorder. *Journal of Substance Abuse Treatment, 21*, 55–64.

Grant, I., Gonzalez, R., Carey, C. L., Natarajan, L., & Wolfson, T. (2003). Non-acute (residual) neurocognitive effects of cannabis use: a meta-analytic study. *Journal of the International Neuropsychological Society, 9*, 679–689.

Haney, M., Bisaga, A., & Foltin, R. W. (2003). Interaction between naltrexone and oral THC in heavy marijuana smokers. *Psychopharmacology, 166*, 77–85.

Haney, M., Hart, C. L., Vosburg, S. K., Nasser, J., Bennett, A., Zubaran, C., & Foltin, R. W. (2004). Marijuana withdrawal in humans: effects of oral THC or Divalproex. *Neuropsychopharmacology, 29*, 158–170.

Hart, C. L., van Gorp, W., Haney, M., Foltin, R. W., & Fischman, M.W. (2001). Effects of acute smoked marijuana on complex cognitive performance. *Neuropsychopharmacology, 25*, 757–765.

Langenbucher, J. W., Labouvie, E., Martin, C. S., Sanjuan, P. M., Bavly, L., Kirisci, L., & Chung, T. (2004). An application of item response theory to alcohol, cannabis, and cocaine criteria in DSM-IV. *Journal of Abnormal Psychology, 113*, 72–80.

Marijuana Treatment Project Research Group (2004). Brief treatments for cannabis dependence: findings from a randomized multisite trial. *Journal of Consulting and Clinical Psychology, 72*, 455–466.

Stephens, R. S., & Roffman, R. A. (2005). Assessment of cannabis dependence. In D. Donovan, & G. A. Marlatt (Eds.), *Assessment of addictive behaviors* (2nd ed., pp. 248–273) New York: Guilford.

Stephens, R. S., Wertz, J. S., & Roffman, R. A. (1995). Self-efficacy and marijuana cessation: a construct validity analysis. *Journal of Consulting and Clinical Psychology, 63*, 1022–1031.

Stephens, R. S., Roffman, R. A., & Curtin, L. (2000). Comparison of extended versus brief treatments for marijuana use. *Journal of Consulting and Clinical Psychology, 68*, 898–908.

Stephens, R. S., Babor, T. F., Kadden, R., Miller, M., & The Marijuana Treatment Project Research Group (2002). The marijuana treatment project: rationale, design and participant characteristics. *Addiction, 97*, 109–124.

# Index

# Index

National Treatment Improvement Evaluation
  Study 278
natural history
  cannabis dependence 89
  clinical features, relation to 89–90
natural recovery studies 208–10, 347
nature
  of cannabis dependence 343–8
  cannabis effects 345
  dependence syndrome concept 22, 343,
    344
  dose–response relationship 346
  endocannabinoid system, identification
    344
  nicotine withdrawal 344
  psychometric studies 344
  treatment studies 347
negative punishment 156
negative reinforcement 156
neuroadaptation 22
neuroadaptive changes
  cannabinoid withdrawal 47
  G-protein activity 46
neurobiological mediators 345
neurochemical mechanism
  CB$_1$ cannabinoid receptor
    mechanisms of action 45–6
    interrelationships 47–8
    CRF 48
    dopamine 47
    mesolimbic system 47
    neuroadaptive changes 46–7
neurochemical processes 346
neurological adaptation 343, 344
neuropsychopharmacology 89
New York Academy of Medicine 10
NHSDA *see* NSDUH
nicotine withdrawal 345
"no problem class"
  cannabis users 63, 64
non-cannabinoid agents 46
non-treatment-seeking populations 291, 351,
  352
"nose-poke" procedure 45
nosological studies 59–64
  alcohol dependence syndrome 60
  cannabis dependence
    clinical features 60–1
    level of 63
  epidemiology uses 61
  opiate dependence 60
  proxy dependence 61
  recent-onset cannabis users
    classes 63
NSDUH 62
nucleus accumbens 44

Office of Applied Statistics
  SAMHSA 69
open-ended questions 133, 186, 302
opioid receptor 49
opioid system modulation
  cannabinoid dependence 49–50
optimal treatment dose 350
oral cancer
  cannabis smokers 110
oral squamous cell carcinoma 109, 110
Outcome Expectancy Scale 185
  costs and benefits (CB) scale 185
outpatient psychotherapy 267

Panama Canal Zone Report, 1925 9
parent–adolescent connection 257
parent/caregiver involvement 254–5
parent–child bonding 83–4
parental consent 283, 289
parents 170, 252, 254, 268, 289
  education sessions 252, 253
  and parenting 85
  self-of-the-parent 257
parents movement 14
partial prohibition policy 75
pathogenesis
  cannabis dependence 87
  exposure opportunity 88
  gateway phenomenon 88
Penn Psychotherapy Project 227
periodic summary of client 134
personal conservatism 84
Personal Feedback Report (PFR) 134–5,
  178, 250, 280
personality traits 77–8
pharmacological effects 37, 41, 117
pharmacological interventions 345
pharmacological treatments 354
pharmacology and physiology 37
  animal studies, implications 50
  cannabinoid and opioid systems, reciprocal
    roles
    interrelationships 48–50
  cannabis effects
    and endocannabinoid system 37–8
  characterization
    cannabinoid self-administration 44–5
    cannabinoid withdrawal 41–4
    cannabis withdrawal symptoms, clinical
      significance 39–40
    overview 38–9
  neurochemical mechanisms
    CB$_1$ cannabinoid receptor 45–6
    neuroadaptive changes 46–7
    neurochemical systems,
      interrelationships 47–8

Printed in the United States
By Bookmasters